Translational Perspectives in Auditory Neuroscience

Translational Perspectives in Auditory Neuroscience

Special Topics

KELLY TREMBLAY, PHD, CCC-A
ROBERT BURKARD, PHD, CCC-A

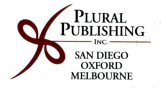

PLURAL
PUBLISHING
INC.

SAN DIEGO
OXFORD
MELBOURNE

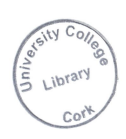
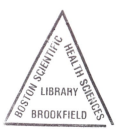

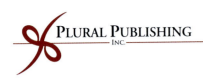

5521 Ruffin Road
San Diego, CA 92123

e-mail: info@pluralpublishing.com
Web site: http://www.pluralpublishing.com

49 Bath Street
Abingdon, Oxfordshire OX14 1EA
United Kingdom

Typeset in 10.5/13 Palatino Book by Flanagan's Publishing Services, Inc.
Printed in Hong Kong by Paramount
Front and back cover images by Kristin Swenson-Lintault. Back cover image is entitled "Ripple."

Library of Congress Cataloging-in-Publication Data

Tremblay, Kelly.
  Translational perspectives in auditory neuroscience / Kelly Tremblay, Robert Burkard.
      p. ; cm.
  Includes bibliographical references and index.
  ISBN-13: 978-1-59756-202-7 (v. 1 : alk. paper)
  ISBN-10: 1-59756-202-5 (v. 1 : alk. paper)
  ISBN-13: 978-1-59756-467-0 (v. 2 : alk. paper)
  ISBN-10: 1-59756-467-2 (v. 2 : alk. paper)
  [etc.]
  I. Burkard, Robert F., 1953- II. Title.
  [DNLM: 1. Hearing—physiology. 2. Auditory Perception—physiology. 3. Hearing Disorders.
4. Translational Medical Research. WV 270]

  612.8'5—dc23
                          2012005803

Contents

Preface

Kelly Tremblay and Robert Burkard

WHY ANOTHER HEARING SCIENCE BOOK?

The term "hearing science" has come to mean many different things. Virtually anything related to hearing that has a scientific basis could be included in a book so labeled, so the term "translational" in the title might help clarify what we intended to include. In the editors' opinion, "translational research" was a term coined to give underrepresented clinical research a chance to develop in a research world that is dominated by two ends of the research continuum: cellular and molecular experiments (i.e., reductionistic work) and (on the other end of the continuum) clinical trials. Our definition hints at the disconnect between basic and clinical scientists that has become a topic of discussion in scientific (Declan, 2008) as well as mainstream media (*Newsweek*, 2010). Despite a common mission to improve hearing health care, basic and clinical scientists ask very different questions, use very different approaches, and belong to very different cultures (Figure P–1). Moreover, even though evidence at the cellular or molecular end could manifest itself into rehabilitation treatments, and observed clinical behaviors could better define biological processes, information can get lost when there is no translation.

This book is part of a mission to improve dialogue between the two cultures of science so that health-related science can translate in many directions: from bench to bedside and vice versa. The editors of this book are two examples of people who have managed to straddle this valley of death (see Figure P–1), but not without struggle. We are clinical audiologists as well as classically trained hearing scientists, who, while putting politics aside for a moment, are committed to the advancement of "translational research." To do this we approached colleagues who work along each step of the scientific continuum, from basic to applied, and asked them to provide information that was theoretically deep, but contextually broad. In some instances this meant pairing authors who would not normally write together and asking them to coauthor chapters. We also included a diverse group of students, post-docs, and scientists to interact with the authors by asking questions and infusing comments during the review process. This process ensured both basic and applied material would be integrated.

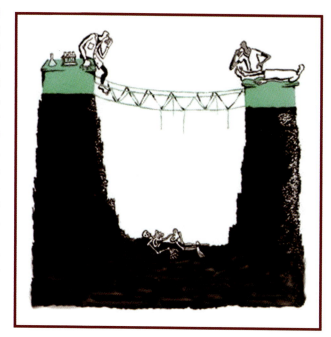

Figure P–1. Translational research: Crossing the valley of death — A chasm has opened up between biomedical researchers and the patients who need their discoveries. *Source:* From B. Declan, 2008, "Translational Research: Crossing the Valley of Death," *Nature, 453,* 840–842. Reprinted with permission from *Nature.*

This compendium has become a three-book series. The first book, *Normal Aspects of Hearing*, is not really translational in nature. It includes acoustics, the anatomy and physiology of the auditory system, and ends with chapters that relate perception to physiologic processes. It serves as foundation for readers who may not be familiar with some of the neural mechanisms underlying topics discussed in the second and third books.

In the second book, entitled *Hearing Across the Life Span—Assessment and Disorders*, we review what is known about the developing auditory system, what happens as we age, as well as a brief synopsis of the disordered auditory system. These aspects of human perception are then extended by the discussion of state-of-the-art noninvasive physiologic measures of hearing. Many of these measures are tools used to assay the auditory system in applied research studies, as well as used in the clinical evaluation of subjects. These chapters truly embrace the "translational" theme of the book series.

This, the third book in the series, entitled *Special Topics*, interweaves both basic and applied research, and hence provides a "translational" perspective on "hot topics" in hearing science. One example is the final chapter, "Current Issues in Auditory Plasticity and Auditory Training." Rather than simply review evidence of experience-related physiological changes documented in animal models, the authors chose to address the functional significance of "auditory plasticity" as it pertains to "auditory learning." By simply revisiting the concepts of "plasticity" in relation to "learning" there has been a resurgence of interest in the area of auditory rehabilitation. For those of us who are monists philosophically, brain function must underlie all behavioral changes, and hence there is no surprise that as long as we can learn, and adapt our behavioral responses, then of course the brain is somehow changing (and hence is "plastic"). So here the challenge was to present the literature in a way that allowed us to ask the tough questions, like "Does a statistically significant change in perception (or biology) necessarily constitute a functionally relevant change in behavior?" More importantly, "Do the observed changes impact a person's ability to communicate? And does it impact their quality of life?"

WHO ARE THESE BOOKS FOR?

Perhaps you are thumbing through this book series, and are trying to figure out if you should buy it. Is this book for you? Should you use it to teach a class on the anatomy/physiology of hearing? The answer to this lies in part in who you are. If you are already a neuroscientist or clinician scientist and interested in cross-training, then these books are for you. The series should serve as a source of knowledge that is both deep and broad; presenting current theory within a clinical context so one can learn to appreciate about what rests on the other side of the "valley of death." The final two books in the series are intended to relate the more basic scientific knowledge about the auditory system to more clinical aspects of the discipline. These books should be used as the basis for detailed class discussions. They should be thought provoking, and (in some instances) controversial. They should serve as a catalyst for term papers, updated literature reviews, and research projects. As these fields mature, no doubt some controversial statements will be proven true or false, or even rendered irrelevant, as the purpose of science is to continually update our current state of knowledge.

Some of the "translational" chapters in the last two books at least briefly extend into the realm of clinical practice. Students from clinical disciplines will note that there is often a dearth of experimental evidence that a specific therapeutic approach actually leads to improved function for a given clinical population. We hope that such gaps in knowledge will be addressed in your future clinical research efforts. The results of these future research efforts will form the basis of truly evidence-based practice in our clinical professions.

Acknowledgments. A few words of thanks are in order here. This book reflects the collective wisdom (and writing skills) of the many authors who contributed to the various chapters. While a textbook is typically poor in character development, it is their efforts that make this book useful (or not) to educate and hopefully inspire those students who read the book.

Several students, post-docs, clinicians, and scientists at the University of Washington read the various chapters, offered editorial comment, and crafted many of the questions posed to the authors at the end of each chapter. A special thanks to Hannah Martin, who assisted with copy editing, and Lindsay DeVries, who provided editorial comments as well as managed many of the administrative duties that are involved with producing a book. We would also like to say a special thanks to Kristin Swenson-Lintualt for creating the cover art used in this book.

REFERENCES

Declan, B. (2008, 12 June). Translational research: Crossing the valley of death [News feature]. *Nature, 453,* pp. 840–842.

Newsweek. (2010). http://www.newsweek.com/2010/05/15/desperately-seeking-cures.html

About the Editors

Kelly Tremblay, PhD, CCC-A, is a Professor in the Department of Speech and Hearing Sciences at the University at Washington. She earned a bachelor's degree in psychology from the University of Western Ontario, Canada, and an MSc in audiology from Dalhousie University in Halifax, Nova Scotia. Her interest in hearing science began in Colorado, as an audiologist who worked with hearing aid and cochlear implant users. Interested in auditory rehabilitation, she returned to school to learn more about the neuroscience underlying rehabilitation. She completed a PhD at Northwestern University, followed by postdoctoral training at the House Ear Institute in Los Angeles, California.

As a clinician and neuroscientist, Kelly Tremblay uses her training in neuroscience to better understand some of the everyday listening difficulties people with hearing loss describe. Because the typical person with a hearing loss is usually older and has been deprived of sound for some time, Dr. Tremblay's scholarly interests include defining the effects of aging and hearing loss on the brain. Another research interest of hers is to determine if auditory training can be used to improve the neural representation of acoustic cues transmitted by the ear to the cortex. She has published numerous papers and book chapters on these topics, and has received grant awards from many organizations including the National Institutes of Health. She has served as an associate editor for the *American Journal of Audiology*, an assistant editor for the *Journal of the American Academy of Audiology*, and a section editor for the journal *Ear and Hearing*.

Robert Burkard, PhD, CCC-A, is Professor and Chair, Department of Rehabilitation Science, at the University at Buffalo. He earned his BS in communication disorders at Buffalo State College, and his MS and PhD in audiology at the University of Wisconsin–Madison. He did a postdoctoral fellowship in the Department of Biology at Washington University. His first faculty position (Assistant then Associate Professor) was in the Department of Communication Disorders at Boston University. He moved to the University at Buffalo, where he was an Associate and then a Full Professor, in the Departments of Communicative Disorders and Sciences, and Otolaryngology. He moved to the Department of Rehabilitation Science, in the School of Public Health and Health Professions, in 2006.

His scholarly interests include acoustics and calibration, auditory physiology, and (more recently) vestibular function and balance. His research in auditory physiology has focused on human and animal auditory evoked potentials, but includes some single-unit electrophysiology and functional imaging studies. He has served as editor for the *American Journal of Audiology*, was the Audiology Co-Chair of the 2007 American Speech-Language-Hearing Association (ASHA) Annual Convention in Boston, has served as Vice Chair and Chair of the American National Standards (ANSI) S3 Bioacoustics Accredited Standards Committee, and currently serves as a member of the ASHA Health Care Economics Committee.

ABOUT THE COVER AND THE ARTIST

The cover art starts with an interesting story that highlights the power of perspective. Some might look at the cover and ask "Why is there an image of a guy who swallowed a mouse?" Perspective is everything. When the first editor saw the image of "ripple" (back book cover), she clearly saw the artist's depiction of hair cells. But when the artist turned it upright (as it was intended to be viewed) she laughed and said, "no," they are actually ripples and roots representing the changes a newborn baby brings to life. Clearly we saw the image from different perspectives, each influenced by our own experiences. And like science, we appreciated the art form and we learned from it. The author shared images and knowledge about the science of hair cells, which the artist unknowingly illustrated so well. In turn the artist taught the scientist about encaustic painting.

The art form used in the cover art work is called encaustic painting. Encaustic painting is an ancient art form notably used in the Fayum mummy portraits from Egypt around 100 to 300 AD. The art form in and of itself is relevant to our mission. It involves heating beeswax to which colored pigments are added. Because wax is used as the pigment binder, other materials can be encased or collaged into the surface, or layered, using the encaustic medium to adhere it to the surface. Our front cover art was created using multiple layers of wax, each composed of figures and concepts that appear throughout the textbook. When viewed as a whole, each micro element contributes to the more macro understanding of human communication.

The artist, Kristin Swenson-Lintault, earned her MFA in fiber/textiles in 1996 and her BA in fine art/drawing in 1993. She has studied painting at Hospitalfield House, a 13th-century studio arts center in Arbroath, Scotland, as well as traditional natural dye and indigo textile dyeing, washi hand papermaking, and wood-fired ceramics in Japan and South Korea. Her paintings have been exhibited nationally and in Nakajo, Japan. She has always been inspired to create work that deals with extracting the essence of some aspect of nature with an emphasis on abstraction, color, surface, and layering. Her current work is part of an ongoing series examining origins, connections, and lifelines. She teaches mixed media encaustic painting workshops at her studio in Seattle, Washington. More information can be found at www.theheatedpalette.blogspot.com and www.ksl-studio.blogspot.com.

Contributors

Jos J. Eggermont, PhD
Campbell Mc Laurin Chair for Hearing
    Deficiencies
Alberta Heritage Medical Scientist
Professor, Department of Physiology and
    Pharmacology
Department of Psychology
University of Calgary
Calgary, Alberta, Canada
Chapter 5

Linda J. Hood, PhD
Professor
Department of Hearing and Speech Sciences
Vanderbilt Bill Wilkerson Center
Vanderbilt University
Nashville, Tennessee
Chapter 2

Clifford R. Hume, PhD, MD
Associate Professor
Virginia Merril Bloedel Hearing Research Center
Department of Otolaryngology—Head and
    Neck Surgery
University of Washington School of Medicine
VA Puget Sound Health Care System
Seattle, Washington
Chapter 4

David Moore
Professor
Director
MRC Institute of Hearing Research
University Park, Nottingham, United Kingdom
Chapter 6

Thierry Morlet, PhD
Head, Auditory Physiology and Psychoacoustics
Research Laboratory
A.I. DuPont Hospital for Children
Adjunct Assistant Professor
Department of Linguistics and Cognitive
    Science
College of Arts and Science

University of Delaware
Wilmington, Delaware
Chapter 2

Kevin K. Ohlemiller, PhD
Associate Research Professor
Program in Audiology and Communication
    Sciences
Washington University
Fay and Carl Simons Ctr. for Biology of Hearing
    and Deafness
Central Institute for the Deaf at Washington
    University
Department of Otolaryngology
Washington University School of Medicine
Saint Louis, Missouri
Chapter 1

Dennis P. Phillips, PhD
Professor, Department of Psychology and
    Neuroscience
Professor, Department of Surgery (Division of
    ENT)
Dalhousie University
Halifax, Nova Scotia, Canada
Chapter 3

Jennifer S. Stone, PhD
Research Associate Professor
Department of Otolaryngology—Head and
    Neck Surgery
Virginia Merrill Bloedel Hearing Research Center
University of Washington School of Medicine
Seattle, Washington
Chapter 4

Kelly Tremblay, PhD, CCC-A
Professor
Department of Speech and Hearing Sciences
Affiliate of the Virginia Merrill Bloedel Hearing
    Research Center
University of Washington
Seattle, Washington
Chapter 6

1

Current Issues in Noise-Induced Hearing Loss

Kevin K. Ohlemiller

LEARNING OBJECTIVES

Upon completion of this chapter, the reader should be able to answer the following:

- What are the OSHA requirements for employers operating work environments in which daily TWA exposures exceed 85 dBA?
- What is the basic assertion of the equal energy hypothesis?
- Define permanent threshold shift (PTS), temporary threshold shift (TTS), compound threshold shift (CTS), and asymptotic threshold shift (ATS). How do TTS and the temporary component of CTS differ?
- What features of an audiogram might indicate that most of the hearing loss observed was caused by noise?
- Name two ways that the temporal structure of noise (e.g., continuous versus interrupted; Gaussian versus kurtotic) may influence the extent of PTS.
- What are the major cellular targets of noise? What anatomical changes best predict the extent of PTS?
- How are auditory neuronal frequency tuning curves altered by outer hair cell loss? What about inner hair cell stereocilia injury?

- Name five possible perceptual effects of PTS.
- Name five types of preconditioning treatments that confer protection against PTS.

Key Words. Standard threshold shift, equal energy hypothesis, audiogram, temporary threshold shift, permanent threshold shift, compound threshold shift, asymptotic threshold shift, critical point, acoustic trauma, half-octave shift, toughening, sound conditioning, acoustic augmentation, excitotoxic, apoptosis, necrosis, frequency tuning curve, frequency difference limens, loudness recruitment

INTRODUCTION

Barring thunderstorms and occasional cataclysms like volcanic eruptions and asteroid strikes, noise sufficient to have psychosocial and physiological effects is entirely a manmade pollutant. For epochal events like asteroids, noise might be the least of one's problems; yet, since the arrival of the industrial age, pervasive environmental noise, particularly occupational noise, has posed a major health issue. About 30 million people in the United States are suggested to be at risk of occupational hearing loss (Henderson et al., 2008). Some estimates place the prevalence of permanent noise induced hearing loss (NIHL) as

1

high as 4% of the population in western cultures, or about 10% worldwide (Hawkins & Schacht, 2005). Such estimates are unlikely to be accurate after middle age, when age-related hearing loss (ARHL, or presbycusis) probably dominates and obscures true NIHL (Dobie, 2008). We are still discovering ways that noise exposure can produce cochlear pathology indistinguishable from ARHL, and ways noise and aging can interact. Thus, it will be difficult to distinguish "pro-NIHL genes," as they are discovered, from putative "pro-ARHL genes." On an evolutionary timescale, the sudden onset of loud non-natural noises has left the tolerance of the auditory system little time to "catch up," nor is it clear how related selection pressures would operate. It is therefore likely that any systems or cellular processes shown to protect the auditory system from NIHL evolved to solve other problems, and have simply been co-opted to meet modern noise challenges.

Since the imposition of workplace hearing conservation programs in the United States, rates of occupational hearing loss appear to be decreasing (Dobie, 2008; Rabinowitz, 2006). However, threats posed by recreational exposure have multiplied. Whereas firearms use remains the riskiest after-work activity for hearing (Clark, 1991), the sheer number and power of other ways we can abuse our ears, concerts and movies, home theaters, video arcades, computer games, and Ipods, have skyrocketed. It does not help that children and young adults, who may make up the very demographic segment most vulnerable to NIHL (see later), are also most likely to turn up the volume. The effects of noise extend beyond hearing (Miller, 1974). Noisy environments generate added stress and alter mood. Even the most pleasant of sounds presented at sufficiently high levels, and for a long enough period, can constitute a form of torture. In addition to NIHL, chronic occupational noise is associated with systemic problems such as hypertension and cardiovascular disease. In this chapter, we create a picture of NIHL in broad, if necessarily shallow, strokes. Major points are drawn from both animal experiments and clinical literature, as these are highly interreliant. Our goal is to impart to the clinician, engineer, and researcher a sense of how acoustics and biology interact at extremes, how effective therapies might work, yet why therapies against NIHL remain so limited.

HISTORY AND THE EMERGENCE OF EXPOSURE STANDARDS

From the earliest records it has been clear that certain occupations (e.g., blacksmiths, millers, boilermakers, artillerymen) were linked to loss of hearing (Hawkins & Schacht, 2005). In 1874, S. J. Roosa, who is also credited with some of the earliest observations on hearing in aging (Ohlemiller & Frisina, 2008), first linked "boilermakers' deafness" to loss of cochlear nerve fibers. The first recorded animal experiments took place in the early 1900s. In 1912, H. Hoosli used an ingenious automatic "Hammerwerk" device to impart noise injury to guinea pigs from automated impact sounds of hammers, and devised within-subject controls by disarticulating the middle ear bones on one side. His illustrations (see Hawkins & Schacht, 2005) clearly show loss of the organ of Corti in the unprotected cochlea. In 1943, H. Davis, one of the most influential early investigators in the area of hearing and deafness, used himself and other volunteers as "guinea pigs," purposely inflicting threshold shifts upon their own ears. The noise levels employed by Davis and colleagues (110 to 140 dB SPL) were not intended to inflict permanent hearing loss. But, at the time, no one knew how much noise the human ear could tolerate. As a result, both temporary and permanent hearing loss were observed and carefully documented (Hawkins, 1976). Many now-established principles, including the 4 kHz "notch," recruitment, and the "half-octave shift" (see below), emerged from this work. In the late 1940s, the rise of new technology for producing and measuring sound, combined with an epidemic of NIHL in returning WWII veterans, launched the field of audiology (Clark, 2008).

The period from about 1950 to 1983 was unique and hugely important for understanding of occupational noise injury. Aided by the availability of new instrumentation during this time, the limits of noise tolerance of the human ear began to be established, yet broad regulatory mechanisms were not yet in place. Study of "preregulated" industrial settings facilitated the study of hearing loss as a function of noise environment and occupation, both in the United States and abroad. A few studies from this period were especially influential, including a large scale longitudinal study by Taylor and colleagues of female jute-weaving plant employees in Scotland (Taylor et al., 1964). Since 1983 the Federal Occupational Safety and Health Administration (OSHA) has required that occupational settings in the United States that subject employees to a time-weighted average (TWA) ≥85 dBA[1] of noise over an 8 hr workday must initiate a hearing conservation program (Rabinowitz, 2006; Rabinowitz et al., 2007). According to OSHA Hearing Conservation Standards, any covered employee exhibiting a **Standard Threshold Shift** (STS) must be counseled and continually monitored. The criterion for STS is an average increase in threshold of 10 dB or more at 2, 3, and 4 kHz in either ear. Assuming the threshold shift is deemed job related, upon notification, any affected employee must begin wearing hearing protection. According to the 2002 OSHA "Record-keeping rule," cases in which employees show an average threshold shift of at least 25 dB at 2, 3, and 4 kHz must be reported as job-related illness or injury. A cornerstone of both noise research and noise regulation is the **equal energy hypothesis**, according to which single exposures having the same energy will generally produce the same amount of injury and hearing loss (Ward et al., 1981; Ward & Turner, 1982). This well-supported principle provides part of the basis for time-versus-intensity trading in occupational exposures, whereby doubling the exposure duration and increasing the level by 5 dB are predicted to yield the same hearing loss, and thus are considered to carry equivalent risk. Note that the previous sentence carries the qualifier "part of the basis," as this rule does not adhere to a strict time/intensity tradeoff which, according to physical acoustics, would equate doubling of the exposure duration with a 3 dB increase in intensity of uncorrelated noise. However, most data suggest that the growth of risk of permanent NIHL is slower than would be predicted by a 3 dB rule. The substitution of 5 dB for 3 dB represents a more conservative approach that effectively protects workers while reducing costs to employers. Since 1983, rates of occupational PTS have declined (Dobie, 2008; Rabinowitz, 2006). Most residual risks have stemmed from: (1) inadequate

worker compliance, (2) effectively unregulated work settings where noise risk is not well characterized, and (3) increased blast exposure risk and weapons system noise in the military. Extra risk to some individuals may be imposed by genetic factors or health conditions that remain little understood.

TYPES OF THRESHOLD SHIFTS AND THEIR SIGNIFICANCE

The effect of noise on the auditory system depends on the type of noise, the region of the cochlea stimulated, and how changes in hearing are assessed. Both physiologically and perceptually, the cochlea and auditory system most resemble a bank of independent frequency filters. The essential dimensions that capture normalcy of hearing therefore entail: (1) the bandwidth of the filters, (2) the temporal fidelity of the filters, (3) the dynamic range of the filters, and (4) how sensitive the filters are to low-level sounds. Sensitivity is most easily assessed, so that threshold shifts provide the primary framework of our discussion.

Measurement of Thresholds

The cochlear spiral comprises a logarithmically spaced frequency map whereby low frequencies are represented near the top (the apex) of the spiral, and high frequencies are represented near the bottom (the base). At least for low-intensity signals, the response threshold for a particular sound frequency therefore indicates the health of a discrete cochlear segment tuned to that frequency. Thresholds can be measured behaviorally, or can be assessed physiologically by placing a recording electrode near the major neural generators of responses to sound. Suitable locations may include the pinna, ear canal, eardrum, or the surface of the head over the brainstem or cortex. The latter locations will emphasize central auditory generators, so that the method will depend on

---

[1] dBA refers to "A-weighted sound pressure level." A-weighting is a filtering method that spectrally shapes sounds similar to the way the human auditory periphery shapes moderately loud sounds. The dB SPL value is then measured for the filtered signal.

the question that is asked. When recorded from the cochlea or brainstem, the shortest latency electrical waves arise from synchronous responses of cochlear neurons to the stimulus onset. The typically micro-volt-range responses emerge from random electrical noise by averaging responses to many stimulus presentations. The lowest level sound that elicits a measurable response is declared threshold. Behaviorally, the lowest level sound that reliably elicits a response "hit" constitutes the threshold. When thresholds are determined across the frequency range of hearing, the resulting graphic relation is termed the **audiogram**. Compared to behavioral methods, physiological methods tend to overestimate thresholds, particularly at high frequencies (Dallos & Cheatham, 1976). One reason is that behavioral judgments take advantage of temporal integration of the stimulus, a perceptual operation to which physiologic measures are not sensitive. In addition, physiologic recordings are limited by electrical noise that obscures the response near threshold. Clinical audiograms and physiologic or behavioral "audiograms" obtained in the laboratory are typically reversed on the y-axis (owing simply to custom), and often use different reference values for 0 dB (dB HL versus dB SPL). Nevertheless, they are generally similar in shape. Regardless of how they are measured, noise-related threshold shifts appear dominated by injury to the cochlea, rather than the middle ear or central auditory system.

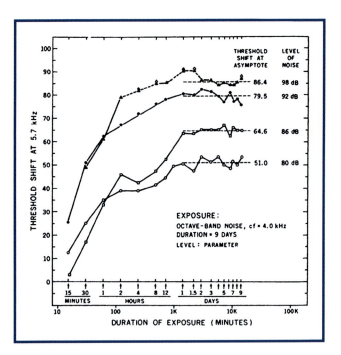

Figure 1–1. The average growth of threshold shifts in chinchillas at 5.7 kHz during noise exposure measured during brief interruptions. In each case, the total exposure duration was 9 days. Each curve represents a single exposure level, as indicated. For each exposure intensity, the shift rises to a constant asymptotic level, although this value increases with noise intensity. The rate of rise and time to asymptote are independent of noise intensity. (From Mills, 1973, *Journal of Speech and Hearing Research*. Reprinted with permission of the American Speech-Language-Hearing Association.)

Definitions of Threshold Shifts

As a moderately intense, continuous, noise exposure progresses, the response threshold will increase until some maximum shift from baseline is reached (Figure 1–1). After the noise ceases, the threshold will decrease, and over days or weeks will eventually return to baseline or settle permanently at some new level indicative of permanent injury (Figure 1–2). If the threshold returns to the initial normal level, the transient shift is termed a temporary threshold shift (**TTS**) (Miller, 1963). If the transient component ultimately leaves a higher permanent baseline, the difference between the final and original baselines

is termed the noise-induced permanent threshold shift (NIPTS or simply PTS). During the time that a transient component masks an eventual permanent component, the summed threshold shift has been termed the compound threshold shift (CTS) (Miller, 1963). There has been an unfortunate trend toward labeling the transient component in each case a TTS. This is perhaps because no economical name has been offered for the transient-threshold-shift-that-ultimately-decays-to-a-PTS. However, the transient part of a CTS (henceforth CTS$_t$ for lack of a better term) and TTS show different frequency distributions, different recovery dynamics, and appear to have different cellular correlates. As we shall see, TTS and PTS appear to have different cellular targets, and to reflect different processes. Thus the time

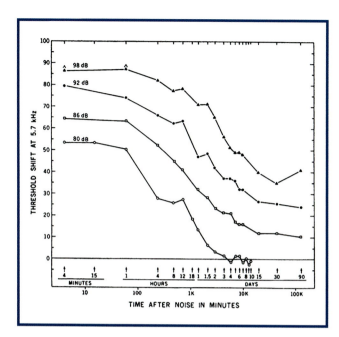

Figure 1–2. The time course of resolution of threshold shifts in chinchillas at 5.7 kHz following 9 days of noise exposure (same experiments as in Figure 1–1) measured for times out to 90 days postexposure. Higher exposure intensities result in permanent threshold shifts (PTS), as exhibited by a final baseline >0 dB. Note that the time to final threshold was greater in cases of PTS, indicating that the processes involved in TTS versus CTS$_t$ (see text) are different. (From Mills, 1973, *Journal of Speech and Hearing Research*. Reprinted with permission of the American Speech-Language-Hearing Association.)

course and extent of CTS$_t$ probably is determined by the partial recovery of the cells and structures underlying the final PTS.

The maximum threshold shift that is measured during exposure has proven a useful metric, and is termed the asymptotic threshold shift (ATS) (Miller, 1963). The ATS is proportional to noise level. For any level, an ATS will be reached within about a day of continuous exposure (see Figure 1–1), but will not increase even with succeeding months or (at least hypothetically) years of exposure. The ATS has been interpreted as the maximum PTS that could result from any given exposure after an infinite duration. Practically, some recovery is nearly always found when continuous noise is finally turned off, or a continual exposure is terminated.

Audiogram Clues to the Presence of PTS

Generally, PTS will not feature sensitivity losses greater than 40 dB at low frequencies, or 75 dB at high frequencies (Miller, 1963). A steeply sloping high frequency hearing loss that creates a >60 dB threshold differential between high and low frequencies is often a sign of traumatic noise injury, such as exposure to explosives or firearms (Clark, 2008). The severity of PTS may not correspond in any simple way with the duration of a long term exposure: In cases of long-term occupational exposure, PTS appears to grow most rapidly over the first 10 to 15 years of exposure, then to increase at a slower rate (Taylor et al., 1964). It is commonly reported that a wide variety of exposures lead to a "notch" in the human audiogram in the 4 to 6 kHz region (Rabinowitz et al., 2006). The notch appears to have an analog in the chinchilla, cat, and gerbil (Schmiedt, 1989). It can appear even while other frequencies are relatively spared, and has been interpreted as a hallmark of noise injury versus other conditions such as ototoxic injury or aging. The notch is most pronounced in younger subjects, and may ultimately be masked as the effects of age become dominant. Its origins may lie in the shape of the normal audiogram, which often shows greatest sensitivity at mid-frequencies, thus reflecting pinna or middle ear transfer characteristics. It may also coincide with processes or features particular to the middle of the cochlea, where distinct low-frequency *temporal* coding processes and high-frequency *firing-rate-based* coding processes meet (Ohlemiller & Siegel, 1994). Thresholds at high frequencies (>9 kHz) are also especially susceptible to noise (Quaranta et al., 1998), but this part of the human hearing range is not yet commonly monitored clinically, and is especially subject to confounding effects of aging.

Predicting PTS from TTS or Otoacoustic Emissions

The primary goal of noise research is, of course, to prevent PTS. However, the risk of PTS to any individual in a particular work or recreational setting will depend on both individual and environmental variables. One area of investigation has addressed the potential for predicting the potential for PTS from an experimental or inadvertent TTS. One might, for example, compare the hearing thresholds of workers at both the beginning and end of a shift to determine TTS, and then track their hearing over months or years to quantify eventual PTS. To date, no practicable approach has emerged from this. As we stated, TTS and PTS appear to reflect different processes, and will probably be differentially genetically modulated across individuals. In chinchillas, the extent of TTS has been argued to reflect mechanical "disconnect" events that are partly protective (Harding et al., 1992; Nordmann et al., 2000). The thinking in these models is that reduced height of the organ of Corti caused by buckling of pillar cells may disengage outer hair cells from mechanical input.

From work in cats (Liberman & Mulroy, 1982) and chinchillas (Hamernik et al., 2002), noise exposures causing less than 40 dB of threshold shift, as measured soon after the exposure, will not usually give rise to PTS. A question that might therefore be posed is, in cases where PTS is anticipated, at what point in time will a measured CTS_t permit the eventual PTS to be predicted? From the chinchilla work, shifts that remain after 24 hrs appear well correlated with the extent of PTS, exhibiting a slope of roughly 0.7 dB of PTS per dB of CTS_t (Hamernik et al., 2002).

Another strategy for predicting PTS attempts to monitor changes in the amplitude of otoacoustic emissions (OAEs). These are sounds measured from the ear canal, whose amplitude is generally positively correlated with the integrity of active outer hair cell (OHC) mechanics. In a healthy ear, presentation of two simultaneous tones (f_1, f_2, with $f_2 > f_1$) will elicit distortion products (DPOAEs, most prominently $2f_1 - f_2$) that reflect nonlinear amplification. A click stimulus will elicit an amplified transient response (TOAE). DPOAEs and TOAEs are quite sensitive to cochlear injury, and may be reduced or even absent in cochleas that show near-normal thresholds. Accordingly, some have attempted to use short-term decrements in these to anticipate eventual PTS. Presently, neither DPOAEs nor TOAEs appear to indicate which people are most vulnerable to noise, nor do they reliably identify those who

are in the initial stages of NIPTS (Müller & Janssen, 2008; Shupak et al., 2007).

Although it is quite an active area of research, there currently exist no objective tests to identify individuals who may be more at risk of PTS in noisy environments. Later we consider whether there could be genetic markers for susceptibility alleles that place some people at risk.

THE IMPORTANCE OF NOISE LEVEL AND TYPE

"Noise" is not a monolithic entity. The interventions we devise must work against real-world noise, and in the conditions under which people are exposed. In the laboratory, it is most practical to present approximately Gaussian noise (in theory, noise having a perfectly flat frequency spectrum, and whose time waveform possesses no internal structure) limited to some frequency band, and to present it one time at moderate-to-high intensity. For study of the biochemical cascades by which noise injury occurs, this has value: At least up to overtly traumatic intensities, fundamental cellular injury processes probably cross exposure conditions. Nevertheless, the extent of injury by area and cell type will vary markedly with level and temporal dynamics of the noise.

Effect of Noise Level

We said that up to a certain noise level, single exposures having the same energy will generally produce the same amount of hearing loss. For any species and noise type, however, there exists an intensity above which PTS and injury (particularly hair cell loss) abruptly accelerate (Figure 1–3). Across this **critical point,** energy equivalence does not apply (Ward et al., 1981; Ward & Turner, 1982). The critical point is suggested to represent the intensity where principally biochemical injury gives way to direct mechanical trauma. Although the term **acoustic trauma** has been used to refer to all PTS, it was originally intended to apply strictly to this case. The prin-

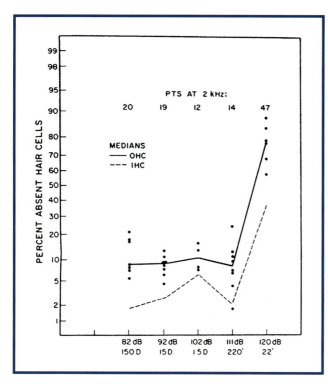

Figure 1–3. Percent inner and outer hair cell loss (IHC, OHC) in chinchillas for five exposure conditions to band-pass noise (0.7 to 2.8 kHz) having the same total energy, but differing durations and levels. Exposure duration/level combinations ranged from 150 days (D) at 82 dB to 22 minutes at 120 dB. Final PTS (*top of graph*) and cell counts were established 30 days after exposure. Note the large increase in PTS and cell loss when the exposure level was increased from 111 to 120 dB. (From Ward et al., 1981, *Annals of Otology.* Reprinted with permission of the Annals Publishing Co.)

Effect of Noise Frequency Band

For both TTS and PTS, sensitivity to high frequencies is generally more affected at any given noise level, and broadband noise will accordingly promote more high frequency TTS than low frequency TTS (Miller, 1963). More so than for PTS, the frequency range of TTS may resemble the frequency band of the noise.

Basal-apical vulnerability differences are more prominent for PTS than for TTS. Accordingly, broadband noise will damage the cochlear base more heavily, perhaps producing only TTS injury in the apex. Low-frequency noise can elicit similar PTS in the cochlear base and apex, whereas high-frequency noise will impact solely the base. This latter observation reflects asymmetry of the basilar membrane traveling wave, whereby the base responds to both high and low frequencies, depending on level, whereas the apex responds only to low frequencies regardless of stimulus level. Nevertheless, there are additional intrinsic differences in the vulnerability of the cochlear base and apex (Altschuler et al., 1992). Such differences may reflect differences in the shape and cellular makeup of the organ of Corti, yet may extend to the very composition and function of the hair cells themselves (Sha et al., 2001). From simple mechanical considerations, since the optimal excitatory frequencies are higher in the base, the velocity of transverse (up and down) movement must also be higher. Thus, for any given amount of basilar membrane displacement, the energy dissipated by the base will be greater than in the apex. This requirement suggests that the cochlear amplifier must generate more power in the base than in the apex, and that the requirements imposed on OHCs render them more vulnerable.

When narrowband noise leads to a discrete frequency range of PTS and spatially restricted cochlear injury, it is often noted that there is approximately a **half-octave shift** between these, with the locus of injury shifted basal to the region tuned to the noise band (Liberman & Kiang, 1978). The half-octave shift may find its origins in the mismatch between cochlear macromechanics (basilar membrane tuning) and micromechanics (OHC responses) (Clark, 2008). The cochlear amplifier relies on spatial interaction, whereby the responses of OHCs tuned to the stimulus frequency depend on a passive mechanical

cipal change in the *form* of injury above the critical point is that holes may appear in the reticular lamina (see upcoming Figure 1–8), or the organ of Corti may even be ripped from the basilar membrane. Breach of scala media boundaries alters qualitatively the stresses to which hair cells and supporting cells are exposed. As we will consider in greater detail, they are also exposed to high K$^+$ endolymph, which appears toxic (Ahmad et al., 2003). As a result, the hair cell injury process may be prolonged, and threshold may actually continue to deteriorate in the hours or days after noise, potentially the temporal "signature" of reticular lamina breach.

contribution from a region of the basilar membrane somewhat more basal. It is this passively responding region that sustains the most injury at high sound levels. It follows that the activity of the cochlear amplifier may not be essential for noise injury. Noise injury occurs at high amplitudes where the amplifier contributes little to hair cell and neural responses.

Temporal Aspects of Noise

The injurious nature of noise will depend on how it is distributed over time. Most real world noise is temporally heterogeneous, varying over time in level and in the content of transient components. Occupational noise exposure will typically be spread over 8 hours per day, 5 days a week. Barring recreational activities that compound weekday exposures, this potentially leaves evenings and weekends for recovery, and the engagement of protective mechanisms.

Interrupted, Intermittent, Time Varying (IITV) Noise

IITV noise, a phrase coined by Hamernik and colleagues (Qiu et al., 2007), captures the varied temporal qualities of occupational noise. The opposite of continuous noise, interrupted and intermittent respectively refer to noise embedded in long or short periods of quiet. Time varying refers to changes in the level of noise over time, but with no periods of complete quiet. Introduction of periods of quiet into an exposure schedule reduces the amount of PTS observed, even while the total energy remains the same. Noncontinuous exposure schedules can lead to progressive *reduction* of the daily effects of the noise (Clark et al., 1987). An exposure causing a 30 to 40 dB threshold shift at the end of the first day may, after a few days, elicit less than 5 dB of acute shift from the new baseline (Figure 1–4). This phenomenon has been termed **toughening**, and seems to be based on activation of cochlear protective or repair mechanisms (Sinex et al., 1987). Toughening involves some amount or permanent injury, but reduces subsequent injury. A related phenomenon that does not require initial injury is **sound conditioning**, whereby sustained moderate but noninjurious noise can protect against subsequent damaging exposures (Niu & Canlon, 2002). Yet another mani-

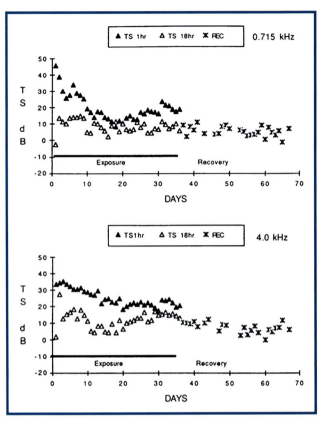

Figure 1–4. Daily changes in hearing thresholds at 0.715 kHz (*top*) and 4.0 kHz (*bottom*) in one chinchilla exposed 6 hrs/day to octave band noise centered at 0.5 kHz at 95 dB SPL for 36 days. Threshold shifts measured 1 hr postexposure gradually decrease, then merge with those measured at 18 hrs, which is indicative of toughening. Recovery data (X's) show that shifts at 18 hrs represent the amount of PTS. (From Clark et al., 1987, *Journal of the Acoustical Society of America*. Reprinted with permission of the American Institute of Physics.)

festation of protection by noise is **acoustic augmentation**, wherein sustained low level exposures can slow the time course of progressive hearing loss in mice that are genetically predisposed (Willott & Turner, 1999). All of these fit into a category of treatments known as preconditioning (see "Preconditioning Phenomena" section, below).

Impact and Impulse Noise

Occupational noise is typically not Gaussian, but instead includes sounds generated by concussive events such as the banging of hammers (impacts), or sudden release of gases under pressure (impulse).

These will occur unpredictably. Analytically, the characteristics that distinguish Gaussian noise from intermittent impact and impulse noise follow higher order noise distribution metrics known as *kurtosis*. In a series of papers, Hamernik and colleagues (Hamann et al., 2004; Hamernik et al., 2003; Hamernik et al., 2007; Qiu et al., 2006) tested in chinchillas the injury potential of noise continua ranging from mostly Gaussian to mostly randomly interspersed impulse/impact noise. For a constant overall energy level, the latter produce more PTS. Presumably, by virtue of their rapid onset, they more readily exceed the natural elastic limits of the inner ear, and are more likely to inflict acoustic trauma. The combination of kurtosis and energy metrics has proven effective in predicting both PTS and hair cell loss from wide variety of exposures that mimic realistic intermediate term occupational exposures.

Traumatic impulsive noise, such as the type associated with gunfire or the improvised explosive devices (IEDs) made infamous by recent military operations, are increasingly of interest to investigators working to prevent the ensuing PTS and tinnitus. It merits mention here that these are prohibitively difficult to model in the laboratory. If one wishes to record and replay blast noise through a speaker, at least two problems may be encountered. First, the dynamic range of the microphone may not allow accurate recording of the event. Many published characterizations of impulsive sounds are likely compromised by peak-clipping by the recording microphone that could have been diagnosed by looking at the output waveform. Second, the inertial mass and dynamic range of a conventional speaker often cannot reproduce the steep initial rise of the original event, even if it was properly recorded. Although one can use a speaker to present some impulsive sounds to characterize acoustic trauma and its treatment, it may literally require creation of blast events in the lab to closely model blast injury.

Question 1

In loud settings sound is often conducted via bone conduction. What is the impact of this type of exposure in comparison to air conducted sound?

Answer 1

Acoustic injury will reflect the energetically dominant input. The pressure gain in cochlear fluids owed to pinna and middle ear amplification is typically 30 to 40 dB. Hence, with the exception of blast shockwave trauma to the head, airborne sound will be the dominant influence in NIHL.

ANATOMIC EFFECTS OF NOISE ON THE COCHLEA

For decades, study of cochlear noise injury has focused on hair cell loss. Indeed, in some models and for some cochlear locations, hair cell loss reasonably predicts PTS. In some models, however, nonlethal hair cell injury and injury to supporting cells and neurons best account for PTS for most "real world" exposures. There is also growing interest in events in the cochlear lateral wall (stria vascularis and spiral ligament) (Figure 1–5) as influences on the degree of PTS, and perhaps its stability. Due to limited availability for study of human temporal bones with well characterized exposure histories, it is not completely clear which noise effects consistently apply to humans and explain human PTS. The anatomic correlates of a particular noise exposure vary even within a species according to genetic makeup (Ohlemiller & Gagnon, 2007), so that there may be no single answer for any species. Although we will employ the economy of referring to "the chinchilla," "the guinea pig," "humans," and so on, it should be recognized that this is an oversimplification.

Correlates of TTS

TTS is generally greatest near the frequencies of noise exposure, and peaks near the center frequency of narrow band noise. Although the correlates of TTS may vary by species, the cochlear regions tuned to the noise may show reversible injury to hair cell stereociliary bundles, conformational changes within

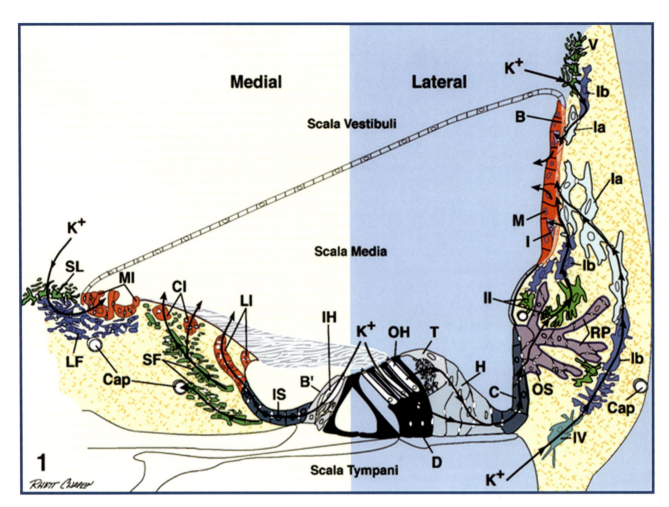

Figure 1–5. Cochlear operation depends on dozens of cell types, some whose functions are not well understood. Shown is schematic radial view of the organ of Corti and adjacent lateral wall. Arrows indicate posited medial and lateral transcellular routes for K⁺ effluxed from inner and outer hair cells (IH, OH) during auditory transduction. B, strial basal cell; B′, border cell; Cap, capillary; C, Claudius cell; CI, central interdental cell; D, Deiters cell; H, Hensen cell; I, strial intermediate cell; IS, inner sulcus cell; M, strial marginal cell; MI, medial interdental cell; LF, light fibrocyte; LI, lateral interdental cell; OS, outer sulcus cell; RP, root process of outer sulcus cell; SF, stellate fibrocyte; SL, supralimbal fibrocyte; T, tectal cell; Ia, Ib, II, IV, and V, types of spiral ligament fibrocytes. (From Spicer and Schulte, 1998, *Hearing Research*. Reprinted with permission Elsevier Publishing.)

the organ of Corti (particularly pillar cell buckling), and excitotoxic injury to radial afferent neuronal dendrites (Nordmann et al., 2000; Wang et al., 2002; Zhao et al., 1996). Excitotoxic injury to neurons was until recently thought to be reversible. However, as we will revisit, TTS may signal injury to cochlear neurons that has no threshold component, and may take years to manifest (Kujawa & Liberman, 2006).

Correlates of PTS

Although injury to the organ of Corti is generally the best predictor of PTS, injury often extends to afferent neurons, lateral wall, spiral limbus, even Reissner's membrane (Liberman & Beil, 1979; Liberman & Mulroy, 1982; Salvi et al., 1982; Wang et al., 2002; Ward & Duvall, 1971). Given a severe enough exposure, almost any cell or structure one might name will be affected. This includes literally dozens of cell types whose functions are not well understood. Such broad injury emphasizes the "communal" nature of cochlear function, and the complexity of its homeostatic processes (see Figure 1–5). What may separate different cell types in their effects on PTS is how many can be lost before hearing is affected. We have more "extra" supporting cells, fibrocytes, marginal cells, and so forth than we have extra hair cells. Yet every cell type must serve a unique function, and cannot be lost entirely without cost.

Hair Cells and Neurons

The most general correlate of PTS is OHC loss and injury, especially injury to OHC stereocilia bundles (Figure 1–6). Inner hair cell (IHC) stereocilia are also affected, and more severe exposures can cause IHC loss. Unlike the hair bundles on IHCs, however, the bundles of OHCs are embedded directly into the tectorial membrane. This feature appears pivotal to the ability of OHCs to exert force on the basilar membrane as part of active mechanics, but also subjects the embedded bundles to injury.

The relative contributions of hair cell loss versus permanent hair cell injury appear to vary with noise level, cochlear location, and species. For subcritical exposures, hair cell loss in CBA/CaJ mice (a standard "good hearing" strain) occurs principally in the most basal 20%, largely independent of the noise band (see Figure 1–6) (Wang et al., 2002). Above-critical-level exposures in mice, however, dramatically redistribute hair cell loss, along with other aspects of injury. Rats and cats more readily show hair cell loss in the most basal 50% (Chen & Fechter, 2003; Liberman & Kiang, 1978). Guinea pigs, chinchillas, and potentially humans, seem more prone to hair cell loss that corresponds to the location of the noise band (allowing for a half-octave shift) (Figure 1–7) (Altschuler et al., 1992; Hamernik et al., 1989). Upon detailed examination, frequency-matched hair cell loss in chinchillas appears to coincide with holes in the reticular lamina where OHCs had been (Figure 1–8) (Ahmad et al., 2003). Although the general phenomenon of reticular lamina breach appears universal at high noise levels, its details may vary with species. Supercritical levels of noise may lead to

large tears in the reticular lamina, and thereby large areas of endolymph entry. Such dramatic injury may, however, not be required for endolymph entry into the organ of Corti to play a significant factor in PTS. In chinchillas, levels of noise near the critical level may be associated with ejection of dead OHCs from the reticular lamina, leaving holes where endolymph can infiltrate. These holes remain until scars can form between adjacent Deiters' cells, or between Deiters' and pillar cells, and may require days to resolve (Ahmad et al., 2003). By contrast, studies in guinea pigs indicate that dead and dying OHCs are removed in such a way as to preserve the continuity of the lamina (Altschuler et al., 1992; Raphael et al., 1993). It is not clear whether the chinchilla organ of Corti is especially fragile, or whether the process of hair cell loss and scar formation in the chinchilla is simply qualitatively different from that in some other models. It remains a vital unresolved issue whether pronounced hair cell loss reliably signals breach of the reticular lamina, what form it takes (holes versus tears), and how readily it occurs in humans. The critical exposure level for disruption of the reticular lamina depends on the type of noise, but for any type, may be low in chinchillas versus other models (Ward et al., 1981). Identifying reticular lamina holes requires tedious analysis of recently noise-exposed material. One indicator of their formation may be reduction of the endocochlear potential (EP). The EP, a positive electrical potential (+80 to 100 mV, depending on species) that exists within scala media, is generated by the stria vascularis, and provides much of the electrochemical driving force for K^+ flow during transduction (see Figure 1–5) (Wangemann, 2006). The EP depends on the integrity of tight junctions between cells that form the boundary of the endolymphatic space. In chinchillas, the EP is transiently reduced while holes in the reticular lamina remain open (Ahmad et al., 2003). As we will see, however, results from mouse models show that EP reduction by noise can independently reflect either injury to the organ of Corti or to the lateral wall.

When hair cells die, their postsynaptic neurons eventually die too, although supporting cells that remain may also promote neuronal survival (Sugawara et al., 2005). Neuronal loss probably reflects the

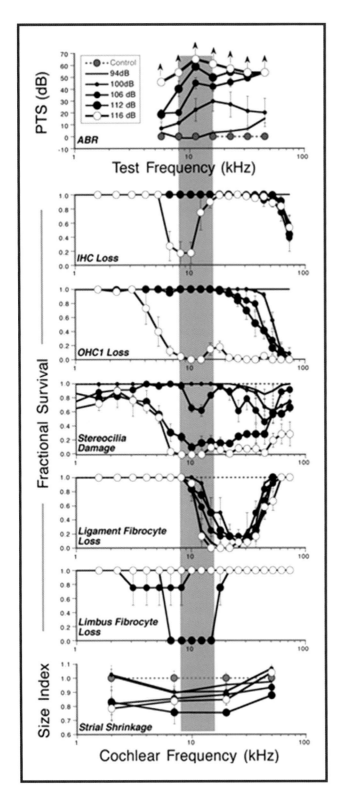

Figure 1–6. Spatial distribution of permanent noise injury to the CBA/CaJ mouse cochlea (determined 2 wks postexposure) as a function exposure level (see key in top panel). All exposures were 2 hrs in duration, and covered the band indicated by gray shading (8–16 kHz octave band). Top panel shows threshold shifts. Note that hair cell loss matched to the noise band occurred only at the highest exposure level, so that stereocilia damage better explained PTS. Ligament fibrocyte loss refers to type IV cells adjacent to the basilar membrane (see Figure 1–5). Spiral limbus and stria vascularis sustained permanent injury, but the injury did not grow monotonically with noise level, and was not considered to predict PTS. Error bars are SEM. (From Wang et al., 2002, *Journal of the Association for Research in Otolaryngology*. Reprinted with permission of the Association for Research in Otolaryngology.)

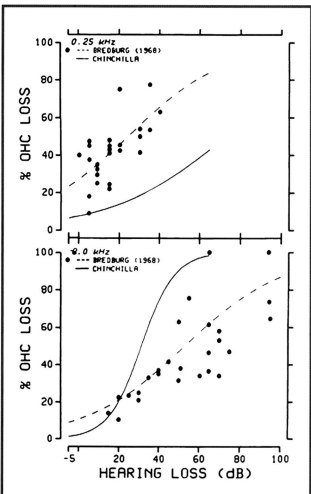

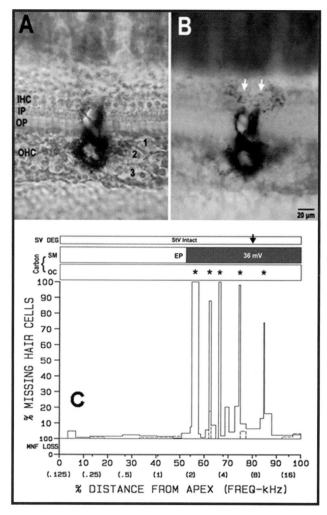

Figure 1–7. The relation between OHC loss and hearing loss in noise exposed chinchillas and humans, compared for two cochlear locations. Chinchilla data were derived from a large sample and are rendered as fitted curves (*solid lines*). Individual data from human temporal bones are shown, along with fitted curves (*dashed lines*). Correlations are apparent in each case, although moderate cell loss is not necessarily associated with hearing loss at the 0.25 kHz place in humans, and the relation is shallower in humans at the 8.0 kHz place. (Human data are replotted from Bredberg, 1968). (From Hamernik et al., 1989, *Hearing Research*. Reprinted with permission Elsevier Publishing.)

Figure 1–8. Phase contrast microscope view (**A**) and bright-field view (**B**) of a segment of the organ of Corti in a chinchilla showing noise-induced breach of the reticular lamina. The noise was octave band centered at 4.0 kHz, delivered at 108 dB SPL for 1.75 hrs. The breach has been demonstrated by injection of carbon tracer particles, which line the hole and permeate the surrounding extracellular space in the organ. **C.** Superimposed plots of cochlear injury versus frequency-place in the same chinchilla. Although the endocochlear potential was abnormally low (*36 mV, measured at point indicated by arrow*), the stria vascularis appeared normal (*top*). Injury to the organ of Corti consisted of 5 focal lesions (*asterisks*) in which most or all OHCs had degenerated, leaving OHC-sized holes in the reticular lamina. There was no loss of myelinated neuronal processes (MNF, bottom). IP: Inner pillar cells; OP: Outer pillar cells (From Ahmad et al., 2003, *Hearing Research*. Reprinted with permission Elsevier Publishing.)

loss of excitatory drive and loss of trophic interactions between IHCs and afferent dendrites, as approximately 95% of afferent neurons innervate IHCs (Spoendlin, 1978). To some extent, however, it may also reflect injury stemming from **excitotoxic** effects of glutamate release during the exposure (Puel et al., 1998). Glutamate, the principal neurotransmitter released by hair cells, is toxic to neurons when released in large quantities. Excitotoxic processes generate active intermediates such as nitric oxide and peroxynitrite that may also mediate injury to other cells in the organ of Corti and lateral wall. Although excitotoxic injury may be reversible, recent work suggests that it can disrupt IHC/afferent interactions in a way that promotes delayed neuronal loss resembling *neural* presbycusis (Kujawa & Liberman, 2006). Even more surprisingly, this process need not be associated with measurable PTS. Although this may seem nonintuitive, lesion data show that moderate loss of neurons and even IHCs may not greatly affect ABR response thresholds (El-Badry & McFadden, 2009). Behavioral detection of tones in quiet is also relatively insensitive to moderate neuronal loss, so that detection of tones in noise and identification of speech provide more sensitive indicators. The roughly 30,000 afferent neurons we normally possess in each cochlea were not an evolutionary response to simple detection needs. For that, we could probably get by with 5% of that total (Pauler et al., 1986). Instead, they evolved to mediate fine judgments of spectral shape against noisy backgrounds.

It should be mentioned that human cochlear neurons appear unique with regard to the near complete absence of myelination of cell bodies in Rosenthal's canal (Ota & Kimura, 1980). Although the myelination of both central and peripheral processes appear like that in other species, human neurons often form clusters that are ensheathed by a single glial cell. The close apposition this affords is attended by junctions, both between cell bodies and between passing axons and cell bodies. The former suggests that the neurons are electrically coupled, whereas the latter may demarcate a stage of efferent feedback that is not present in other species. The arrangement of neurons in humans may help account for the surprising ability of human neurons to survive hair cell loss, in that neurons that have lost their targets may receive trophic support from adjacent neurons, or even be electrically driven by adjacent neurons. Electrically linked clusters may compose "functional units" that give synchronized responses to signal periodicity. Although animal cochleas generally differ from human cochleas in relatively minor, quantitative ways, the lack of myelination and cell-cell junctions that distinguish human cochlear neurons may limit what can be generalized from animals.

Supporting Cells

In addition to a normal complement of hair cells, proper function of the organ of Corti requires the contributions of a host of supporting cell types. In the medial organ of Corti (near IHCs) these include inner and outer border cells (see Figure 1–5). Laterally, near OHCs, they include inner and outer pillars, and Deiters' cells. More lateral still are tectal cells, Hensen cells, Claudius cells, Boettcher cells, and outer sulcus cells. It can be difficult to distinguish between some of these (e.g., Hensen versus tectal, Claudius), and their densities appear highly variable. Counts of supporting cells are impractical and not very informative, since we do not know the relative contribution of each cell.

Some general supporting cell functions have been identified. To minimize levels of extracellular glutamate and the prospect of excitotoxic injury, some supporting cells express glutamate transporters. During transduction, K^+ accumulates in the area around hair cells. If it is allowed to remain, it can alter ion gradients and interfere with hair cell responses, and as we considered, may be toxic. To minimize the problem of K^+ buildup, and probably also to maximize the efficiency of K^+ homeostasis, the system has evolved an elaborate network of gap junctions that electrically couple the cells of the lateral organ of Corti. Junctions composed of the proteins termed connexin 26 and 30 (Cx26, Cx30) appear to join most cells of the lateral organ, so that K^+ taken up by Deiters' cells is conveyed into the spiral ligament via the root processes of outer sulcus cells (Zhao et al., 2006). Ultimately, this K^+ reaches the stria vascularis, for "recycling" back into the endolymphatic space. An additional route for K^+ may depend on diffusion through perilymph to the cells of the inferior spiral ligament (Type IV fibrocytes)

(Wangemann, 2002). Potassium released by IHCs may principally move medially via gap junctions through border cells, inner sulcus cells, and the spiral limbus, either for transport into the perilymph of scala vestibuli, or into the endolymphatic space via the epithelium that lines the limbus (see Figure 1–5) (Spicer & Schulte, 1998).

Although the advisability and gained efficiency of conveying K^+ away from the organ of Corti and back to the stria seem clear, just how high K^+ levels in the organ of Corti can become during noise exposure is not clear. Obvious toxicity has only been shown for endolymphatic K^+ levels, whereas values that are actually reached are likely to be lower. However, deleterious effects of elevated K^+ in the organ of Corti may not be based solely on toxicity to cells. The "conduit" role of gap junctions is now known to extend beyond K^+ to include important signaling molecules such as Ca^{++}, ATP, and inositol triphosphate (IP_3) (Ohlemiller, 2008). Two-way passage of these, both along the cochlear tonotopic gradient and between the organ of Corti and spiral ligament, may coordinate stress responses during noise exposure. Both oxidative stress, which is known to mediate noise injury, and changes in the extracellular medium can reduce the conductance of gap junctions. Noise injury models that invoke K^+ toxicity may not require frank holes in the reticular lamina; even modest increases in K^+ may be enough to impair gap junction-based communication, and thereby increase PTS.

Spiral Ligament, Stria Vascularis, and Spiral Limbus

The spiral ligament is not technically a ligament, but is composed principally of cartilage that is produced and maintained by several distinct classes of fibrocytes (Types I–V, with additional subtypes) (see Figure 1–5). Noise exposure can cause partial loss of most fibrocyte types (Ohlemiller & Gagnon, 2007; Wang et al., 2002), but Type IV fibrocytes may be decimated. It has been asserted that this pathology contributes to PTS, perhaps through disruption of ion and metabolite traffic between the organ of Corti and lateral wall.

We said that formation and repair of holes in the reticular lamina is associated with temporary EP reduction (Ahmad et al., 2003). EP reduction can also purely reflect lateral wall events, so that there may be two independent processes at work. Work in mice (Ohlemiller & Gagnon, 2007; Wang et al., 2002) has revealed reversible EP decline that gives way to characteristic permanent changes in the stria vascularis and spiral ligament. Acute signs of permanent damage from subcritical exposures may include vacuolization or shrinkage of fibrocytes and vacuolization of strial basal cells. Damage from supercritical exposures may extend to strial marginal cells. About 12 to 24 hrs after exposure, the appearance of the stria may change even more dramatically, swelling to more than twice its normal thickness (Figure 1–9). This swelling reverses, leaving a stria that is thinner, with fewer capillaries and constituent cells. All major ligament cell types are also reduced in number. At least in mice, these changes show strong genetic control that appears independent of overall genetic predisposition to PTS (Ohlemiller & Gagnon, 2007).

The constituent fibrocytes of the spiral limbus are highly vulnerable to noise (Liberman & Kiang, 1978; Wang et al., 2002). It is not unusual for the limbus to become nearly acellular (except for its epithelial surface) after even modest exposure in some models. All the roles of the limbus have not yet been revealed. It may mediate passage of ions and metabolites from scala tympani to scala vestibuli, channel K^+ away from the organ of Corti, and potentially maintain the tectorial membrane (Spicer et al., 1999). The tectorial membrane (TM) is altered by noise in ways that are likely to be permanent (Tsuprun et al., 2003). Long ignored as a noise target, the TM does more than simply give OHC stereocilia something to push against. Its physical properties appear to be matched to the resonant frequency of each location. It is quite difficult to observe this acellular, collagen-based structure without artifact, and changes are hard to quantify. Its density, size, and apparent fragility vary along the apical-basal axis. It is presently unclear to what extent it can be repaired.

In summary, the cochlear lateral wall and limbus show noise-related degeneration whose relation to PTS remains in dispute. These structures initially develop with a surfeit of cells, followed by steady decline throughout life (Ohlemiller & Frisina, 2008). This decline may be partially tempered by cell replacement. Because neighboring regions may be able to compensate for focal degeneration, and

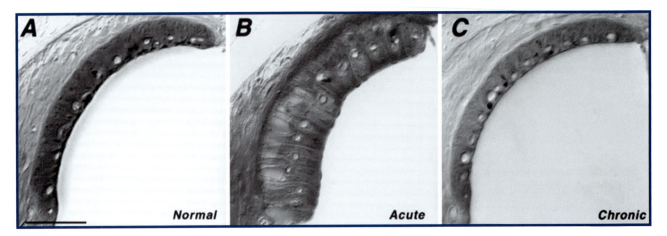

Figure 1–9. Stria vascularis in the cochlear upper basal turn of CBA/CaJ mice exposed to 8-16 kHz band noise at 116 dB SPL for 2 hrs. **A.** Normal control. **B.** 24 hrs after noise the stria is grossly swollen and the EP (not shown) is reduced. **C.** Two weeks after noise in a different mouse, the stria has regained its overall normal appearance, but is thinner due to cell loss and loss of interdigitating cell processes. Scale bar: 50 μm (From Wang et al., 2002, *Journal of the Association for Research in Otolaryngology*. Reprinted with permission of the Association for Research in Otolaryngology.)

because there may be some redundancy of function among fibrocyte types, the range of possible effects of degeneration on PTS extends from no effect at all to exacerbation of a progressive decline of hearing. This is an increasingly active area of study.

Question 2

The purpose of amplification through the use of hearing aids is to make sounds louder. Aren't we damaging hearing even further by delivering intense sounds to a damaged ear?

Answer 2

There is no evidence that a damaged ear is more vulnerable to noise than a normal ear. Moreover, elevated thresholds effectively reduce the level of noise inputs, reducing any additional NIHL from a given exposure.

CELL DEATH AND SURVIVAL MECHANISMS

Dying cells, including hair cells, are generally considered to follow one of two "death pathways": **apoptosis** or **necrosis** (oncosis), depending on the severity of injury (Henderson et al., 2006; Van De Water et al., 2004). Apoptosis, commonly referred to as **programmed cell death**, is a process whereby cells actively engage enzymes that dismantle DNA, proteins, and membranes. Necrosis represents a largely uncontrolled process wherein cells spill their contents into the extracellular space. Necrosis appears dominant in overt trauma, whereas apoptosis may dominate in the case of subtler injury. Often, both mechanisms may operate, so that a focal area of necrosis may be surrounded by a ring of apoptotic death. In apoptosis, degraded cell components are packaged into large membrane-bound vesicles that are scavenged by resident or invading macrophages. The process seems to have evolved to avoid influx of inflammatory cells and possible development of autoimmune reactions.

Two major apoptotic pathways are recognized: extrinsic and intrinsic (or mitochondrial) (Van De Water et al., 2004). Both of these involve enzymes known as caspases. Mitochondria, the cells' primary ATP "power" generators, initiate the intrinsic form by releasing cytochrome C (which engages caspases), apoptosis-inducing factor (AIF), and endonuclease G (endoG) into the cytoplasm (Han et al., 2006; Yamashita et al., 2004). One or both of the latter then migrate into the cell nucleus and initiate DNA fragmentation. The mechanism linking cell stress to the mitochondrial response may depend on dysregulation of cytosolic calcium and subsequent activation of Bcl-2-associated death promoter (BAD) (Vicente-Torres & Schacht, 2006). BAD is thought to migrate into mitochondria and sequester anti-apoptotic proteins, leading to permeabilization of the mitochondrial membrane, followed by cytochrome C, AIF, and endoG release. Nitric oxide (NO), produced either in the cytosol of OHCs or within mitochondria, may also initiate the caspase-independent mitochondrial pathway (Shi et al., 2007).

Studies in cats suggest that IHCs can survive for months or years with damaged stereociliary bundles (Liberman, 1987). Once IHCs are lost, there appears to be a great deal of species variation in the length of time (relative to life span) that de-afferented spiral ganglion cells survive. In humans they may last years, buying vital time for the benefits of cochlear implantation. It is generally observed that dysfunctional OHCs cells tend to die. Gene mutations that do not clearly disrupt basic cell house-keeping functions in OHCs nevertheless often lead to their death. A bit of thought reveals that this need not have been the case. It might be deemed evolutionarily advantageous if dysfunctional hair cells did not die, but instead survived to help maintain ionic boundaries. Or why not endow these critical cells with highly effective repair mechanisms? Oddly, it seems that when cells are "given a reason" not to die, they not only survive, but can also recover some receptor function. This surprise has emerged from work involving anti-apoptotic drugs (Matsui et al., 2003). These have opened up a new and exciting therapeutic avenue, particularly for application *after* an exposure.

NOISE-RELATED CHANGES IN BLOOD FLOW

The role in PTS of changes in cochlear blood flow has been an area of intense speculation and confusion, and merits its own discussion. The process of transduction places rigorous requirements on ion homeostasis. Without the proper gradients for K^+, Na^+, Ca^{++}, and Cl^-, transduction will not occur. Much of the control of ion flow can be accomplished

passively, that is, using voltage-gated channels and ion exchange pumps (Wangemann, 2002). However, somewhere in the system there must be active pumping that moves ions up their concentration and voltage gradients, expending ATP in the process. Evolution has moved this task largely to the lateral wall: Most Na^+/K^+-ATPase and Ca^{++}-ATPase function resides in the lateral wall, particularly within Type II fibrocytes and strial marginal cells. This significantly reduces the energy load on hair cells, and ostensibly their vulnerability to metabolic injury during prolonged exposure. Retention of the most energetically expensive operations to the lateral wall coincides with most of the microvasculature in the cochlear duct also being restricted to the lateral wall (Axelsson, 1988). All blood supplying the cochlea travels through the modiolus, entering with the auditory nerve through the internal auditory meatus, then traveling apically via the spiral modiolar artery. In each cochlear turn, vessels split into two major circuits: a modiolar loop that supports neurons and spiral limbus, and a lateral loop that supports the lateral wall. In most mammals, the latter is presumed to support the operation of the organ of Corti, and has been the subject of most experiments. Arterioles travel through the bony septa that separate the cochlear turns, and then enter the spiral ligament from the scala vestibuli side where they branch into somewhat independent ligament and strial networks. Within any turn, these recombine in the inferior ligament and drain into the spiral modiolar vein. A potentially important difference in humans is the reported consistent presence of a vessel on the scala tympani side of the basilar membrane, unsurprisingly termed the vessel of the basilar membrane (VBM). The VBM is not present in all adult mammals, or even all primates (Axelsson, 1988). Any significant role for this vessel in humans in meeting the metabolic needs of the organ of Corti during stress may ultimately limit the generalization of cochlear blood flow results from lower mammals.

Although regulation of the VBM is largely uncharacterized, blood flow in the lateral wall has been extensively studied. Regulation of cochlear blood flow by vasoconstriction takes place both within the modiolus and the lateral wall. Reduction of blood flow in the lateral wall could therefore reflect vasoconstriction in the modiolus, lateral wall, or both. Ideally, an increase in metabolic activity should be echoed by increased blood flow in the lateral wall, as determined by faster movement of red blood cells and increased vessel diameter. Depending on species and condition, however, blood flow during noise can either decrease or increase (Nakashima et al., 2003; Quirk & Seidman, 1995), and may be accompanied by increased vessel permeability. Although increased permeability might sound like a good thing, it actually refers to unregulated and maladaptive flow of ions and solutes across vessel walls. This phenomenon may take the form of gaps between endothelial cells that can be observed by electron microscopy. It can also be diagnosed using "tracer" molecules (such as horseradish peroxidase) or abnormal immunoglobulin deposits in strial pericapillary spaces (Duvall et al., 1974). Reversible perivascular swelling within the stria, seen in more extreme noise exposures, may reflect either increased pressure in constricted capillaries, or water movement following ion dysregulation. Such swelling may be most prominent in the hours after exposure, and may be associated with "shorting out" of the EP across strial microcapillary walls. Potentially central to the kinds of changes exhibited by strial and ligament capillaries are pericytes, a specialized cell type that surround capillary endothelial cells, and along with endothelial cells, produce and maintain the basement membrane (Edelman et al., 2006). A wide range of roles have been suggested for pericytes, including that of macrophage, stem cell, and regulator of capillary permeability.

The literature is fairly consistent in demonstrating that magnesium and compounds that reduce vasoconstriction within the stria vascularis and spiral ligament can decrease PTS (Le Prell et al., 2007b). Nevertheless, there has remained a logical "disconnect" between asserted changes in cochlear blood flow due to noise, and how this should impact cochlear function temporarily or permanently. Most studies have focused on alterations of strial capillaries, which can be shown to constrict during exposure. This constriction may reflect local effects of reactive oxygen species (ROS) generation on endothelial cells (Miller et al., 2003). Unlike microcapillaries in the ligament, however, strial microcapillaries do not possess a means of active vasoconstriction, so it may simply reflect colloidal pressure disruption

and passive fluid dynamics. The intrastrial space does not freely communicate with either endolymph or the spiral ligament, but transfer of metabolites from the stria to the organ of Corti could be facilitated by the same gap junctional network that guides K^+ in the opposite direction (Chang et al., 2008). Nutrients delivered by strial or ligament capillaries could thus potentially reach the organ either via perilymph or gap junctional networks. If these are "shut down" by noise exposure, it could help explain why these junctions are crucial to hair cell survival.

In summary, how noise impacts cochlear blood flow, and precisely how this is supposed to mediate PTS requires more study and clearer models. Nevertheless, evidence for reduction in PTS by compounds that enhance blood flow is fairly strong. How and why these compounds really work, and how they might be improved, is an area fairly begging for innovative ideas and experiments.

EFFECTS OF NOISE ON COCHLEAR FUNCTION

As radial afferent neurons provide the cochlear output underlying perception, we will consider how noise injury alters their responses in the frequency and intensity domains. Because IHCs drive these neurons, changes in their responses represent a direct reflection of alterations in the operation of hair cells, and in turn, the basilar membrane. The frequency response of cochlear neurons is typically characterized by their **frequency tuning curve (FTC)**, which defines across many frequencies the minimum sound level needed to elicit a criterion increase in spike (action potential) rate (Figure 1–10). Depending on the frequency to which they are tuned (the characteristic frequency, or CF), FTCs resemble band-pass filters, or "hybrid" low-pass/band-pass combination filters. The FTCs of neurons tuned to higher frequencies possess two segments: a sharp "tip" at the CF, and a less sensitive "tail" plateau below the CF. The tail region is the manifestation of the traveling wave asymmetry and the fact that any cochlear region will respond best to its own frequency as well as all lower frequencies. The shape and sensitivity of the FTC near the tip is determined

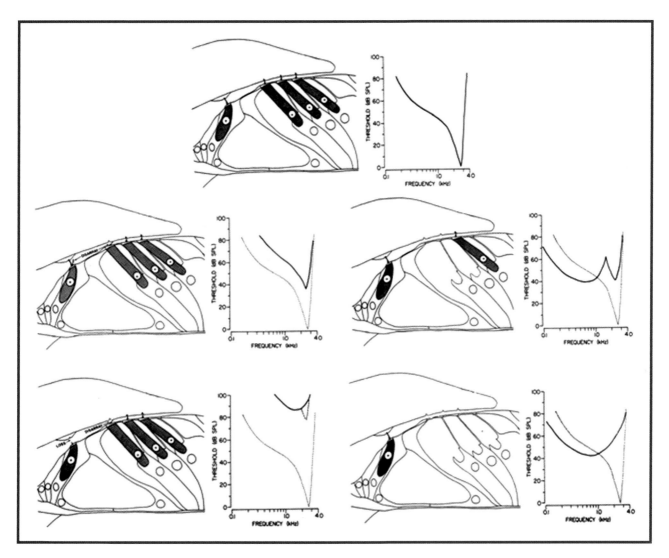

Figure 1–10. Schematic illustration of the relation between the nature of noise injury to the organ of Corti and the effects on frequency tuning of afferent neurons. Top shows normal cell conformation and normal tuning. Middle left shows result of injury to IHC stereocilia. The tuning curve is elevated, but remains sharp. Middle right shows result of partial OHC loss. The tuning curve tail becomes hypersensitive, while the tip is greatly elevated. Bottom left shows result of injury to stereocilia of both IHCs and OHCs. Both tail and tip are elevated; tip is minimal. Bottom right shows result of complete OHC loss. Tuning curve tail becomes hypersensitive; Tip is completely absent. (From Liberman and Dodds, 1984, *Hearing Research*. Reprinted with permission Elsevier Publishing.)

by the contribution of OHCs and active mechanics. Injury to the stereocilia of the presynaptic IHC will not affect the shape of the curve, but rather will shift the entire curve upward. Typical changes in tuning due to noise are illustrated in Figure 1–10. FTCs are most altered in the frequency range of largest PTS. The most prominent changes in these curves at the peak of noise damage is loss of tip sensitivity and

sharpness, while the tail region (dominated by passive mechanics) is less affected.

With increasing sound intensity, the spike rate of cochlear neurons typically steadily increases, then plateaus at higher levels. PTS generally shifts these curves to the right, but does not alter the shape of the relation (Henderson & Salvi, 1998). Other response characteristics, such as the temporal pattern of spikes and "phase-locking" to the stimulus frequency, are similarly maintained, although higher sound intensities are needed.

CENTRAL AUDITORY AND PERCEPTUAL CONSEQUENCES OF PERIPHERAL INJURY

The perceptual deficits that result from cochlear noise injury could hypothetically arise purely as a reflection of the type and extent of the cochlear injury. Alternatively, they could be exacerbated by additional changes that occur in the auditory central nervous system (ACNS). There is also a third possibility, that the net effects on perception will reflect adaptive "plastic" changes within the ACNS that compensate for the peripheral injury. As we will see, cochlear noise injury can lead to surprising additional ACNS changes, some of which are clearly degenerative. Although the term plasticity has been used a great deal in the context of PTS, it is not clear that any truly adaptive changes take place in the brain.

Perceptual Effects

The effects of cochlear noise injury on sound perception resemble those due to aging and ototoxins, because noise targets many of the same cells and processes. To a significant extent, they can be predicted by the effects of PTS on afferent FTCs. Loss of OHCs and active mechanics needed for the cochlear amplifier will lead to loss of sensitivity and broadened tuning. Perceptually, this is associated with increased **frequency difference limens**, the smallest change in stimulus frequency that can be detected. A related ability is frequency resolution, that is, the smallest frequency difference between two simultaneous stimuli that can be resolved. The latter ability is important for pitch discrimination, which in turn is related to the ability to determine the fundamental frequency in a spoken vowel and identify a speaker.

Loss of the tips of afferent FTCs means that neurons will respond to stimuli lying in the tail region nearly as well as to stimuli near the CF (see Figure 1–10). As the cochlear base is most readily affected by noise, principally basal OHC injury will result in afferent neurons that should be sharply tuned to high frequencies responding broadly to frequencies below their CF. As a consequence, as the intensity of a low or mid-frequency stimulus is increased, there will be a narrow range of intensities over which most basal neurons are suddenly activated. This **loudness recruitment** sensation is unpleasant or even painful, and is associated with diminution of the useful dynamic range of the auditory system. A perhaps surprising additional deficit that may stem from the same process is loss of temporal acuity, the ability to follow rapid frequency and amplitude changes in the stimulus. Loss of the ability to use fine temporal information has been associated with a loss of speech reception in noise backgrounds (Hopkins & Moore, 2008).

PTS is usually bilaterally symmetric, but can be asymmetric owing to the nature of some noise sources such as firearms. There is also some evidence that the left ear is inherently more vulnerable to noise than the right (Henderson et al., 1993; Ward, 1995). In instances of marked PTS asymmetry, the ability to localize sounds, particularly at higher frequencies, may be compromised.

Tinnitus, the perception of sound where there is none, is a frequent consequence of noise injury (Bauer, 2004; Noble & Tyler, 2008). Tinnitus is usually constant, but in intermittent cases may have environmental triggers such as noise and drugs, even particular somatosensory stimuli. Its percept is usually tonal, but may more resemble a buzz or noise.

Cell Loss and Changes in Neurochemistry

When cochlear afferent neurons die, so do their axonal processes extending into the cochlear nucleus (Kim et al., 1997; Morest et al., 1998). Surprisingly, this may trigger "transneuronal" death of cochlear nucleus neurons, their targets in the inferior colliculus, and even further beyond, into the auditory thalamus (Basta et al., 2005). Two basic processes have been proposed. The first is cell death following the loss of excitatory drive. The second invokes excitotoxicity, and is based on evidence for heightened ACNS activity after noise exposure (Salvi et al.,

2000). For a given surviving ACNS neuron, loss of projecting neurons from lower centers is expected to alter the balance of excitatory and inhibitory influences. As a result, characteristics of spontaneous firing rate, driven firing rate, input/output curve shape, and frequency tuning may change. Enhancement of evoked potentials in the auditory brainstem that can be observed in animals after noise exposure is a suggested correlate of tinnitus (Salvi et al., 2000), and has been interpreted to reflect an increase in the "gain" within auditory relay stations.

Plasticity in the Auditory Thalamus and Cortex

In adult animals, loss of excitatory drive from a delimited region of the cochlea is associated with broadened tuning and loss of sensitivity of neurons in the brainstem that derive their main inputs from the affected region. In the thalamic medial geniculate body (MGB) and auditory cortex, the effect may be qualitatively different: The affected areas become retuned to the frequencies lying at the borders of the injured cochlear segment, yet with normal tuning to these "edge" frequencies (Irvine, 2007; Rajan, 2001). The effect thus superficially resembles learning-based plasticity in both auditory and somatosensory systems, whereby dynamic and reversible remapping appears foundational to enhanced discrimination abilities. Since, in adults, this effect is limited to the thalamus and cortex, it seems to suggest an adaptive mechanism, and perhaps similar plastic changes. The term "plastic" is generally used to indicate an active, rather than passive, process. But do these changes yield improved or preserved perceptual abilities? In fact, little evidence has been presented associating central auditory remapping at any level with significant gains in detection or discrimination. Exceptions include modest improvement in frequency difference limens at the low frequency edge of the cochlear lesion (Thai-Van et al., 2007), as might be expected to result from broadened spatial representation. Perhaps relatedly, subjects with cochlear "dead regions" show may show a slight advantage in perceiving low-pass filtered speech sounds (Hopkins & Moore, 2008).

INNATE PROTECTIVE AND REPAIR PROCESSES

Noise exposure simultaneously engages both protective/repair processes and cell death cascades. Protective and repair processes exist at the system level, intercellular level (paracrine signaling among cochlear cells), and subcellular level. We said that these processes probably did not evolve to meet the challenges of noise injury, and just how and when they are protective remains under debate. Indeed, some inter- and intracellular molecular cascades seem to compete in a manner that is not obviously adaptive. Does such competition represent evolutionary "fine-tuning" or a kind of democratic chaos, in which stability is maximized by having every reaction balanced by an opposing reaction? As evidence accrues, putative causal chains become more like spider webs, so that the best molecular target for intervention becomes a matter of trial and error.

Intracellular and Intercellular Signaling

Within cells there exist a host of stress-related cascades. These are activated by immediate byproducts of noise injury, prominently including ROS (such as superoxide, peroxide, and hydroxyl radical), reactive nitrogen species (e.g., peroxynitrite), and elevated Ca^{++}. On the downstream end of the cascades are transcription factors that promote the synthesis of protective factors, including antioxidants, heat shock proteins, and trophic factors. Factors that reduce ROS generation, a nearly universal consequence of stress, may act primarily within cells. Others may be produced primarily for release into the extracellular medium to act on other cells. A given cascade may engage both pro-survival and pro-death mechanisms, and there is often substantial antagonism between cascades. Further complicating matters, the protective or harmful character of some factor may depend both on *how much* and *where* it is generated. For example, noise-related activation of NFκB can upregulate inducible nitric oxide synthase (iNOS). The resulting NO generation may preserve cochlear blood flow in the lateral wall, but may also promote peroxynitrite production in both the lateral wall and organ of Corti (Shi et al., 2007). By contrast, NFκB activation within radial afferent dendrites may aid Ca^{++} regulation and reduce excitotoxic injury (Tahera et al., 2006a). Noise-related NFκB activation in the lateral wall would be expected to promote vasodilation, but in doing so apparently also promotes inflammation that may exacerbate injury (Shi & Nuttall, 2007).

One important family of feedback loops involves intercellular signaling by purines. Noise exposure promotes the release into endolymph of adenosine and adenosine triphosphate (ATP) (Ford et al., 1997; Munoz et al., 2001). These act in paracrine manner on cells lining the endolymphatic space, both by direct gating of ion currents, and via G-protein-coupled cascades. Adenosine receptors are widely distributed in the organ of Corti, spiral ganglion, and lateral wall (Vlajkovic et al., 2007), and are upregulated by noise (Ramkumar et al., 2004). Application of adenosine analog R-phenylisopropylanosine (R-PIA) has been shown to reduce PTS in chinchillas (Hu et al., 1997), and may also effect protection by activating antioxidant systems (Ramkumar et al., 2001). The primary source of noise-elicited ATP release into endolymph appears to be marginal cells of stria vascularis (Munoz et al., 2001; White et al., 1995). Like adenosine receptors, ATP receptors are widely distributed around the luminal surfaces of the endolymphatic space (Lee et al., 2001; Mockett et al., 1995; Mockett et al., 1994). Ca^{++} waves transmitted through gap junctions within the organ of Corti (and perhaps lateral wall) facilitate rapid ATP movement, potentially as part of a response to noise injury (Gale et al., 2004; Piazza et al., 2007). ATP in the organ may in part act directly on mechanics to reduce cochlear amplification (Bobbin & Salt, 2005) (assuming of course that active processes enhance noise injury). Another way to reduce the responsivity of the cochlea in order to gain protection is to reduce the currents that drive hair cell receptor potentials. Additional protective effects of ATP are thought to arise from its activation of a K$^+$ shunt conductance that lowers the input resistance of scala media and reduces the EP (Thorne et al., 2004). In summary, purinergic regulatory systems in the cochlea can protect against noise, although the need for feedback control of cochlear fluid homeostasis and to maintain constancy of hearing sensitivity may have been the driving pressures.

Cochlear Efferents

Evidence indicates that the strength of the medial olivocochlear (MOC) efferent reflex can account for some interindividual differences in noise susceptibility (Maison and Liberman, 2000). In support of this idea, genetically engineered strengthening of the MOC reflex in mice by increasing the density of key membrane receptors appears protective against both TTS and PTS (Maison et al., 2002). Other work (Darrow et al., 2007) also implicates the lateral (IHC afferent) olivocochlear (LOC) system in resistance to TTS. It was suggested that LOC activity reduces excitotoxic injury to afferent dendrites. There remains some doubt that resistance to noise injury would have presented the most significant selective pressure on the evolution of cochlear efferent systems (Kirk and Smith, 2003). Protection from noise may only be a by-product of selective pressures for improved signal detection in noisy backgrounds.

Preconditioning Phenomena

As we will consider further, pharmacologic approaches to preventing PTS have been only somewhat successful. This may reflect a tendency of exogenous agents to throw complex endogenous feedback loops out of balance. An alternative approach may emerge from discoveries involving *preconditioning*, that is, engaging innate protection using mild stress, thereby conferring protection against later, more severe stress. Preconditioning has the potential to activate multiple endogenous mechanisms in a coordinated manner and thus produce clearer net benefits. In animal experiments, preconditioning protection in the cochlea has been shown to accrue from briefly increasing body temperature (heat stress) (Yoshida et al., 1999b), exposure to moderate nondamaging noise (Canlon, 1997; Niu & Canlon, 2002; Yoshida & Liberman, 2000), physical restraint (which presumably engages broad stress reactions) (Wang & Liberman, 2002), mild hypoxia (Gagnon et al., 2007), and low-dose aminoglycosides (Fernandez et al., 2010). Canlon and colleagues (Tahera et al., 2006a; Tahera et al., 2006b; Tahera et al., 2007) have proposed that glucocorticoids mediate protection by sound and restraint, although most of these data have been obtained in the context of neuronal injury during TTS. Hypoxia, heat stress, loud sound, and so forth, are not immediately convertible to practical therapies, of course, and have not been tested in humans. Nevertheless, the underlying principles are highly likely to apply to humans. Pharmacologic mimicry of preconditioning stimuli by pharmacologically initiating upstream events may ultimately show clinical advantages versus other agents.

Noise-Evoked Phagocyte Invasion

Repair and partial restoration of function to the organ of Corti after noise injury requires re-establishment of boundaries and removal of dead cells. Both resident and non-resident macrophages may participate in this process (Abrashkin et al., 2006; Fredelius & Rask-Andersen, 1990). Deiters' cells in particular may ingest debris from dying OHCs. Also, recent experiments (Hirose et al., 2005; Tornabene et al., 2006) have revealed large scale influxes of mononuclear phagocytes into the spiral limbus and ligament, peaking about 7 days after a single damaging exposure. Phagocytes may be drawn to the ligament by cytokines such as CCL2 (MCP-1), IL-6, IL-1β, and TNFα (Fujioka et al., 2006; Ichimiya et al., 2000; Yoshida et al., 1999a), all known to be expressed by fibrocytes and fibroblasts upon sensing stress-related changes in their surroundings (Gallit & Clark, 1994; Schonherr & Hausser, 2000). Within the cochlea, conditions to which these cells react may include hypoxia/ischemia, osmotic stress, and changes in tensile stress exerted by the collagen scaffold to which they attach (Grinnell, 2000). Capillary endothelial cells within the ligament may also secrete chemotactic factors (Shi & Nuttall, 2007). Once released, cytokines appear to act in both autocrine and paracrine fashion to promote further cytokine release (Ichimiya et al., 2000; Yoshida et al., 1999a). Invading phagocytes may primarily be removing debris. The

largest mobilization of phagocytes is seen in regions of the ligament where noise-related cell loss is most evident (Hirose et al., 2005; Ohlemiller & Gagnon, 2007; Wang et al., 2002). Another process that may operate in parallel is for migratory hematopoietically derived cells to serve as progenitors to replace lost fibrocytes (Lang et al., 2006a). The protective value of fibrocyte replacement, via natural or clinical means, remains to be clarified. Notably, recruited macrophages are typically not seen in the organ of Corti. Thus, if their arrival helps to preserve hearing, any positive effects on the organ of Corti must be indirect.

Question 3

When I wear earplugs I occlude my ears. Does this enhance bone conduction? Does this make a drummer or other type of musician more susceptible to noise damage?

Answer 3

The pressure gain in cochlear fluids owed to pinna and middle ear amplification is typically 30 to 40 dB, so that airborne sound will be the dominant influence in NIHL. Also, occlusion effects are minimal for frequencies over 500 Hz.

RISK FACTORS FOR NIPTS

Environmental and Systemic Factors in Adults

Oxidative stress and hypoxia/ischemia are implicated in PTS. Environmental factors that amplify cochlear oxidative stress and impair blood flow might therefore be anticipated to exacerbate noise injury. Evidence supports such an effect by volatile industrial compounds such as toluene and ethylbenzene (Fechter et al., 2007). This interaction, in turn, may be amplified by behaviors such as smoking

(Uchida et al., 2005; Wild et al., 2005) and by systemic conditions such as diabetes, microvascular pathology, and blood conditions like hyperlipidemia (Chang et al., 2007).

Prenatal and Epigenetic Factors

Human and animal evidence indicates that environmental stress on the mother during pregnancy adversely impacts the development and stress responses of her offspring (Barker, 1998). Stress-related chronic elevation of glucocorticoids in utero may favor the growth of some organs and systems at the expense of others. "Losers" may include inner ear tissues, which might end up with fewer blood vessels and progenitor cells. Prenatal stress in humans is suggested to lead to a combination of depressed birth weight, short adult stature, elevated hearing thresholds (Barrenäs et al., 2005), and sensitivity to noise (Canlon et al., 2003; Kadner et al., 2006).

The prenatal environment may exert its effects in part through epigenetic modifications to DNA. In utero and early life events can modify gene expression via methylation of DNA and resulting histone repression of transcription, and also posttranscriptionally through de-methylation and activation of microRNAs (Feil, 2006; Gallou-Kabani et al., 2007). This process governs tissue differentiation during development, but only recently has its influence beyond developmentally regulated genes been recognized. Based on a mix of environment (uterine and postnatal) and stochastic processes, anyone may effectively become hemizygous or genetically null for many genes. Cell epigenotypes are passed on in somatic cell mitosis *and* can be passed to offspring. Even more surprisingly, epigenotype can be inherited in patterns that seem to violate Mendel's laws (e.g., imprinting and transgenerational inheritance). Hearing-related genes are not immune to this process, so that epigenetic principles seem likely to complicate human and animal studies of genetic influences on acquired hearing loss.

Genes That May Impact NIPTS

The popular press often refers to the "gene for" a disease. What is actually meant when one of these is found is that a particular DNA base sequence in some region of the genome is found to associate with increased risk of a disease. The kinds of sequence differences that are sought are typically either single bases (single nucleotide polymorphisms, or SNPs) or short repeating sequences of bases (short sequence length polymorphisms, or SSLPs) that are known to vary across the population (thus "polymorphic"). All polymorphisms begin as mutations, that is, random changes that occur during DNA copying (either meiosis or mitosis). These changes may be harmful, beneficial, or neutral. Now that the entire human and mouse genomes have been sequenced, literally hundreds of thousands of SNPs and SSLPs (collectively called "markers") have been catalogued in both species. Thus, it is often possible to determine in association studies exactly where a polymorphism is, what the gene normally does, and how the mutation affects gene function. Genes that affect hearing may be generally divided into those that act alone to cause "monogenic" hearing loss, and those that may only add to the risk of acquired hearing loss due to noise, ototoxins, or aging. Either type of gene is worth investigating — particularly as a way to avoid having to test all ~20,000 genes in the human genome. Genes that cause typically early and severe monogenic hearing loss may have variants that impose much more mild, delayed effects. To find genes that may *primarily* promote acquired hearing loss, we may select genes known to impact cell repair, antioxidant defenses, or ion homeostasis. This approach has delivered several candidate "pro-PTS" genes.

Mouse studies have been extremely important in the hunt for human pro-PTS genes, as variations of particular genes — and particular classes of genes — have been shown to promote PTS in mice. Best studied among these is $Cdh23^{ahl}$, first shown to promote both presbycusis-like pathology and PTS in C57BL/6 (B6) mice (Johnson et al., 1997). This protein is part of the tip linkage of hair cell stereocilia, and interacts with Ca^{++}. The *ahl* allele of the cadherin 23 gene has illustrated several useful principles. One is apparent overlap of processes that impact presbycusis and PTS risk. Homozygosity for the *ahl* allele also amplifies hearing loss caused by other stereociliary mutations, other proteins that interact with Ca^{++}, and at least one mitochondrial gene. Finally, what range of pathology might be caused by malfunction of a hair cell–specific gene that kills hair cells? Should it somehow also cause pathology of the spiral ligament or stria vascularis? The answer seems to be "no," at least insofar as these contribute to hearing loss (Ohlemiller, 2009).

Hypotheses about the kind of genes and alleles that might promote NIPTS often involve genetically engineered "knockout" (KO) mice, in which a specific gene is rendered inactive, and transgenic mice (in which extra copies of a gene have been inserted). Alleles that promote TTS in mice include knockout alleles for NFκB (Lang et al., 2006b), for estrogen receptor β (ERβ) and aromatase (Meltser et al., 2008), and for orphan glutamate receptor δ1 subunit (GluRδ1) (Gao et al., 2007). GluRδ1 deficiency may promote reversible EP reduction. NFκB deficiency may magnify excitotoxic injury to afferent dendrites (Tahera et al., 2006a), and appears to promote a degenerative process that resembles neural presbycusis (Lang et al., 2006b). ERβ and aromatase deficiency may similarly magnify excitotoxic injury, perhaps by reducing levels of brain-derived neurotrophic factor (BDNF). Mutations affecting hair cell ion channels could also impact noise vulnerability. Accordingly, increased PTS has been now found for mice deficient in the BK calcium-activated K^+ channel expressed by basal OHCs (Engel et al., 2006).

Based on work in mice, genes mediating cochlear protection may operate as pro-PTS alleles (Fairfield et al., 2005; Ohlemiller et al., 2000a; Ohlemiller et al., 1999; Sugahara et al., 2003) in humans. Certain alleles of genes encoding heat shock protein HSP70 isoforms (Yang et al., 2006), and antioxidants paraoxonase, manganese superoxide dismutase (SOD2) (Fortunato et al., 2004), and glutathione S-transferase (Rabinowitz et al., 2002) may promote PTS. Some alleles of *KCNE1*, which encodes a potassium channel regulatory subunit, may also worsen PTS (Van Laer et al., 2006). The major cochlear function of this protein is to impart control of K^+ flow from strial marginal cells into the endolymphatic space, perhaps as part of a protective feedback loop involving ATP and Ca^{++} (Housley et al., 2002; Lee & Marcus, 2008).

The role of strial pigmentation has long been of interest because of suggested protective effects of melanin against noise and ototoxins (Meyer zum Gottesberge, 1988). Although animal studies of this issue can be based upon direct characterization of strial melanin, human studies have had to rely on proxy measures of skin and eye color. Except in the case of albinism, skin color seems a poor indicator of the amount of strial pigment (Bonaccorsi, 1965; Tota & Bocci, 1967). Eye color may represent a better index of the amount of strial melanin, but not necessarily of type (Barrenäs, 1997; Bartels et al., 2001), as there is more than one form. Retrospective human studies of noise-exposed workers stratified by eye color have produced quite mixed results (Attias & Pratt, 1985; Cunningham & Norris, 1982). One study of a large sample of metal workers (Da Costa et al., 2008) obtained a ~9 dB sensitivity difference between "dark-eyed" and "fair-eyed" subjects having a history of moderate work-related noise exposure. Animal data bearing on this issue are inconclusive, and often have relied on suboptimal genetic controls. In one well-controlled study (Bartels et al., 2001), the absence of melanin in C57BL/6-*Tyr^{c-2J}* (albino) congenic mice had no influence on the extent of PTS. Comparisons of the effects of broadband noise and aging on the EP in B6 and the C57BL/6-*Tyr^{c-2J}* albino congenic mice (Ohlemiller, 2009; Ohlemiller and Gagnon, 2007) revealed modest but statistically significant (~10 mV) reductions for both conditions only in the albinos. While the EP probably recovers from noise, the common thread linking these findings to positive results in humans may be reduced resilience of the non-pigmented stria. The larger principle clearly is not whether albinism (a rare condition in humans) can promote cochlear noise injury. Rather, it is whether any of the many genes that impact the amount, type, or distribution of strial melanin can, for some allele combinations, render some individuals more susceptibility to PTS.

INTERACTION BETWEEN AGE AND NOISE INJURY

It is an old question in ARHL whether an old ear is a more fragile ear (Ward, 1995). Apparent aging processes may accelerate over time due to progressive dysfunction of homeostatic, repair, and protective mechanisms. The potential interactions between age, ARHL, and noise injury fall under headings covering influences in both directions, that is, how age affects PTS and whether early noise exposure affects apparent cochlear aging.

Age Versus Susceptibility to Noise

Evidence from mice and other models supports two windows of increased susceptibility to noise exposure: early in life and late in life. In cats (Price, 1976), hamsters (Bock & Seifter, 1978), guinea pigs (Falk et al., 1974) and mice (Henry, 1982; Ohlemiller et al., 2000b; Saunders & Hirsch, 1976), the period up through adolescence into early adulthood is a time of heightened vulnerability. In mice, this early window extends up to about four months of age (Henry, 1983). It is not clear what process distinguishes this period. The increased PTS is associated with greater OHC loss when mice of different age but similar hearing loss are compared (Ohlemiller et al., 2000b). The mechanisms involved therefore may be local to the organ of Corti. The early period overlaps only partially with early vulnerability to ototoxins (Chen & Saunders, 1983; Henry et al., 1981), suggesting it is not based on downstream cellular injury pathways common to noise and ototoxins. Such findings suggest that some observations on PTS for young adult animals and humans may not generalize to older adults, and vise versa. They also suggest heightened risk of hearing loss to children and young adults from loud toys and CD players, and in common recreational venues.

The study of noise vulnerability late in life is often complicated by ceiling effects posed by preexisting hearing loss (Glorig & Linthicum, 1998). Moderate sensorineural hearing loss due to any cause will render the cochlea less sensitive to noise injury (Boettcher, 2002; Mills et al., 1997). Miller and colleagues (Miller et al., 1998) showed that 21-month-old CBA/CaJ mice with near-normal initial hearing sustain more PTS than younger mice. Studies in humans that have reasonably separated noise injury from aging support similar conclusions (Toppila et al., 2001). Such results raise the possibility that apparent aging processes gain momentum late in life through more rapid accumulation of injury. This is consistent with notions of aging as progressive impairment of stress responses (Ohlemiller & Frisina, 2008).

Effects of Noise Exposure on Apparent ARHL

It is often assumed that any threshold shift remaining after 2 to 3 weeks resolves to a stable permanent component. An exception already noted is work by Kujawa and Liberman (Kujawa & Liberman, 2006) showing that early noise exposure in CBA/CaJ mice can trigger progressive neuronal loss. The stability of PTS may also depend on systemic and genetic factors. For example, spontaneously hypertensive rats (a genetically disposed experimental strain) show PTS that seems to worsen over time (Borg, 1983). This progressive character is evident without regard to the age of exposure, but may progress more rapidly in animals exposed at older ages.

PREVENTION AND TREATMENT OF NIPTS

Clearly, the best approach to preventing PTS is not to be exposed to noise. For both recreational and occupational exposures, education about the danger represents the first line intervention. The slow cumulative nature of PTS ("I go to loud concerts all the time and I can hear just fine.") can combine with attitudinal and cultural biases ("Nobody else is wearing hearing protection, so it must be okay.") to keep many from using HPDs. In the workplace, ever improving HPDs, active noise cancellation, and engineering approaches that reduce noise hazards at their source represent cost effective strategies. However, there will always be work environments that are not suitable, and there will always be employees, audiophiles, and gun enthusiasts who are not compliant. And increasingly, there will be new guns, tanks, and airplanes that no ear can withstand, HPD or not. For those situations, conditioning paradigms, therapeutic agents, and (if it's too late) stem cell and gene therapies remain worthwhile goals.

Pharmacologic Approaches

Many studies have tested the protective ability of a wide variety of compounds against NIPTS. Given that benefit accrues from application of many types of antioxidants, growth factors, calcium antagonists, and anti-apoptotics, there is hope that some combination of these can ultimately be shown practical in humans, assuming they can be applied orally or aurally, and in time. Because PTS encompasses multiple, and somewhat independent injury pathways, the efficacy of any single agent may be limited. Antioxidants represent the largest single class of therapeutics tested (Le Prell et al., 2007b; Ohlemiller, 2008); yet, their success when applied alone may be limited by access to cellular compartments, action against only few forms of ROS, interference with redox-based signaling, or a tendency to throw innate ROS protections out of balance. Thus, therapies combining multiple antioxidants, or antioxidants plus other agents, may have advantages over single-agent approaches (Choi et al., 2008; Le Prell et al., 2007a).

Gene and Stem Cell Therapy

Noise affects many interdependent cell types. Even if we could replace lost hair cells or neurons in an extensively damaged organ of Corti, the new cells might not survive in such an abnormal environment. Gene therapy generally seeks to add genes to existing cells in order to impart the capacity to: (1) produce vital molecules that were never present (as in the case of genetic disorders), (2) produce molecules that have ceased to be produced in adequate amounts (due to injury or aging), or (3) replace missing cells by reprogramming resident cells. The fluid spaces that surround cochlear neurons, hair cells, and supporting cells openly communicate with perilymphatic spaces. If the goal is to increase levels of a diffusible survival factor whose target lies within the organ of Corti, any resident cell type could be transfected to act as a secretory "factory" for antioxidants, trophins, or other factors in an attempt to mitigate noise injury. Targets for added genes could even include fairly nonspecialized cells such as mesothelial cells that line the perilymphatic scalae or fibrocytes in the spiral ligament. If, as some suggest (Lang et al., 2003), the latter are renewed from bone marrow-derived cells, the cochlea need not be the site where genes are introduced.

Gene therapy has already been shown to be feasible as a means of introducing essential diffusable enzymes (Ohlemiller et al., 2001), boosting survival factor levels (Green et al., 2008), and even replacing lost hair cells (Heller & Raphael, 2008; Kawamoto et al., 2003). The latter work, in which hair cell "fate determining" gene *Atoh1* (or *Math1*) was introduced using viral vectors injected into scala media, has garnered a great deal of interest. In those experiments, several supporting cell types acquired hair cell–like features. Nevertheless, such successes have not yet resolved the question of how long any new hair cells can survive in an organ of Corti lacking many of the normal cell-cell adjacencies and chemical interactions. Stem cell therapy has yet to produce in the cochlea any successes rivaling those from gene therapy. However, theoretically, stem cells could solve problems just posed if they can be made to "recognize" what cells are missing, and then repopulate the organ of Corti or lateral wall accordingly. In the long run, stem cell therapy may hold more promise for restoring that which was lost, but many technical problems must first be solved.

SUMMARY: CRITICAL UNKNOWNS FOR PREVENTING OR TREATING PTS

It remains to be seen just how effective pharmacotherapies against NIPTS therapies can be. Genetic variation at many loci, some of which are known, will render some individuals more susceptible to noise or less protected by any particular drug or preconditioning paradigm. Assuming issues of privacy and genetic discrimination can be surmounted, it may eventually be possible to identify those inherently more at risk in noisy environments. Very likely, however, association studies will produce a long list of genes, each of which contributes a few percent of added PTS risk. Any individual may carry multiple pro-PTS polymorphisms, and it will often be unclear what to do with this information. The genetics of acquired hearing loss share this limitation with virtually every other acquired health condition.

If extensive injury cannot be prevented, reconstitution of sensory cells becomes the primary goal. Although the success of cochlear implants is phenomenal, these devices convey only a shadow of the acoustic information available. They represent merely a stop-gap approach while our understanding of inner ear cell biology remains rudimentary. Despite the nearly universal effect of noise on cell types in the cochlear duct, the most prominent form of permanent cochlear injury appears to be loss or dysfunction of OHCs. If the organ of Corti is intact, replacing outer hair cells *should* restore most lost function. Although stem cell and vector-mediated gene therapies may yet solve this problem, this potential has not been realized. The hope that OHC restoration equals hearing restoration presumes: (1) that the new OHCs can situate in the organ of Corti so as to recreate the cochlear amplifier, and (2) that new OHCs become innervated, or that their afferent and efferent innervation are not vital. Another issue is whether the organ of Corti environment is altered by noise in such a way that new OHCs have no long-term viability. Among tissue repair strategies, stem cell therapy may hold the greatest promise, given the ability of stem cells to integrate into an epithelium and assume the full array of characteristics of resident cells. The key may be to turn back the clock to a developmental stage where cell identities and spatial relationships in the organ of Corti are not yet fixed.

Acknowledgments. Thanks to Drs. W. Clark and B. Bohne for critical comments, and to A. Rosen, A. Schrader, and P. Gagnon for assistance with figures. Supported by P30 DC004665 (R. Chole), P30 NS057105 (D. Holtzman), R01 DC03454 (KKO), R01 DC08321 (KKO), WUSM Department of Otolaryngology.

FURTHER READINGS

Clark, W. W. (1991). Recent studies of temporary threshold shift (TTS) and permanent threshold shift (PTS) in animals. *Journal of the Acoustical Society of America, 90,* 155–163.

Clark, W. W. (2008). Chapter 18: Noise-induced hearing loss In W. W. Clark & K. K. Ohlemiller (Eds.), *Anatomy and physiology of hearing for audiologists* (pp. 321–343). Clifton Park, NY: Thomson Delmar Learning.

Gates, G. A. (2006). The effect of noise on cochlear aging. *Ear and Hearing, 27,* 91.

Hawkins, J. E., & Schacht, J. (2005). Sketches of Otohistory. Part 10: Noise-induced hearing loss. *Audiology and Neurotology, 10,* 305–309.

Henderson, D., Hu, B. H., & Bielefeld, E. (2008). Patterns and mechanisms of noise-induced cochlear pathology.

In J. Schacht, A. N. Popper & R. R. Fay (Eds.), *Auditory trauma, protection, and repair* (pp. 195–217). New York, NY: Springer Science.

Le Prell, C. G., Yamashita, D., Minami, S. B., Yamasoba, T., & Miller, J. M. (2007b). Mechanisms of noise-induced hearing loss indicate multiple methods of prevention. *Hearing Research, 226,* 22–43.

Ohlemiller, K. K. (2008). Recent findings and emerging questions in cochlear noise injury. *Hearing Research, 245,* 5–17.

Quaranta, A., Portalatini, P., & Henderson, D. (1998). Temporary and permanent threshold shifts: An overview. *Scandinavian Audiology, 27*(Suppl. 48), 75–86.

Saunders, J. C., Cohen, Y. E., & Szymko, Y. M. (1991). The structural and functional consequences of acoustic injury in the cochlea and peripheral auditory system. *Journal of the Acoustical Society of America, 90,* 136–146.

Schmiedt, R. A. (1984). Acoustic injury and the physiology of hearing. *Journal of the Acoustical Society of America, 76,* 1293–1317.

Talaska, A. E., & Schacht, J. (2007). Mechanisms of noise damage to the cochlea. *Audiological Medicine, 5,* 3–9.

REFERENCES

Abrashkin, K. A., Izumikawa, M., Miyazawa, T., Wang, C.-H., Crumling, M. A., Swiderski, D. L., . . . Raphael, Y. (2006). The fate of outer hair cells after acoustic or ototoxic insults. *Hearing Research, 218,* 20–29.

Ahmad, M., Bohne, B. A., & Harding, G. W. (2003). An in vivo tracer study of noise-induced damage to the reticular lamina. *Hearing Research, 175,* 82–100.

Altschuler, R. A., Raphael, Y., Prosen, C., Dolan, D. F., & Moody, D. B. (1992). Acoustic stimulation and overstimulatoni in the cochlea: A comparison between basal and apical turns of the cochlea. In A. L. Dancer, D. Henderson, R. J. Salvi, & R. P. Hamernik (Eds.), *Noise-induced hearing loss* (pp. 60–73). St. Louis, MO: Mosby Year Book.

Attias, J., & Pratt, H. (1985). Auditory-evoked potential correlates of susceptibility to noise-induced hearing loss. *Audiology, 24,* 149–156.

Axelsson, A. (1988). Comparative anatomy of cochlear blood vessels. *American Journal of Otolaryngology, 9,* 278–290.

Barker, D. J. P. (1998). In utero programming of chronic disease. *Clinical Sciences, 95,* 115–128.

BBarrenäs, M. (1997). Hair cell loss from acoustic trauma in chloroquine-treated red, black and albino guinea pigs. *Audiology, 36,* 187–201.

arrenäs, M.-L., Bratthall, A., & Dahlgren, J. (2005). The association between short stature and sensorineural hearing loss. *Hearing Research, 205,* 123–130.

Bartels, S., Ito, S., Trune, D. R., & Nuttall, A. L. (2001). Noise-induced hearing loss: The effect of melanin in the stria vascularis. *Hearing Research, 154,* 116–123.

Basta, D., Tzschentke, B., & Ernst, A. (2005). Noise-induced cell death in the mouse medial geniculate body and primary auditory cortex. *Neuroscience Letters, 381,* 199–204.

Bauer, C. A. (2004). Mechanisms of tinnitus generation. *Current Opinion in Otolaryngology-Head and Neck Surgery, 12,* 413–417.

Bobbin, R. P., & Salt, A. N. (2005). ATP-γ-S shifts the operating point of outer hair cell transduction towards scala tympani. *Hearing Research, 205,* 35–43.

Bock, G. R., & Seifter, E. J. (1978). Developmental changes of susceptibility to auditory fatigue in young hamsters. *Audiology, 17,* 193–203.

Boettcher, F. A. (2002). Susceptibility to acoustic trauma in young and aged gerbils. *Journal of the Acoustical Society of America, 112,* 2948–2955.

Bonaccorsi, P. (1965). Il colore dell'iride come "test" di valutazione quantiatativia, nell'uomo, della concentrazzione di melania nella stria vascolare. *Della concentrazzione di melania nella stria vascolare, 64,* 725–738.

Borg, E. (1983). Delayed effects of noise on the ear. *Hearing Research, 9,* 247–254.

Bredberg, G. (1968). Cellular pattern and nerve supply of the human organ of Corti. *Acta Oto-laryngologica (Suppl.), 236*(236), 1–135.

Canlon, B. (1997). Protection against noise trauma by sound conditioning. *Ear, Nose, and Throat Journal, 76,* 248–255.

Canlon, B., Erichsen, S., Nemlander, E., Chen, M., Hossain, A., Celsi, G., . . . Ceccatelli, S. (2003). Alterations in intrauterine environment by glucocorticoids modifies the developmental programme of the auditory system. *European Journal of Neuroscience, 17,* 2035–2041.

Chang, N.-C., Yu, M. L., Ho, K.-Y., & Ho, C. K. (2007). Hyperlipidemia in noise-induced hearing loss. *Otolaryngology-Head and Neck Surgery, 137,* 603–606.

Chang, Q., Tang, W., Ahmad, S., Zhou, B., & Lin, X. (2008). Gap junction mediated intercellular metabolite transfer in the cochlea in compromised in connexin 30 null mice. *Public Library of Science, PloS One, 3,* e4088.

Chen, C.-S., & Saunders, J. C. (1983). The sensitive period for ototoxicity of kanamycin in mice: Morphological evidence. *Archives of Otorhinolaryngology, 238,* 217–223.

Chen, G.-D., & Fechter, L. D. (2003). The relationship between noise-induced hearing loss and hair cell loss in rats. *Hearing Research, 177,* 81–90.

Choi, C. H., Chen, K., Vasquez-Weldon, A., Jackson, R. L., Floyd, R. A., & Kopke, R. D. (2008). Effectiveness of 4-hydroxy phenyl *N-tert*-butylnitrone (4-OHPBN) alone and in combination with other antioxidant drugs in the treatment of acute acoustic trauma in chinchilla. *Free Radical Biology and Medicine, 44,* 1772–1784.

Cunningham, D. R., & Norris, M. L. (1982). Eye color and noise-induced hearing loss: A population study. *Ear and Hearing, 3,* 211–214.

Da Costa, D. A., Castro, J. C., & Macedo, M. E. G. (2008). Iris pigmentation and susceptibility to noise-induced hearing loss. *International Journal of Audiology, 47,* 115–118.

Dallos, P., & Cheatham, M. A. (1976). Compound action potential (AP) tuning curves. *Journal of the Acoustical Society of America, 59,* 591–597.

Darrow, K. N., Maison, S. F., & Liberman, M. C. (2007). Selective removal of lateral olivocochlear efferents increases vulnerability to acute acoustic injury. *Journal of Neurophysiology, 97,* 1775–1785.

Dobie, R. A. (2008). The burdens of age-related and occupational noise-induced hearing loss in the United States. *Ear and Hearing, 29,* 565–577.

Duvall, A. J., Ward, W. D., & Lauhala, K. E. (1974). Stria ultrastructure and vessel transport in acoustic trauma. *Annals of Otology, 83,* 498–514.

Edelman, D. A., Jiang, Y., Tyburski, J., Wilson, R. F., & Steffes, C. (2006). Pericytes and their role in microvasculature homeostasis. *Journal of Surgical Research, 135,* 305–311.

El-Badry, M. M., & McFadden, S. L. (2009). Evaluation of inner hair cell and nerve fiber loss as sufficient pathologies underlying auditory neuropathy. *Hearing Research, 255,* 84–90.

Engel, J., Braig, C., Ruttiger, L., Kuhn, S., Zimmermann, U., Blin, N., . . . Knipper, M. (2006). Two classes of outer hair cells along the tonotopic axis of the cochlea. *Neuroscience, 143,* 837–849.

Fairfield, D. A., Lomax, M. I., Dootz, G. A., Chen, S., Galecki, T. A., Benjamin, I. J., . . . Altschuer, R. A. (2005). Heat shock factor 1-deficient mice exhibit decreased recovery of hearing following noise overstimulation. *Journal of Neuroscience Research, 81,* 589–596.

Falk, S. A., Cook, R. O., Haseman, J. K., & Sanders, G. M. (1974). Noise-induced inner ear damage in newborn and adult guinea pigs. *Laryngoscope, 84,* 444–453.

Fechter, L. D., Gearhart, C., Fulton, S., Campbell, J., Fisher, J., Na, K., . . . Pouyatos, B. (2007). Promotion of noise-induced cochlear injury by toluene and ethylbenzene in the rat. *Toxicological Sciences, 98,* 542–551.

Feil, R. (2006). Environmental and nutritional effects on the epigenetic regulation of genes. *Mutation Research, 600,* 46–57.

Fernandez, E. A., Ohlemiller, K. K., Gagnon, P. M., & Clark, W. W. (2010) Protection against noise-induced hearing loss in young CBA/J mice by low-dose kanamycin. *Journal of the Association for Research in Otolaryngology, 11,* 235–244.

Ford, M. S., Maggirwar, S. B., Rybak, L. P., Whitworth, C., & Ramkumar, V. (1997). Expression and function of adenosine receptors in the chinchilla cochlea. *Hearing Research, 105,* 130–140.

Fortunato, G., Marciano, E., Zarrilli, F., Mazzaccara, C., Intrieri, M., Calcagno, G., . . . Sacchetti, L. (2004). Paraoxonase and superoxide dismutase gene polymorphisms and noise-induced hearing loss. *Clinical Chemistry, 50,* 2012–2018.

Fredelius, L., & Rask-Andersen, H. (1990). The role of macrophages in the disposal of degeneration products within the organ of Corti after acoustic overstimulation. *Acta Oto-laryngologica, 109,* 76–82.

Fujioka, M., Kanzaki, S., Okano, H. J., Masuda, M., Ogawa, K., & Okano, H. (2006). Proinflammatory cytokines expression in noise-induced damaged cochlea. *Journal of Neuroscience Research, 83*, 575–583.

Gagnon, P. M., Simmons, D. D., Bao, J., Lei, D., Ortmann, A., J., & Ohlemiller, K. K. (2007). Temporal and genetic influences on protection against noise-induced hearing loss by hypoxic preconditioning in mice. *Hearing Research, 226*, 79–91.

Gale, J. E., Piazza, V., Ciubotaru, C. D., & Mammano, F. (2004). A mechanism for sensing noise damage in the inner ear. *Current Biology, 14*, 526–529.

Gallit, J., & Clark, R. A. (1994). Wound repair in the context of extracellular matrix. *Current Opinion in Cell Biology, 6*, 717–725.

Gallou-Kabani, C., Vige, A., Gross, M.-S., & Junien, C. (2007). Nutri-epigenomics: Lifelong remodelling of our epigenomes by nutritional and metabolic factors and beyond. *Clinical Chemistry and Laboratory Medicine, 45*, 321–327.

Gao, J., Maison, S. F., Wu, X., Hirose, K., Jones, S. M., Bayazitov, I., . . . Zuo, J. (2007). Orphan glutamate receptor δ1 subunit required for high-frequency hearing. *Molecular and Cellular Biology, 27*, 4500–4512.

Glorig, A., & Linthicum, F. E. (1998). The relations of noise-induced hearing loss and presbycusis. *Journal of Occupational Hearing Loss, 1*, 51–60.

Green, S. H., Altschuler, R. A., & Miller, J. M. (2008). Cell death and cochlear protection. In J. Schacht, A. N. Popper & R. R. Fay (Eds.), *Auditory trauma, protection, and repair* (pp. 275–319). New York, NY: Springer Science.

Grinnell, F. (2000). Fibroblast-collagen-matrix contraction. growth-factor signalling and mechanical loading. *Trends in Cell Biology, 10*, 362–365.

Hamann, I., Gleich, O., Klump, G. M., Kittel, M. C., & Strutz, J. (2004). Age-dependent changes of gap detection in the Mongolian gerbil (Meriones unguiculatus). *Journal of the Association for Research in Otolaryngology, 5*, 49–57.

Hamernik, R. P., Ahroon, W. A., Patterson, J. H., & Chiu, W. (2002). Relations among early postexposure noise-induced threshold shifts and permananent threshold shifts in chinchillas. *Journal of the Acoustical Society of America, 111*, 320–326.

Hamernik, R. P., Patterson, J. H., Turrentine, G. A., & Ahroon, W. A. (1989). The quantitative relation between sensory cell loss and hearing thresholds. *Hearing Research, 38*, 199–212.

Hamernik, R. P., Qiu, W., & Davis, B. (2003). Cochlear toughening, protection, and potenition of noise-induced hearing loss by non-Gaussian noise. *Journal of the Acoustical Society of America, 113*, 969–976.

Hamernik, R. P., Qui, W., & Davis, R. (2007). Hearing loss from interrupted, intermittent, and time varying non-Gaussian noise exposure: The applicability of the equal energy hypothesis. *Journal of the Acoustical Society of America, 122*, 2245–2254.

Han, W., Shi, X., & Nuttall, A. L. (2006). AIF and endoG translocation in noise exposure induced hair cell death. *Hearing Research, 211*, 85–95.

Harding, G. W., Baggot, P. J., & Bohne, B. A. (1992). Height changes in the organ of Corti following noise exposure. *Hearing Research, 63*, 26–36.

Hawkins, J. E. (1976). Experimental noise deafness: Recollections and ruminations. In S. K. Hirsh, D. H. Eldredge, I. J. Hirsh, & S. R. Silverman (Eds.), *Hearing and Davis: Essays honoring Hallowell Davis* (pp. 73–84). St. Louis, MO: Washington University Press.

Henderson, D., Bielefeld, E. C., Harris, K. C., & Hu, B. H. (2006). The role of oxidative stress in noise-induced hearing loss. *Ear and Hearing, 27*, 1–19.

Henderson, D., Subramaniam, M., & Boettcher, F. A. (1993). Individual susceptibility to noise-induced hearing loss: An old topic revisited. *Ear and Hearing, 14*, 152–168.

Henry, K. R. (1982). Influence of genotype and age on noise-induced auditory losses. *Behavior Genetics, 12*, 563–573.

Henry, K. R. (1983). Lifelong susceptibility to acoustic trauma: Changing patterns of cochlear damage over the life span of the mouse. *Audiology, 22*, 372–383.

Henry, K. R., Chole, R. A., McGinn, M. D., & Frush, D. P. (1981). Increased ototoxicity in both young and old mice. *Archives of Otolaryngology, 107*, 92–95.

Hirose, K., Discolo, C. M., Keasler, J. R., & Ransohoff, R. (2005). Mononuclear phagocytes migrate into the murine cochlea after acoustic trauma. *Journal of Comparative Neurology, 489*, 180–194.

Hopkins, K., & Moore, B. C. J. (2008). Effects of moderate cochlear hearing loss on the ability to benefit from temporal fine structure information in speech. *Journal of the Acoustical Society of America, 123*, 11450–11153.

Housley, G. D., Jagger, D. J., Greenwood, D., Raybould, N. P., Salih, S. G., Jarlebark, L. E., . . . Munoz, D. J. M. (2002). Purinergic regulation of sound transduction and auditory neurotransmission. *Audiology and Neurotology, 7*, 55–61.

Hu, B. H., Zheng, X. Y., McFadden, S., & Henderson, D. (1997). The protective effects of R-PIA on noise-induced hearing loss. *Hearing Research, 113*, 198–206.

Ichimiya, I., Yoshida, K., Hirano, T., Suzuki, M., & Mogi, G. (2000). Significance of spiral ligament fibrocytes with cochlear inflammation. *International Journal of Pediatric Otorhinolaryngology, 56*, 45–51.

Irvine, D. R. F. (2007). Auditory cortical plasticity: Does it provide evidence for cognitive processing in the auditory processing in the auditory cortex? *Hearing Research, 229*, 158–170.

Johnson, K. R., Erway, L. C., Cook, S. A., Willott, J. F., & Zheng, Q. Y. (1997). A major gene affecting age-related hearing loss in C57BL/6J mice. *Hearing Research, 114*, 83–92.

Kadner, A., Pressimone, V. J., Lally, B. E., Salm, A. K., & Berrebi, A. S. (2006). Low-frequency hearing loss in prenatally stressed rats. *NeuroReport, 17*, 635–638.

Kawamoto, K., Ishimoto, S.-I., Minoda, R., Brough, D. E., & Raphael, Y. (2003). Math1 gene transfer generates new cochlear hair cells in mature guinea pigs in vivo. *Journal of Neuroscience, 23*, 4395–4400.

Kim, J., Morest, K., & Bohne, B. A. (1997). Degeneration of axons in the brainstem of the chinchilla after auditory overstimulation. *Hearing Research, 103*, 169–191.

Kirk, E. C., & Smith, D. W. (2003). Protection from acoustic trauma is not a primary function of the medial olivocochlear system. *Journal of the Association for Research in Otolaryngology, 4*, 445–465.

Kujawa, S. G., & Liberman, M. C. (2006). Acceleration of age-related hearing loss by early noise: Evidence of a misspent youth. *Journal of Neuroscience, 26*, 2115–2123.

Lang, H., Ebihara, Y., Schmiedt, R. A., Minamiguchi, H., Zhou, D., Smythe, N., M., . . . Schulte, B. A. (2006a). Contribution of bone marrow hematopoietic stem cells to adult mouse inner ear: Mesenchymal cells and fibrocytes. *Journal of Comparative Neurology, 496*, 187–201.

Lang, H., Schulte, B. A., & Schmiedt, R. A. (2003). Effects of chronic furosemide treatment and age on cell division in the adult gerbil inner ear. *Journal of the Association for Research in Otolaryngology, 4*, 164–175.

Lang, H., Schulte, B. A., Zhou, D., Smythe, N., M., Spicer, S. S., & Schmiedt, R. A. (2006b). Nuclear factor κB deficiency is associated with auditory nerve degeneration and increased noise-induced hearing loss. *Journal of Neuroscience, 26*, 3541–3550.

Lee, J. H., Chiba, T., & Marcus, D. C. (2001). P2X$_2$ receptor mediates stimulation of parasensory cation absorption by cochlear outer sulcus cells and vestibular transitional cells. *Journal of Neuroscience, 21*, 9168–9174.

Lee, J. H., & Marcus, D. C. (2008). Purinergic signaling in the inner ear. *Hearing Research, 235*, 1–7.

Le Prell, C. G., Hughes, L. F., & Miller, J. M. (2007a). Free radical scavengers vitamins A, C, and E plus magnesium reduce noise trauma. *Free Radical Biology and Medicine, 42*, 1454–1463.

Liberman, M. C. (1987). Chronic ultrastructural changes in acoustic trauma: Serial section reconstruction of stereocilia and cuticular plates. *Hearing Research, 26*, 65–88.

Liberman, M. C., & Beil, D. G. (1979). Hair cell condition and auditory nerve response in normal and noise-damaged cochleas. *Acta Otolaryngologica, 88*, 161–176.

Liberman, M. C., & Dodds, L. W. (1984). Single neuron labeling and chronic cochlear pathology. III. Stereocilia damage and alterations of threshold tuning curves. *Hearing Research, 16*, 55–74.

Liberman, M. C., & Kiang, N.-Y. S. (1978). Acoustic trauma in cats: Cochlear pathology and auditory nerve activity. *Acta Otolaryngologica (Suppl.), 358*, 1–63.

Liberman, M. C., & Mulroy, M. J. (1982). Acute and chronic effects of acoustic trauma: Cochlear pathology and auditory nerve pathophysiology. In R. P. Hamernik, D. Henderson, & R. Salvi (Eds.), *New perspectives on noise-induced hearing loss* (pp. 105–135). New York, NY: Raven Press.

Maison, S. F., & Liberman, M. C. (2000). Predicting vulnerability to acoustic trauma with a noninvasive assay of olivocochlear reflex strength. *Journal of Neuroscience, 20*, 4701–4707.

Maison, S. F., Luebke, A. E., Liberman, M. C., & Zuo, J. (2002). Efferent protection from acoustic injury is mediated via alpha9 nicotinic acetylcholine receptors on outer hair cells. *Journal of Neuroscience, 22*, 10838–10846.

Matsui, J. I., Haque, A., Huss, D., Messana, E. P., Alosi, J. A., Roberson, D. W., . . . Warchol, M. E. (2003). Caspase inhibitors promote vestibular hair cell survival and function after aminoglycoside treatment in vivo. *Journal of Neuroscience, 23*, 6111–6122.

Meltser, I., Tahera, Y., Simpson, E. M., Hultcrantz, M., Charitidi, K., Gustafsson, J.-A., . . . Canlon, B. (2008). Estrogen receptor β protects against acoustic trauma in mice. *Journal of Clinical Investigation, 118*, 1563–1570.

Meyer zum Gottesberge, A. M. (1988). Physiology and pathophysiology of inner ear melanin. *Pigment Cell Research, 1*, 238–249.

Miller, J. D. (1963). Deafening effects of noise on the cat. *Acta Oto-Laryngologica*, (Suppl. 176), 1–91.

Miller, J. D. (1974). Effects of noise on people. *Journal of the Acoustical Society of America, 56*, 729–764.

Miller, J. M., Brown, J. N., & Schacht, J. (2003). 8-iso-prostglandin F(2alpha), a product of noise exposure, reduces inner ear blood flow. *Audiology and Neurotology, 8*, 207–221.

Miller, J. M., Dolan, D. F., Raphael, Y., & Altschuler, R. A. (1998). Interactive effects of aging with noise induced hearing loss. *Scandinavian Audiology, 27*, 53–61.

Mills, J. H. (1973). Threshold shifts produced by exposure to noise in chinchillas with noise-induced hearing loss. *Journal of Speech and Hearing Research, 16*, 700–708.

Mills, J. H., Boettcher, F. A., & Dubno, J. R. (1997). Interaction of noise-induced permanent threshold shift and age-related threshold shift. *Journal of the Acoustical Society of America, 101*, 1681–1686.

Mockett, B. G., Bo, X., Housley, G. D., Thorne, P. R., & Burnstock, G. (1995). Autoradiographic labelling of P$_2$ purinoceptors in the guinea-pig cochlea. *Hearing Research, 84*, 177–193.

Mockett, B. G., Housley, G. D., & Thorne, P. R. (1994). Fluorescence imaging of extracellular purinergic sites and putative ecto-ATPase sites on isolated cochlear hair cells. *Journal of Neuroscience, 14*, 1692–1707.

Morest, D. K., Kim, J., Potashner, S. J., & Bohne, B. A. (1998). Long-term degeneration in the cochlear nerve and cochlear nucleus of the adult chinchilla following acoustic overstimulation. *Microscopy Research and Technique, 41*, 205–216.

Müller, J., & Janssen, T. (2008). Impact of occupational noise on pure-tone threshold and distortion procudt otoacoustic emissions after one workday. *Hearing Research, 246*, 9–22.

Munoz, D. J. B., Kendrick, I. S., Rassam, M., & Thorne, P. R. (2001). Vesicular storage of adenosine triphosphate in the guinea-pig cochlear lateral wall and concentration of ATP in the endolymph during sound exposure and hypoxia. *Acta Otolaryngologica, 121*, 10–15.

Nakashima, T., Naganawa, S., Sone, M., Tominaga, M., Hayashi, H., Yamamoto, H., . . . Nuttall, A. L. (2003). Disorders of cochlear blood flow. *Brain Research Reviews, 43,* 17–28.

Niu, X., & Canlon, B. (2002). Protective mechanisms of sound conditioning. *Advances in Otorhinolaryngology, 59,* 96–105.

Noble, W., & Tyler, R. (2008). Physiology and phenomenology of tinnitus: Implications for treatment. *International Journal of Audiology, 46,* 569–574.

Nordmann, A. S., Bohne, B. A., & Harding, G. W. (2000). Histopathological differences between temporary and permanent threshold shift. *Hearing Research, 139*(1–2), 13–30.

Ohlemiller, K. K. (2009). Mechanisms and genes in human strial presbycusis from animal models. *Brain Research, 1277,* 70–83.

Ohlemiller, K. K., & Frisina, R. D. (2008). Age-related hearing loss and its cellular and molecular bases. In J. Schacht, A. N. Popper, & R. R. Fay (Eds.), *Auditory trauma, protection, and repair* (pp. 145–194). New York, NY: Springer.

Ohlemiller, K. K., & Gagnon, P. M. (2007). Genetic dependence of cochlear cells and structures injured by noise. *Hearing Research, 224,* 34–50.

Ohlemiller, K. K., McFadden, S. L., Ding, D.-L., Lear, P. M., & Ho, Y.-S. (2000a). Targeted mutation of the gene for cellular glutathione peroxidase (Gpx1) increases noise-induced hearing loss in mice. *Journal of the Association for Research in Otolaryngology, 1,* 243–254.

Ohlemiller, K. K., McFadden, S. L., Ding, D.-L., Reaume, A. G., Hoffman, E. K., Scott, R. W., . . . Salvi, R. J. (1999). Targeted deletion of the cytosolic Cu/Zn-superoxide dismutase gene (SOD1) increases susceptibility to noise-induced hearing loss. *Audiology and Neurotology, 4,* 237–246.

Ohlemiller, K. K., & Siegel, J. H. (1994). Cochlear basal and apical differences reflected in the effects of cooling on responses of single auditory nerve fibers. *Hearing Research, 80,* 174–190.

Ohlemiller, K. K., Vogler, C. A., Daly, T. M., & Sands, M. S. (2001). Chapter 37. Preventing sensory loss in a mouse model of lysosomal storage disease. In J. F. Willott (Ed.), *Handbook of mouse auditory research: From behavior to molecular biology* (pp. 581–601). New York, NY: CRC Press.

Ohlemiller, K. K., Wright, J. S., & Heidbreder, A. F. (2000b). Vulnerability to noise-induced hearing loss in "middle-aged" and young adult mice: A dose-response approach in CBA, C57BL, and BALB inbred strains. *Hearing Research, 149,* 239–247.

Ota, C. Y., & Kimura, R. S. (1980) Ultrastructural study of the human spiral ganglion. *Acta Oto-Laryngologica, 89,* 53–62.

Pauler, M., Schuknecht, H. F., & Thornton, A. R. (1986). Correlative studies of cochlear neuronal loss with speech discrimination and pure-tone thresholds. *Archives of Otolaryngology, 243,* 200–206.

Piazza, V., Ciubotaru, C. D., Gale, J. E., & Mammano, F. (2007). Purinergic signalling and intercellular Ca^{++} wave propagation in the organ of Corti. *Cell Calcium, 41,* 77–86.

Price, G. R. (1976). Age as a factor in susceptibility to hearing loss: Young versus adult ears. *Journal of the Acoustical Society of America, 60,* 886–892.

Puel, J.-L., Ruel, J., Gervais d'Aldin, C., & Pujol, R. (1998). Excitotoxicity and repair of cochlear synapses after noise-trauma induced hearing loss. *NeuroReport, 9,* 2109–2114.

Qiu, W., Davis, B., & Hamernik, R. P. (2007). Hearing loss from interrupted, intermittent, and time varying Gaussian noise exposures: The applicability of the equal energy hypothesis. *Journal of the Acoustical Society of America, 121,* 1613–1620.

Qiu, W., Hamernik, R. P., & Davis, B. (2006). The kurtosis metric as an adjunct to energy in the prediction of trauma from continuous, nonGaussian noise exposure. *Journal of the Acoustical Society of America, 120*(Suppl.), 3901–3906.

Quirk, W. S., & Seidman, M. D. (1995). Cochlear vascular changes in response to loud noise. *American Journal of Otology, 16,* 322–325.

Rabinowitz, P. M. (2006). Trends in the prevalence of hearing loss among young adults entering an industrial workforce 1985 to 2004. *Ear and Hearing, 27,* 369–375.

Rabinowitz, P. M., Galusha, D., Ernst, C. D., & Slade, M. D. (2007). Audiometric "early flags" for occupational hearing loss. *Journal of Occupational and Environmental Medicine, 49,* 1310–1316.

Rabinowitz, P. M., Galusha, D., Slade, M., Dixon-Ernst, C., Sircar, K. D., & Dobie, R. A. (2006). Audiogram notches in noise-exposed workers. *Ear and Hearing, 27,* 742–750.

Rabinowitz, P. M., Wise, J. P., Mobo, B. H., Antonucci, P. G., Powell, C., & Slade, M. (2002). Antioxidant status and hearing function in noise-exposed workers. *Hearing Research, 173,* 164–171.

Rajan, R. (2001). Plasticity of excitation and inhibition in the receptive field of primary auditory cortical neurons after limited receptor organ damage. *Cerebral Cortex, 11,* 171–182.

Ramkumar, V., Hallam, D. M., & Nie, Z. (2001). Adenosine, oxidative stress and cytoprotection. *Japanese Journal of Pharmacology, 86,* 265–274.

Ramkumar, V., Whitworth, C., Pingle, S. C., Hughes, L. F., & Rybak, L. P. (2004). Noise induces A$_1$ adenosine receptor expression in the chinchilla cochlea. *Hearing Research, 188,* 47–56.

Raphael, Y., Athey, B. D., Wang, Y., & Hawkins, J. E. (1993). Reticular lamina structure and repair after noise injury. *Reviews in Laryngology, Otology, Rhinology, 114,* 171–175.

Salvi, R., Perry, J., Hamernik, R. P., & Henderson, D. (1982). Relationships between cochlear pathologies and auditory nerve and behavioral responses following acoustic trauma. In R. P. Hamernik, D. Henderson, & R. Salvi (Eds.), *New perspectives in noise-induced hearing loss* (pp. 165–188). New York, NY: Raven Press.

Salvi, R. J., Wang, J., & Ding, D. (2000). Auditory plasticity and hyperactivity following cochlear damage. *Hearing Research, 147,* 261–274.

Saunders, J. C., & Hirsch, K. A. (1976). Changes in cochlear microphonic sensitivity after priming C57BL/6J mice at various ages for audiogenic seizures. *Journal of Comparative and Physiological Psychology, 90,* 212–220.

Schmiedt, R. A. (1989). Spontaneous rates, thresholds and tuning of auditory nerve fibers in the gerbil: Comparison to cat data. *Hearing Research, 42,* 23–46.

Schonherr, E., & Hausser, H.-J. (2000). Extracelular matrix and cytokines: A functional unit. *Developmental Immunology, 7,* 89–101.

Sha, S., Taylor, R., Forge, A., & Schacht, J. (2001). Differential vulnerability of basal and apical hair cells is based on intrinsic susceptibility to free radicals. *Hearing Research, 155,* 1–8.

Shi, X., Han, W., Yamamoto, H., Omelchenko, I., & Nuttall, A. L. (2007). Nitric oxide and mitochondrial status in noise-induced hearing loss. *Free Radical Research, 41,* 1313–1325.

Shi, X., & Nuttall, A. L. (2007). Expression of adhesion molecular proteins in the cochlear lateral wall of normal and PARP-1 mutant mice. *Hearing Research, 224,* 1–14.

Shupak, A., Tal, D., Sharoni, Z., Oren, M., Ravid, A., & Pratt, H. (2007). Otoacoustic emissions in early noise-induced hearing loss. *Otology and Neurotology, 28,* 745–752.

Sinex, D. G., Clark, W. W., & Bohne, B. A. (1987). Effects of periodic rest on physiologic measures of auditory sensitivity following exposure to noise. *Journal of the Acoustical Society of America, 82,* 1265–1273.

Spicer, S. S., Salvi, R. J., & Schulte, B. A. (1999). Ablation of inner hair cells by carboplatin alters cells in the medial K$^+$ route and disrupts tectorial membrane. *Hearing Research, 136,* 139–150.

Spicer, S. S., & Schulte, B. A. (1998). Evidence for a medial K$^+$ recycling pathway from inner hair cells. *Hearing Research, 118,* 1–12.

Spoendlin, H. (1978). The afferent innervation of the cochlea. In R. F. Naunton & C. Fernandez (Eds.), *Electrical activity of the auditory nervous system.* New York, NY: Academic Press.

Sugahara, K., Inouye, S., Izu, H., Katoh, Y., Katsuki, K., Takemoto, T., . . . Nakai, A. (2003). Heat shock transcription factor HSF1 is required for survival of sensory hair cells against acoustic overexposure. *Hearing Research, 182,* 88–96.

Sugawara, M., Corfas, G., & Liberman, M. C. (2005). Influence of supporting cells on neuronal degeneration after hair cell loss. *Journal of the Association for Research in Otolaryngology, 6,* 136–147.

Tahera, Y., Meltser, I., Johansson, P., Bian, Z., Stierna, P., Hansson, A. C., . . . Canlon, B. (2006a). NF-κB mediated glucocorticoid response in the inner ear after acoustic trauma. *Journal of Neuroscience Research, 83,* 1066–1076.

Tahera, Y., Meltser, I., Johansson, P., Hansson, A. C., & Canlon, B. (2006b). Glucocorticoid receptor and nuclear factor-κB interactions in restraint stress-mediated protection against acoustic trauma. *Endocrinology, 147,* 4430–4437.

Tahera, Y., Meltser, I., Johansson, P., Salman, H., & Canlon, B. (2007). Sound conditioning protects hearing by activating the hypothalamic-pituitary-adrenal axis. *Neurobiology of Disease, 25,* 189–197.

Taylor, W., Pearson, J., Mair, A., & Burns, W. (1964). Study of noise and hearing in jute weaving. *Journal of the Acoustical Society of America, 38,* 113–120.

Thai-Van, H., Micheyl, C., Norena, A. J., Veuillet, E., Gabriel, D., & Collet, L. (2007). Enhanced frequency discrimination in hearing-impaired individuals: A review of perceptual correlates of central neuronal plasticity induced by cochlear damage. *Hearing Research, 233,* 14–22.

Thorne, P. R., Munoz, D. J. B., & Housley, G. D. (2004). Puinergic modulation of cochlear partition resistance and its effect on the endocochlear potential in the guinea pig. *Journal of the Association for Research in Otolaryngology, 5,* 58–65.

Toppila, E., Pyykko, I., & Starck, J. (2001). Age and noise-related hearing loss. *Scandinavian Audiology, 30,* 236–244.

Tornabene, S. V., Sato, K., Pham, L., Billings, P., & Keithley, E. M. (2006). Immune cell recruitment following acoustic trauma. *Hearing Research, 222,* 115–124.

Tota, G., & Bocci, G. (1967). Importance of colour of the iris on the evaluation of resistance to auditory fatigue. *Revista Oto-neuro-oftalmologica y Cirugia Neurologica Sudamericana, 42,* 183–192.

Tsuprun, V., Schachern, P. A., Cureoglu, S., & Paparella, M. M. (2003). Structure of the stereocilia side links and morphology of auditory hair bundle in relation to noise exposure in the chinchilla. *Journal of Neurocytology, 32,* 1117–1128.

Uchida, Y., Nakashima, T., Ando, F., Niino, N., & Shimokada, H. (2005). Is there a relevant effect of noise and smoking on hearing? A population-based aging study. *International Journal of Audiology, 44,* 86–91.

Van De Water, T. R., Lallemend, F., Eshraghi, A. A., Ahsan, S., He, J., Guzman, J., . . . Balkany, T. J. (2004). Caspases, the enemy within, and their role in oxidative stress-induced apoptosis of inner ear sensory cells. *Otology and Neurotology, 25,* 627–632.

Van Laer, L., Carlsson, P. I., Ottschytsch, N., Bondeson, M.-L., Konings, A., Vandevelde, A., . . . Van Camp, G. (2006). The contribution of genes involved in potassium-recycling in the inner ear to noise-induced hearing loss. *Human Mutation, 27,* 786–795.

Vicente-Torres, M. A., & Schacht, J. (2006). A BAD link to mitochondrial cell death in the cochlea of mice with noise-induced hearing loss. *Journal of Neuroscience Research, 83,* 1564–1572.

Vlajkovic, S. M., Abi, S., Wang, C. J. H., Housley, G. D., & Thorne, P. R. (2007). Differential distribution of adenosine receptors in rat cochlea. *Cell and Tissue Research, 328,* 461–471.

Wang, Y., Hirose, K., & Liberman, M. C. (2002). Dynamics of noise-induced cellular injury and repair in the mouse cochlea. *Journal of the Association for Research in Otolaryngology, 3,* 248–268.

Wang, Y., & Liberman, M. C. (2002). Restraint stress and protection from acoustic injury in mice. *Hearing Research, 165,* 96–102.

Wangemann, P. (2002). K$^+$ recycling and the endocochlear potential. *Hearing Research, 165,* 1–9.

Wangemann, P. (2006). Supporting sensory transduction: cochlear fluid homeostasis and the endocochlear potential. *Journal of Physiology, 576*(1), 11–21.

Ward, W. D. (1995). Endogenous factors related to susceptibility to damage from noise. *Occupational Medicine: State of the Art Reviews, 10,* 561–575.

Ward, W. D., & Duvall, A. J. (1971). Behavioral and ultrastructural correlates of acoustic trauma. *Annals of Otology, 80,* 881–896.

Ward, W. D., Duvall, A. J., Santi, P. A., & Turner, C. W. (1981). Total energy and critical intensity concepts in noise damage. *Annals of Otology, 90,* 584–590.

Ward, W. D., & Turner, C. W. (1982). The total energy concept as a unifying approach to the prediction of noise trauma and its application to exposure criteria. In R. P. Hamernik, D. Henderson, & R. Salvi (Eds.), *New perspectives on noise-induced hearing loss* (pp. 423–435). New York, NY: Raven Press.

White, J. A., Burgess, B. J., Hall, R. D., & Nadol, J. B. (2000). Pattern of degeneration of the spiral ganglion cell and its processes in the C57BL/6J mouse. *Hearing Research, 141,* 12–18.

White, P. N., Thorne, P. R., Housley, G. D., Mockett, B., Billett, T. E., & Burnstock, G. (1995). Quinacrine staining of marginal cells in the stria vascularis of the guinea-pig cochlea: A possible source of extracellular ATP? *Hearing Research, 90,* 97–105.

Wild, D. C., Brewster, M. J., & Banerjee, A. R. (2005). Noise-induced hearing loss is exacerbated by long-term smoking. *Clinical Otolaryngology, 30,* 517–520.

Willott, J. F., & Turner, J. G. (1999). Prolonged exposure to an augmented acoustic environment ameliorates age-related auditory changes in C57BL/6J and DBA/2J mice. *Hearing Research, 135,* 78–88.

Yamashita, D., Miller, J. M., Jiang, H.-Y., Minami, S. B., & Schacht, J. (2004). AIF and EndoG in noise-induced hearing loss. *NeuroReport, 15,* 2719–2722.

Yang, M., Tan, H., Yang, Q., Wang, F., Yao, H., Wei, Q., . . . Wu, T. (2006). Association of hsp70 polymorphisms with risk of noise-induced hearing loss in Chinese automobile workers. *Cell Stress and Chaperones, 11,* 233–239.

Yoshida, K., Ichimiya, I., Suzuki, M., & Mogi, G. (1999a). Effect of proinflammatory cytokines on cultured spiral ligament fibrocytes. *Hearing Research, 137,* 155–159.

Yoshida, N., Kristiansen, A., & Liberman, M. C. (1999b). Heat stress and protection from permanent acoustic injury in mice. *Journal of Neuroscience, 19,* 10116–10124.

Yoshida, N., & Liberman, M. C. (2000). Sound conditioning reduces noise-induced permanent threshold shift in mice. *Hearing Research, 148,* 213–219.

Zhao, H.-B., Kikuchi, T., Ngezahayo, A., & White, T. W. (2006). Gap junctions and cochlear homeostasis. *Journal of Membrane Biology, 209,* 177–186.

Zhao, Y.-D., Yamoah, E. N., & Gillespie, P. G. (1996). Regeneration of broken tip links and resoration of mechanical transduction in hair cells. *Proceedings of the National Academy of Sciences, 94,* 15469–15475.

2

Current Issues in Auditory Neuropathy Spectrum Disorder

Linda J. Hood and Thierry Morlet

LEARNING OBJECTIVES

After reading this chapter, readers will be able to:

- Appropriately identify and evaluate individuals with auditory neuropathy spectrum disorder.
- Appropriately apply and interpret auditory physiologic tests.
- Distinguish cochlear from neural responses.
- Make appropriate recommendations for intervention.
- Apply appropriate methods in the management of auditory neuropathy/dys-synchrony.

Key Words. Auditory brainstem response, auditory neuropathy, auditory dys-synchrony, auditory neuropathy spectrum disorder, cochlear implant, cochlear microphonic, FM system, genetic, hearing aid, inner hair cells, late latency response, middle ear muscle reflex, middle latency response, medial olivocochlear reflex, otoacoustic emissions, outer hair cells, otoferlin, syndromes

LIST OF ABBREVIATIONS

ABR	Auditory brainstem response
AN	Auditory neuropathy
AN/AD	Auditory neuropathy/auditory dys-synchrony
ANSD	Auditory neuropathy spectrum disorder
APD	Auditory processing disorder
ASSR	Auditory steady-state response
CAEP	Cortical auditory evoked potential
CAP	Compound action potential

CM	Cochlear microphonic
CMT	Charcot-Marie-Tooth disease
CT	Computed tomography
EcochG	Electrocochleography
EVA	Enlarged vestibular aqueduct
FA	Friedreich ataxia
HMSN	Hereditary motor sensory neuropathy
IHC	Inner hair cells
LHON	Leber's hereditary optic neuropathy
LLR	Late latency response
MEMR	Middle ear muscle reflex
MLD	Masking level difference
MLR	Middle latency response
MMN	Mismatch negativity
MOCR	Medial olivocochlear reflex
MRI	Magnetic resonance imaging
OAE	Otoacoustic emissions
OHC	Outer hair cells
OTOF	Otoferlin
SNHL	Sensorineural hearing loss
SP	Summating potential

INTRODUCTION AND GENERAL DESCRIPTION

Patients ranging in age from infants to adults are described with an auditory disorder variably termed auditory neuropathy (AN; Starr et al., 1996), auditory neuropathy/dys-synchrony (AN/AD; Berlin et al., 2001) and more recently, auditory neuropathy spectrum disorder (ANSD; Gravel, 2008). For purposes of the discussion that follows and with the caveats and knowledge of the inherent problems discussed later, we use the term ANSD.

ANSD is characterized by evidence of intact outer hair cell (OHC) function as shown by otoacoustic emissions (OAEs) and/or cochlear microphonics (CM) that is accompanied by poor VIIIth nerve-brainstem responses demonstrated by absent or highly abnormal auditory brainstem responses (ABRs) (Berlin et al., 1998). Further evidence of effects on neural function are demonstrated by generally absent or sometimes elevated middle ear muscle reflexes (Berlin et al., 2005) and abnormal medial olivocochlear reflexes, measured via efferent stimulation effects on OAEs (Hood et al., 2003). Although understanding of speech in noise is below expected levels (re: normal hearing and SNHL), word recognition in quiet and thresholds for pure tones can range from near normal to profound loss ranges. Most ANSD patients show bilateral characteristics, though function may be asymmetric between ears, and cases of unilateral ANSD have been documented.

Despite fairly similar findings from physiologic measures in current clinical use, there is considerable variation in characteristics and functional communication abilities across patients (e.g., Berlin et al., 2010; Starr et al., 2000). Clinical presentation typically, but not always, includes difficulty listening in noise, may include fluctuation in hearing ability, and, in the case of infants and children, most often involves delayed or impaired development of speech and language. ANSD may or may not be accompanied by neural problems in other systems. Patients with ANSD typically demonstrate timing problems (Zeng et al., 1999), which suggest a disturbance in neural synchrony. This variation impacts both evaluation and management of ANSD.

Brief History and Earlier Studies

ANSD is not a new disorder, although patients have only recently been diagnosed with this disorder. What is new is the ability to clinically identify patients and distinguish ANSD from other disorders. Earlier reports, such as those from Worthington and Peters (1980) and Kraus et al. (1984), described patients who, for various reasons, displayed very poor ABRs despite better pure tone thresholds than would be expected. Their observed results were consistent with the presence of some type of neural dysfunction at the level of the brainstem. Patients in these studies most likely included some patients with auditory neuropathy and/or auditory dyssynchrony. However, OAEs were not available at the time these patients were evaluated.

Subsequent to these reports, Starr et al. (1991) described a patient with present OAEs and CM, but no recordable ABR. They demonstrated poor behavioral responses to temporal cues in this patient and ascribed decreased temporal-processing ability to possible changes in temporal encoding of acoustic signals, perhaps occurring at the synapse between hair cells and VIIIth nerve dendrites. Berlin et al.

(1993), in a study focusing on auditory efferent function and suppression of OAEs, reported a lack of OAE suppression in several patients with no ABRs and hypothesized Type I auditory nerve dysfunction as the basis for this observation.

The term AN was applied by Starr et al. (1996) to a group of 10 patients who displayed dyssynchronous ABRs despite evidence of intact OHC function. While such patients undoubtedly existed prior to this time, the advent of clinical use of OAEs precipitated a better understanding of the characteristics of this class of patients by clinicians and researchers. This is consistent with other reports of patients with absent ABRs and present OAEs that identify patients with the characteristics of AN/AD (e.g., Berlin et al., 1993a; Gorga et al., 1995; Gravel & Stapells, 1993; Starr et al., 1991).

The Use of Varying Terminology to Describe AN, AN/AD, and ANSD

Starr et al. (1996) coined the term auditory neuropathy based on their cohort of ten patients. These patients ranged in age from 4 to 49 years and the majority of them demonstrated the presence of neural abnormalities in systems other than the auditory pathways. For example, 3 patients in this group had diagnoses of Charcot-Marie-Tooth disease, a hereditary motor sensory neuropathy that involves the motor systems as well as some sensory pathway (see later discussion). Although not all patients with Charcot-Marie-Tooth disease have accompanying auditory problems, auditory function in these particular patients, and others subsequently reported, is consistent with the pattern of AN.

Later, the term auditory dys-synchrony was suggested as a more comprehensive term than auditory neuropathy (Berlin, Hood, & Rose, 2001). The rationale for this suggestion is based on the possibility of a sensory rather than neural disorder, or a combination of disorders. It was recognized that a number of factors may be found in these patients, including the lack of a compound action potential (CAP) in the electrocochleogram (ECochG) and missing ABR, absence of neuropathy in other than the auditory system in many patients, and human and animal temporal bones showing specific inner hair cell (IHC) loss. Second, there was concern that the term auditory neuropathy and its connotation of pathology of the nerve might lead clinicians to discount cochlear implants as a management option even though cochlear implants have proven beneficial in ANSD patients (Rapin & Gravel, 2003). Most recently, the term ANSD was suggested (Gravel, 2008) to further acknowledge the wide variation observed among patients with performance on clinical tasks and communication abilities ranging from mild to profound impairment.

All of these terms are in current use and each can be associated with certain characteristics of this disorder. From a historical perspective, each descriptive term might be thought to progressively broaden the characterization of the disorder. However, despite use of any of these terms, it should be noted that none of these terms may be preferred in the long run and, in fact, we hope that is the case. Perhaps the original term, AN, will maintain accuracy when we can, indeed, properly identify those patients with true disorders of the auditory nerve. Until we have the knowledge and technical capability to non-invasively (clinically) differentiate among IHC, synaptic, and neural disorders, we shall continue with the more operational (test outcome-based) definitions that AN/AD and ANSD denote. The hope is that we shall soon be able to move to accurate descriptions that might involve hair cell versus neural versus synaptic disorders. As discussed below, progress is being made in this direction that should allow more accurate description and also may provide more accurate guidance toward appropriate intervention.

Incidence of ANSD

Estimates of the incidence of ANSD suggest that it occurs at a rate of about 10% in those individuals who have a dys-synchronous ABR, or an ABR result consistent with a severe or profound estimate of hearing sensitivity. This rate is based on evidence from several sources. Berlin et al. (2000) screened over 1000 hearing-impaired children in schools for the Deaf in the United States and found that 1 to 2% had robust OAEs and 10 to 12% had evidence of residual OHC function shown by presence of OAEs

in limited frequency bands. A similar smaller scale study in schools for hearing-impaired children in Hong Kong found similar results (Lee et al., 2001). Rance et al. (1999) reported that 1 in 9 infants with severe or profound permanent hearing loss shown by ABR had CMs. Sininger (2002) reported that approximately 10% of infants enrolled in the NIH-NIDCD Multicenter Newborn Hearing Screening Study had OAEs and no ABR, consistent with ANSD.

Higher incidence of ANSD has been reported as well. Ngo et al. (2006) and Kirkim et al. (2008) found an ANSD incidence of 17.3% and 15.4%, respectively, among children with hearing loss following newborn hearing screening. In the NICU, Berg et al. (2005) observed that about 24% of 477 infants failed their ABR in one or both ears, while passing OAEs bilaterally. A similar observation was made earlier by Rea and Gibson (2003) in 40% of their NICU patients.

CLINICAL PRESENTATION

ANSD is characterized by intact responses from cochlear OHCs and abnormal neural responses from the VIIIth nerve and brainstem. Thus, clinical findings in patients with an ANSD are most accurately described with physiologic measures that assess cochlear hair cell and peripheral neural function. Normal OHC function is evidenced by the presence of OAEs and CMs. Clinical tests that are specifically sensitive to auditory nerve dysfunction are ipsilateral and contralateral middle ear muscle reflexes (MEMRs), ABR, masking level difference (MLD), the medial olivocochlear (MOC) reflex measured by suppression of OAEs, and to a limited extent, word recognition with an ipsilateral competing noise or message. Of the above measures, OAEs and ABR, when used together, provide insight into preneural as well as neural function in the auditory system and thus may form the most sensitive combination. A summary of physiologic and behavioral audiologic test results in patients with ANSD is shown in Table 2–1.

On behavioral measures, patients with ANSD show variable pure-tone thresholds ranging from normal sensitivity to the severe or profound hearing loss range (e.g., Berlin et al., 1993a, 1994; Gorga

Table 2–1. "Typical" Physiologic and Behavioral Audiologic Test Results in ANSD Patients

Test	Outcome
Otoacoustic emissions	Normal
Middle ear muscle reflexes	
Ipsilateral	Absent
Contralateral	Absent
Cochlear microphonic	Present (Inverts with stimulus polarity reversal)
ABR	Absent (or severely abnormal)
Pure-tone thresholds	Normal to severe/profound hearing loss (Any configuration; can be asymmetric)
Word recognition in quiet	Variable; slightly reduced to greatly reduced
Word recognition in noise	Generally poor
Masking level difference (MLD)	No MLD (i.e., 0 dB)
Efferent suppression of TEOAEs	No suppression

et al., 1995; Kaga et al., 1996; Starr et al., 1991, 1996, 2000). The wide variation among patients is likely a reflection of different underlying causes and mechanisms. Speech recognition is quite variable, though generally much poorer than expected, particularly in noise (Hood et al., 2004; Starr et al., 1996). ANSD patients generally show no MLD, which is consistent with abnormalities in processing of timing and phase information.

Hair Cell Responses: OAEs and CM

Accurately characterizing cochlear responses and distinguishing them from neural responses are important facets of ANSD differential diagnosis. Cochlear responses that are clinically measurable and most valuable in documenting cochlear function are OAEs and CM. These measures and findings in patients with ANSD are discussed in the following sections.

The most direct measure of cochlear function related to the outer hair cell (OHC) system is OAEs and the presence of ANSD is generally initially established based on presence of these responses when neural responses are absent or significantly reduced. Documenting the presence of OAEs is gen-

erally desired, although Starr et al. (2000) report that patients without evidence of OAEs, but presence of intact CM responses, may relate to a form of hereditary ANSD.

The CM is a gross potential generated by cochlear hair cells that can be recorded at several sites. It is believed to result from the vector sum of the extracellular components of receptor potentials arising in IHCs and OHCs, with the latter contributing more to CM generation on account of their greater number (Dallos, 1983). In normal individuals and standard clinical ABR techniques, CMs are typically limited in duration and sometimes obscured by the N1 response of the auditory nerve (ABR wave I). In ANSD patients, CMs can be quite robust and continue over several milliseconds, which may be due to a lack of time-locked neural activity (Berlin et al., 1998). A need remains for further investigation of patients where the CM is only observed for the highest intensity stimuli. For example, CMs to high level stimuli have been reported in patients diagnosed with severe/profound peripheral hearing loss (Aran & de Sauvage, 1976; Santarelli & Arslan, 2002). It may be possible that some of the patients in the Aran and de Sauvage report may have been ANSD patients, had OAEs been available at that time to identify them. Further delineation of specific characteristics of CM in ANSD and their significance remains an area for continued investigation.

In the absence of middle ear disorders, resulting in conductive hearing losses, OAEs are most often present in patients with ANSD. However, middle ear problems can reduce OAE amplitude or prevent the OAE from being recorded. The effect of even minor middle ear problems and the high incidence of otitis media in infants and children can therefore make identification of ANSD problematic. Furthermore, cases are reported where OAEs decline or disappear over time in the absence of middle ear problems. In many of these cases CMs remain.

If middle ear problems prevent measurement of OAEs, then it may be possible to evaluate OHC function using the CM. Because the CM is an electrical response from the cochlea recorded by electrodes attached to the scalp, it is less vulnerable to mild middle ear problems than OAEs (Berlin et al., 1998; Rance et al., 1999). A conductive hearing loss affecting the middle ear attenuates sound transmitted to the cochlea and also attenuates a returning OAE. As OAEs are low amplitude acoustic signals, even a small middle ear problem can be sufficient to reduce OAE amplitude or prevent the OAE from being recorded. Since the CM is an electrical response, it is not dependent on reverse transmission back through the middle ear system. In patients with middle ear problems where OAEs are absent, it is often possible to record the CM.

The CM may be small in surface-recorded responses in some patients, but is more easily recorded with insert than supra-aural earphones since the stimulus artifact is more separated in time from the biological response with insert earphones (Berlin et al., 1998). The CM has been found to be large in amplitude and with normal thresholds with transtympanic ECochG (Santarelli and Arslan, 2002). Transtympanic ECochG, and possibly TM-electrode ECochG methods, are likely to be helpful in understanding underlying conditions, as discussed later in this chapter.

Neural Responses: ABR

ABRs are typically absent in patients with ANSD, although some patients demonstrate small responses for high-level stimuli. In the germinal paper defining AN, Starr et al. (1996) reported absent ABRs in nine of ten patients (aged 4 to 49 years) and an abnormal ABR characterized by wave V responses only to high intensity stimuli in one of their patients. Berlin et al.'s (2010) review of ABR data for 260 patients with ANSD ranging in age from infants through adults indicated that 74% of patients had absent ABRs whereas 26% showed abnormal responses characterized by presence of low amplitude wave V only at high stimulus levels of 75 to 90 dB nHL. An example of an ANSD patient with a high-level wave V only is shown in Figure 2–1 (left ear). This distribution of responses is very similar to that reported by Starr et al. (2000) for 52 patients where 73% had no ABR and 27% had abnormal responses.

The absence or abnormality of all components of the ABR including wave I suggests that the most distal portion of the VIIIth nerve is affected, either directly or indirectly, in ANSD. This characteristic distinguishes ANSD patients from most patients with space-occupying lesions affecting the VIIIth nerve, where often wave I of the ABR is seen in recordings obtained with surface electrodes. Results of radiologic (magnetic resonance imaging: MRI and computed tomography: CT) evaluation are more often normal in ANSD patients, though conditions such as cochlear nerve deficiency may present with an ANSD pattern, as discussed later. Furthermore, the CAP is generally present in patients with space-occupying lesions or multiple sclerosis, but the CAP is typically absent or highly abnormal in ANSD patients.

Characteristics of the ABR, along with other measures, are consistent with a disorder that affects the response of the VIIIth nerve as well as brainstem pathways. Starr et al. (1991) suggested that the abnormal ABR seen in the patient who was the subject of that paper reflected altered temporal synchrony of auditory nerve afferent discharges. In the case of a demyelinating neuropathy, nerve impulses slow when a demyelinated segment of an axon is encountered and then return to a normal conduction velocity when the affected segment is passed (McDonald, 1980). Such neural conduction changes would also affect input to brainstem pathways and auditory reflexes such as the MEMR and MOC reflex, consistent with observations in ANSD patients. Starr

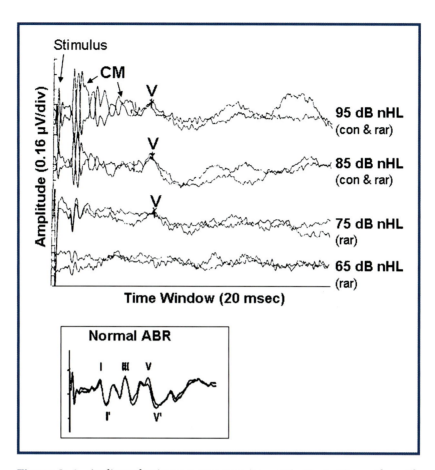

Figure 2–1. Auditory brainstem response in a patient age 12 months with ANSD and residual neural synchrony reflected in a present but abnormal ABR. Cochlear microphonics invert with stimulus polarity changes whereas neural responses do not. For reference, a normal ABR is shown in the box in the lower part of the figure.

et al. (1996) also observed absent ABRs in a patient with an axonal neuropathy, demonstrating that a dys-synchronous ABR may result from such disorders as described later in this chapter.

An important consideration in evaluating ABRs in newborns and infants is the neuromaturation of the ABR after birth that continues through 12 to 18 months of age (see more information later in this chapter). Although the ABR is typically present at birth, it is possible that factors such as premature birth, risk factors, or other trauma surrounding birth may delay development of synchronous neural responses. More information is needed to adequately understand the reasons for poor synchrony and the factors that may contribute to later development of the ABR in some infants who initially present with the signs of ANSD. At present, there are little data on which to base estimates of the number of newborn infants who present with dys-synchronous ABRs and later develop a normal ABR . In the meantime, it is important to closely monitor infants over the first year of life both with ABR and with other indices of auditory development, continually modifying management plans as needed.

Cochlear Microphonics Versus ABR

Several distinct differences exist between cochlear responses, such as the CM, and neural responses, such as the ABR. Distinguishing between these responses can be achieved by using appropriate recording methods. The most direct method of separating the CM and ABR is to compare responses obtained with rarefaction polarity stimuli (usually clicks) to those obtained with condensation stimuli. CM follows the acoustic waveform of the external stimulus; thus, the direction of the CM reverses with a change in polarity of the stimulus. For higher-frequency stimuli (~2 kHz and above) and clicks, neural responses such as the ABR in normal individuals may show slight latency shifts with polarity changes but do not invert. Therefore, cochlear and neural components can be distinguished based on whether or not the peaks invert with reversing stimulus polarity. The tracings in Figure 2–2 show ABRs obtained in an ANSD patient to condensation and rarefaction polarity stimuli. In this example, the CM is clearly seen in the early part of the tracings and there is no neural response. Because the entire response inverts with polarity changes, this confirms that it is CM and not ABR activity. Use of alternating polarity stimuli (to obtain one averaged response) is not helpful in identifying the CM since the CM will cancel, becoming invisible in the averaged response.

Cochlear and neural responses differ in two additional ways. First, ABR waves increase in latency and decrease in amplitude as stimulus intensity is lowered. In contrast, CMs do not increase in latency as the stimulus intensity decreases. If responses are obtained without reversing stimulus polarity, but at several stimulus intensities, it still may be possible to distinguish cochlear from neural components since cochlear components maintain constant latencies, while neural responses do not.

Second, cochlear and neural responses differ in the effects of masking. CM does not change in latency with broadband masking noise presented to the same ear, while the CAP and ABR peaks show amplitude reduction and latency increases during simultaneous masking to the same ear (Dallos, 1993). For an in-depth discussion of this topic and examples of responses showing these characteristics, the reader is referred to Berlin et al. (1998).

Efferent Acoustic Reflexes: MEMR and MOCR

Two reflex responses to acoustic stimuli are measurable noninvasively which allows their assessment in clinical settings. The MEMR assesses responses to higher-intensity tones and noise, based on contraction of the stapedius muscle of the middle ear. The medial olivocochlear reflex (MOCR) is assessed by measuring alterations in OAEs when additional stimuli are introduced that activate the olivocochlear neural pathway which terminates at the cochlear OHCs. Both of these efferent acoustic reflexes are abnormal in ANSD patients.

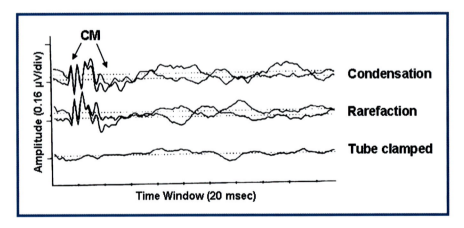

Figure 2–2. Auditory brainstem responses to condensation and rarefaction polarity click stimuli at 90 dB nHL in an ANSD patient age 3 years. Cochlear microphonics invert for condensation versus rarefaction stimuli and disappear when the earphone tube is clamped.

MEMRs, both ipsilaterally and contralaterally elicited, are most often absent, although a small percentage of patients display some MEMR responses (Berlin et al., 2005; Stein et al., 1996). Berlin et al. (2010) extracted MEMR data for 148 patients who had normal tympanograms and/or present OAEs. MEMRs were absent for all frequencies and conditions tested in 90% of the patients. Ten percent of the patients showed some MEMR responses; however, it should be noted that no ANSD patient had normal MEMRs at all frequencies. Those with MEMR responses showed elevated thresholds and/or combinations of present (elevated) and absent reflexes.

Although patients with ANSD typically demonstrate presence of OAEs, they consistently show no or minimal suppression of transient OAEs for binaural, ipsilateral, and contralateral suppressor stimuli (Berlin et al., 1994; Hood et al., 2003a; Starr et al., 1996). Suppression of OAEs involves the reduction in amplitude and/or change in phase of emissions resulting from the addition of another stimulus (Berlin et al., 1995; Collet et al., 1990; Hood et al., 1996). A lack of suppression of DPOAEs has also been demonstrated in ANSD patients (Abdala et al., 2000).

The lack of suppression may reflect efferent pathway dysfunction and/or a compromise of access to the efferent system via the afferent pathway. Although it is difficult to separate possible contributions of afferent and efferent pathways in patients with bilateral ANSD, cases of unilateral neuropathy can shed light on this question. Observations in patients with unilateral ANSD suggest a primarily afferent disorder in that suppression recorded from the side with ANSD can be partially activated by a suppressor to the normal ear. However, when the ANSD side is stimulated, no efferent function in either ear is recordable (Hood et al., 2003a). This pattern of suppression in unilateral ANSD suggests that the lack of suppression is likely due to a primary afferent effect.

Behavioral Findings: Pure-Tone Thresholds and Speech Recognition

Pure-tone thresholds and speech recognition, particularly in quiet, are the least informative measures in the evaluation of ANSD. Patients with ANSD show variable pure-tone thresholds ranging from normal auditory sensitivity to severe or profound hearing loss (Berlin et al., 1993a, 1994; Gorga et al., 1995; Kaga et al., 1996; Starr et al., 1991, 1996). Some patients show rising or unusual configurations, and pure-tone thresholds may or may not be symmetric between ears (Berlin et al., 2010). The variability in pure-tone threshold patterns clearly limits the utility of pure-tone testing by itself to distinguish ANSD. In cases where pure-tone thresholds exceed 30 to 40 dB HL and OAEs are present, the disagreement between these two tests may provide a clue to the presence of ANSD or another type of neural disorder that warrants further investigation.

Many patients with ANSD display some awareness of sound around them but are unable to discriminate speech sounds sufficiently to understand words and sentences. In the majority of ANSD patients, word recognition in quiet is poorer than one would predict from the pure-tone audiogram. In the patients with AN described by Starr et al. (1996), word recognition in quiet in 12 of 16 ears was poorer than would be predicted using the norms for cochlear hearing loss reported by Yellin et al. (1989). Generally, ANSD patients with some word recognition ability in quiet have great difficulty understanding speech, including sentences, when there is even a small amount of background noise.

Speech recognition scores for monosyllables in quiet were greater than 0% for 25 of the 62 patients tested aged 4 years and older (Berlin et al., 2010; Hood et al., 2004). Younger patients were excluded due to differences in procedures and use of nonstandardized test materials. Word recognition scores in quiet for these 25 patients averaged 49% and 45% correct for the right and left ears, respectively, and typically were poorer than audiometric thresholds would predict, based on the Yellin et al. (1989) norms. Word recognition in noise was measurable in only 5 patients (meaning that scores were greater than 0%). These patients represent the "best" performers in speech recognition and, in general, in their communication abilities without intervention. For these 5 patients, word recognition in quiet was 86 to 87% and was 48 to 64% in noise (+8 or +10 signal-to-noise ratio). Speech recognition ability, particularly in noise, is below normal in most ANSD patients and consistent with other patient populations where neural function is affected.

Behavioral Assessment of Neural Function: Masking Level Difference (MLD)

The MLD relies on accurate input to the lower brainstem and is sensitive to neural abnormalities of the VIIIth nerve and lower brainstem. It is based on the principle that a signal buried in noise is more detectable when either the signal or the noise is out of phase in one ear in relation to a simultaneous signal in the other ear (Hirsh, 1948; Licklider, 1948). This neural cancellation effect is not seen unless the input to the lower brainstem pathways is transmitted accurately. ANSD patients demonstrate no MLD effect, as demonstrated by lack of improvement in detection of stimuli in the out-of-phase condition, which supports evidence of compromised temporal processing (Berlin et al, 1994; Kraus, 2000).

Auditory Steady-State Responses in ANSD Patients

Auditory steady-state responses (ASSR) using 80 to 100 Hz modulation rates are typically absent in patients with ANSD (Picton et al., 2003), although present ASSRs have been reported in some patients with ANSD (Attias et al., 2006). Agreement between threshold estimates with ASSR and behavorial thresholds is poorer than observed in patients with sensorineural hearing loss (SNHL). In another study that included 19 pediatric subjects with ANSD, Rance et al. (2005) found that ASSR thresholds in children with ANSD-type hearing loss did not accurately reflect the behavioral audiogram. There presently is not a clear explanation of why ASSRs are present under some conditions in patients with dys-synchronous/absent ABRs. Possible explanations may relate to influence of cortical activity on ASSRs even at the higher modulation rates, or other unknown factors related to the generation of ASSRs.

Question 1

Do you think children with suspected APD are possibly children with ANSD? If so, do you recommend including OAEs, CM, and ABRs (with alternating clicks) as part of the basic test battery for children with suspected APD?

Answer 1

Some of the children (and adults) whom we have identified with ANSD were, indeed, first suspected of having an auditory processing disorder (centrally based APD). This is typically based on problems listening in noise, difficulty in school, sporadic inattention: all signs that accompany both ANSD and APD. We prefer to clearly distinguish ANSD and APD because the test results are quite different and some of the management options also differ. We have included Table 2–2, which outlines these distinctions.

When we evaluate patients who are suspected of having a centrally based APD, the first thing we want to do is rule out ANSD. We begin with OAEs, tympanograms, and middle ear muscle reflexes, as we do with every new patient. If we get a pattern of normal OAEs and elevated or absent MEMRs, then that suggests the possibility of some type of neural problem and would then lead us to do an ABR. For the ABR, as always, we would compare response obtained to rarefaction and condensation clicks to distinguish the CM from the neural response (ABR). By evaluating OAEs and MEMRs, we can gain insight in a way that often has greater feasibility in a public school setting. In our own clinical practice, the workup for APD typically includes a series of auditory evoked potentials that would include the ABR prior to cortically based responses. This provides a way to rule out problems, working from the periphery to more central areas.

Table 2–2. Typical Findings in ANSD and (Central) APD

	ANSD	APD
Test results		
Otoacoustic emissions	Present	Present
Cochlear microphonic	Present	Present
Middle ear muscle reflexes	Absent, abnormal	Normal, near normal
Auditory brainstem response	Absent, abnormal	Normal, near normal
Management		
Cochlear implants	Successful in many	Not appropriate

PUTATIVE SITES OF LESION AND UNDERLYING MECHANISMS

Although the specifics underlying the absent or severely disrupted auditory nerve activity in ANSD are not entirely known, it is presently established that ANSD accompanies disorders of the auditory nerve, or the IHCs and/or their synapses with auditory nerve terminals.

Inner Hair Cell Loss, Inner Hair Cell Malfunction

ANSD can be caused by partial or complete loss of IHC and also IHC malfunction. IHC malfunction caused by genetic mutations is now well documented and abundant research links the otoferlin (*OTOF*) gene to nonsyndromic recessive ANSD (Rodriguez-Ballesteros et al., 2003; Rodriguez-Ballesteros et al., 2008; Varga et al., 2003; Yasunaga et al., 1999). The *OTOF* gene encodes otoferlin, a transmembrane protein belonging to the ferlin protein family involved in calcium binding. Studies in mice indicate that otoferlin plays a crucial role in vesicle release at the synapse between IHCs and auditory nerve fibers. When the *OTOF* gene is mutated, the neurotransmitter release is adversely affected which results in absent ABRs, consistent with a functional loss of auditory nerve input. A CM with normal amplitude, as well as OAEs can be found in most of these patients (Rodriguez-Ballesteros et al., 2008; Santarelli et al., 2009). At least 42 pathogenic mutations of *OTOF* have been identified so far, all resulting in a homogeneous phenotype of prelingual profound hearing loss (Rodriguez-Ballesteros et al., 2008). Recent genetic studies estimated that mutations in *OTOF* account for at least 3% of cases of prelingual nonsyndromic hearing impairment in the Spanish population (Santarelli et al., 2009). Other evidence that synapses between IHC and auditory nerve fibers may be affected in some instances of ANSD derives from ABR studies where the rate of stimulation was varied. In several ANSD patients, wave V was found to be absent at stimulus rate of 20/s and higher but present when the rate was slowed down to 10/s. Such a change does not occur in a normally functioning auditory system and is attributed to decreased synaptic efficacy (Starr et al., 2000).

ANSD is also thought to originate from IHC loss in some instances. Lack of IHCs could result from a delay in development, some traumatic insult, or a loss over some period of time. Selective IHC loss among several premature newborns who failed their ABRs has been observed (Amatuzzi et al., 2001). OAEs were not obtained in these patients. The IHC loss seems to have occurred in utero, and in the absence of significant neuronal loss at the time of the infants' death. While the reasons for such a loss remain unknown, the IHCs are known to be particularly sensitive to hypoxia (Shirane & Harrison, 1987), compared to the OHCs, and to some toxic insults such as carboplatin (though this

IHC-carboplatin effect has only been demonstrated in chinchillas), a widely used platinum-based chemotherapy agent (Takeno et al., 1994).

Neural Disorders

In the germinal paper defining auditory neuropathy (Starr et al., 1996), 8 out of the 10 patients presented with a peripheral neuropathy in the body, which supported the presence of a concomitant neuropathy of the auditory nerve. Cases of ANSD have since been observed with both the absence and the presence of other neural disorders in the body. ANSD has been described in Charcot-Marie-Tooth disease, Mohr-Tranebjaerg syndrome (Starr et al, 1996; Merchant et al, 2001), mitochondrial diseases (Ceranic & Luxon, 2004; Corley & Crabbe, 1999; Forli et al, 2006), and other disorders. Absence of or deficiency in the VIIIth nerve also has been found in patients presenting as ANSD (Buchman et al, 2006).

Definition of Neuropathy

Neuropathy refers to disorders of the nerves of the peripheral nervous system. Peripheral neuropathies vary in their presentation and origin, and may affect the nerve or the neuromuscular junction. There are more than 100 known types of peripheral neuropathy, with the etiology unknown for a significant number of them. One (mononeuropathy) or more (polyneuropathies) types of nerves may be affected. Some neuropathies are distal when the disease progresses from the center toward the periphery and others are proximal when the disease progresses from the periphery toward the center. The form of neuropathy may be further broken down by cause, the speed of progression, the parts of the body involved, or the size of predominant fiber involvement, that is, large fiber or small fiber peripheral neuropathy. Neuropathies are also usually defined according to the part of the nerve that is being affected, that is, the axon, the myelin, or the cell body.

Charcot-Marie-Tooth disease (demyelinating and axonal neuropathy with genetic causes), Guillain-Barré syndrome (inflammatory disease affecting the myelin) and Leber's hereditary optic atrophy are among the peripheral neuropathies already known to engender the symptoms of ANSD. More will likely be identified in the near future.

ANSD Accompanying Other Neuropathies—Hereditary Motor Sensory Neuropathies (HMSN)

Several of the first patients diagnosed with ANSD clearly presented a neural disorder which was not limited to the peripheral auditory pathways. In some study groups, up to 40% of patients with ANSD presented with other peripheral neuropathies in the body (Starr et al., 2000). Interestingly, although the hearing disorder seems to be present as early as birth in most patients, none of the children examined in the Starr et al. (2000) study showed clinical evidence of a peripheral neuropathy before the age of 5 years, whereas 80% of the patients examined after the age of 15 years showed both clinical and nerve-conduction evidence of a peripheral neuropathy. The presence of a peripheral neuropathy did not correlate with the presence of ABR components in these patients.

Charcot-Marie-Tooth Disease

Charcot-Marie-Tooth disease (CMT) is one of the most common inherited neurological disorders, affecting approximately 1 in 2,500 people in the United States. The disease is named for the three physicians who first identified it in 1886: Jean-Martin Charcot and Pierre Marie in Paris, France, and Howard Henry Tooth in Cambridge, England. CMT, also known as hereditary motor and sensory neuropathy or peroneal muscular atrophy, comprises a group of disorders that affect peripheral nerves. CMT is caused by mutations in genes that produce proteins involved in the structure and function of either the peripheral nerve axon or the myelin sheath. Although different proteins are abnormal in different forms of CMT disease, all of the mutations affect the normal function of the peripheral nerves. Consequently, these nerves slowly degenerate and lose the ability to communicate with their distant targets.

The neuropathy of CMT affects both motor and sensory nerves. Onset of symptoms is most often in adolescence or early adulthood; however, presentation may be delayed until mid-adulthood. The severity of symptoms is quite variable in different patients and even among family members with the disease. Progression of symptoms is gradual. Although in rare cases patients may have respiratory muscle weakness, CMT is not considered a fatal disease and people with most forms of CMT have a normal life expectancy.

There are many forms of CMT disease, including CMT1, CMT2, CMT3, CMT4, and CMTX and various subtypes composed of each of these forms. Hearing loss has been found in the primary demyelinating form in CMT1, due to mutation of *PMP22* gene duplication (Boerkoel et al., 2002; Hattori et al., 2003; Joo et al., 2004; Kovach et al., 2002), in the primary axonal forms (CMT2) due to mutations of *MPZ* gene (Chapon et al., 1999; De Jonghe et al., 1999; Hattori et al., 2003; Misu et al., 2000; Starr et al., 2003), connexin 31 (*GJB3*) gene (Lopez-Bigas et al., 2001), connexin 32 (*Cx32*) gene (Boerkoel et al., 2002; Hattori et al., 2003), in a mixed demyelinating/axonal autosomal recessive motor-sensory neuropathy, particular to Roma populations due to a mutation of the *NDRG1* gene (Butinar et al., 1999; Kalaydjieva et al., 1998; Kalaydjieva et al., 2000) and in the X-linked dominant disease (CMTX) caused by a point mutation in the gap junction protein connexin-32 gene on the X chromosome which is expressed in Schwann cells and oligodendrocytes (Bahr et al., 1999).

Several of these studies (Butinar et al., 1999; Kovach et al., 2002; Starr et al., 2003) revealed that the pattern of ANSD was present in affected individuals and thus attributed the hearing loss to a dysfunction of the auditory nerve. Examination of the temporal bone of one subject with CMT2 due to mutations of the *MPZ* gene revealed marked depletion of auditory ganglion cells and central and peripheral auditory nerve fibers within the cochlea with preservation of both IHCs and OHCs (Starr et al., 2003). All these studies showed that hearing loss in CMT can be attributed to an accompanying neuropathy of the auditory nerve sparing the IHCs. A similar conclusion was drawn by both Spoendlin (1974) and Hallpike et al. (1980) based on cochlear histopathology in subjects with CMT and deafness before the tests used to define ANSD were available. In a more recent study, Butinar et al. (2008) found

that affected members in two families with different point mutations of the *NF-L* gene (CMT2) had abnormal ABRs and absent stapedial muscle reflexes but without symptoms of hearing loss, or more precisely, without the symptoms of an auditory temporal-processing disorder that accompanies ANSD. The authors concluded that the absence of "deafness" may reflect the ability of central mechanisms to compensate for the slowly developing auditory nerve abnormalities.

Friedreich Ataxia

Friedreich ataxia (FA), an autosomal recessive disorder, is the most common inherited ataxia. FA is a progressive neurodegenerative disorder with a prevalence of about 1 in 29,000 persons (Cosse et al., 1997). Patients typically present with difficulty walking, loss of coordination, and dysarthria. Degeneration of the dorsal root ganglion neurons, their axons in the dorsal columns, and the dorsal spinocerebellar pathways gives rise to a loss of proprioception and associated ataxia. A few other nuclei (including the dentate nucleus of the cerebellum) within the central nervous system are affected and contribute to the ataxia. Additional clinical manifestations include cardiomyopathy, diabetes, and scoliosis. Average age at onset of symptoms occurs between 10 and 15 years (Durr et al., 1996; Harding, 1981). Life span is reduced, with the average time from onset of symptoms to death being 36 years (De Michelle et al., 1996).

The natural history of FA is one of slow progression of symptoms over decades with increasing dependence on assistance with activities of daily living. Rate of progression is neither constant nor linear. Multiple areas of the central and peripheral nervous system are affected. The discovery of the abnormal gene in FA and its product (frataxin) has provided insight into possible pathophysiologic mechanisms in this disease (Campuzano et al., 1996). Frataxin is active in the mitochondria, and the pathophysiologic mechanism in FA consists of mitochondrial iron accumulation due to frataxin deficiency. This initiates or propagates free radical reactions leading to cell death.

Hearing abilities can be impaired in FA, although there have been only a few studies focusing on these abilities. Some patients, notably among those with more severe neurological symptoms, complain about auditory difficulties or decreased intelligibility in noise. ABR can be abnormal or absent in these patients (Miyamoto et al., 1999; Rance et al., 2008, 2010). ABR abnormalities appear to be more important in patients with early onset of the disorder and abnormalities progress with the severity of the disease, until the response is totally absent (Amantini et al., 1984; Cassandro et al., 1986; Finocchiaro et al., 1985; Satya-Murti et al., 1980). Temporal bone analysis of 2 siblings with FA revealed selective and extensive damage to the neurons of the VIIIth nerve (Spoendlin, 1974) and impairment of temporal processing abilities in affected patients (Rance et al., 2008, 2010) fits with the characteristics of ANSD. Although there clearly seems to be an involvement of the auditory nerve in FA patients presenting with hearing loss, presence of wave I of the ABR in some of these patients (Rance et al., 2008, 2010) does not fit entirely the germinal definition of ANSD (Berlin et al., 2010). This particular pattern (wave I present) probably represents one step of this progressive disorder but raises the question of when the diagnosis of ANSD can (or should) be made, if mostly based on physiologic recordings (ABR). The ideal management of hearing loss in patients with FA also remains to be studied. There is one reported case of cochlear implantation in a child with FA and diagnosis of ANSD, with an outcome that was reported as unsuccessful (Miyamoto et al., 1999).

Waardenburg Syndrome

Waardenburg syndrome is a group of genetic conditions that can cause hearing loss and changes in pigmentation of the hair, skin, and eyes. Four known types of Waardenburg syndrome are distinguished by their physical characteristics and sometimes by their genetic cause. Waardenburg syndrome affects an estimated 1 in 10,000 to 20,000 people. In schools for the Deaf, 2 to 3% of students have this condition. ANSD has been reported in 2 siblings with Waardenburg type 2 syndrome (Jutras et al., 2003).

Leber's Hereditary Optic Neuropathy

Leber's hereditary optic neuropathy (LHON) is one of the best known forms of hereditary optic neu-

ropathy. LHON involves maternal transmission of a mitochondrial DNA point mutation and men are primarily affected. This disorder is characterized by a sudden, bilateral, sequential loss of central vision, as a result of a peripapillary microangiopathy and subsequent optic atrophy, leading to a permanent bilateral severe visual impairment in most patients. Two reports describe progressive ANSD in patients with Leber's hereditary optic neuropathy (Berlin et al., 2010; Ceranic & Luxon, 2004).

Mohr-Tranebjærg Syndrome

Mohr-Tranebjærg syndrome is an X-linked recessive, syndromic SNHL characterized by childhood onset of deafness followed by progressive neural degeneration affecting the brain and optic nerves later in adult life. Bahmad et al. (2007) studied 4 subjects with this syndrome, who all developed progressive hearing loss early in childhood, becoming profoundly deaf by the age of 10 years. All of these subjects developed language, and at least one subject used amplification in early life. All temporal bones examined showed a near total loss of cochlear neuronal cells (90 to 95% compared to control) and severe loss of vestibular neurons (75 to 85% compared to control). Hearing loss in this disorder is likely to be the result of a postnatal and progressive degeneration of cochlear neurons and probably constitutes a true auditory neuropathy.

Autosomal Dominant Optic Atrophy

Autosomal dominant optic atrophy is a retinal neuronal degenerative disease characterized by a progressive bilateral visual loss and is associated with SNHL that mimics ANSD with preserved OAEs and absent or abnormal ABRs. Hearing loss accompanying a mutation found in the *OPA1* gene suggests altered function of terminal unmyelinated portions of auditory nerve (Amati-Bonneau et al., 2005; Bette et al., 2007; Huang et al., 2009).

Other Neuropathies and Genetic Mutations

Multiple family members with ANSD suggest underlying genetic factors. Families with two or more siblings with ANSD and parents with normal auditory function are consistent with a recessive inheritance pattern. The majority of cases of nonsyndromic ANSD are autosomal recessive, and the pure tone loss is generally severe to profound from infancy. Multiple generations within families also can display ANSD, consistent with a dominant inheritance pattern. Patients with syndromic ANSD may be first diagnosed with peripheral neuropathy followed by auditory complaints several years later, though this is not always the case. Since ANSD clearly has hereditary aspects, it is important to consider family history and consider risk of ANSD for subsequent siblings in families who already have one or more members with ANSD.

Genetic studies of patients and families with ANSD continue to reveal new genes and mutations. Mutation in the *pejvakin* gene causes nonsyndromic, prelingual, severe to profound sensorineural hearing impairment, which fits the diagnostic criteria for ANSD (Delmaghani et al., 2006). The mutation induces dysfunction in neurons along the auditory pathway, which is consistent with the observed distribution of *pejvakin* in the cell bodies of neurons in the spiral ganglion and the brainstem auditory nuclei. Kim et al. (2004) reported a gene responsible for autosomal dominant auditory neuropathy (*AUNA1*). Cx29 is now one of the candidates among other genetic mutations that could explain demyelination in the peripheral auditory system (Tang et al., 2006). Cx29 is strongly and exclusively expressed in the Schwann cells myelinating the auditory nerve within the cochlea. In Cx29$^{-/-}$ mice, the authors observed a delay in development of hearing sensitivities, early high-frequency hearing in the matured cochlea, and distortion of the ABR waveforms. Both the IHC and OHC morphology and function appeared to be normal. The most likely etiology is the severe demyelination found at the soma of the spiral ganglion neurons of affected Cx29$^{-/-}$ mice. Other candidates under review include the misexpression of *Pou3f1* which results in peripheral nerve hypomelination and axonal loss (Ryu et al., 2007).

It is becoming obvious that clinical and subclinical forms of ANSD might also be present in other hereditary neuropathies. For example, the clinical expression of ANSD may also occur when individuals are febrile, as in cases known as temperature sensitive auditory neuropathy (Marlin et al., 2010; Starr et al., 1998). Starr et al. (1998) reported three children who showed a type of transient deafness due to changes in body temperature. Testing of one of these patients documented severe to profound hearing loss with mild elevation (approximately 1 degree Celsius) of her core body temperature, probably due to a demyelinating disorder of the auditory nerve. The site of demyelination is not known but could be in the peripheral or Schwann cell myelinated portion of auditory nerve distal to the dura mater and/or in its central portion proximal to the dura mater where the axons are myelinated by oligodendroglial cells. Some tests were found to be normal when febrile and afebrile (OAEs, CM, and tympanometry), some were mildly abnormal when afebrile and markedly abnormal when febrile (ABRs and pure-tone hearing thresholds) while others were markedly abnormal and did not change with body temperature (MEMRs and suppression of OAEs). More recently, Marlin et al. (2010) linked temperature sensitive ANSD with a novel mutation in *OTOF* in three children from one family.

Methods of Differentiating Sites of Abnormality

Although the test protocols necessary to diagnose ANSD are now well established, one of the major issues facing the clinician afterward is to specify both the degree and the potential site of abnormality. As a matter of fact, dysfunction of the IHCs and/or their synapses can lead to a hearing disorder that is almost impossible to distinguish clinically from a neuropathy of the auditory nerve. Finding concomitant peripheral neuropathies in a patient is currently the best possible way of surmising that the patient has a disorder involving the auditory nerve, although that does not conclusively exclude a disorder of the IHCs and/or their synapses.

Imaging studies are useful in evaluating hearing loss to diagnose inner ear malformations as well as to check for presence and size of the auditory nerve. Absent or hypoplastic auditory nerves are not uncommon (Buchman et al., 2006) and these cases usually resemble ANSD when OHC are present and functioning. Audiologic management in these patients is problematic because a cochlear implant cannot work when the nerve is absent and might not work well when the nerve is hypoplastic (Teagle et al., 2010).

Electrocochleography: Pre- and Postsynaptic ANSD

Presently, one tool with promise to be useful in specifying the site of lesion is receiving a great deal of attention. Although the technique is not new (e.g., Cullen et al., 1972), the use of transtympanic ECochG may prove valuable in separating IHC dysfunction (presynaptic dysfunction) from neural elements (postsynaptic dysfunction) (Gibson & Sanli, 2007; McMahon et al., 2008; Santarelli & Arslan, 2002).

Transtympanic ECochG allows the recording of several electrical events (CM, summating potential (SP) and CAP) that are generated in the cochlea following appropriate stimulation. As defined earlier, the CM is a gross potential generated by hair cells that can be recorded at several sites. The CM recorded at the promontory or in the ear canal is believed to arise primarily from the more basal portions of the cochlea, while the apical regions make a negligible contribution to its generation (Withnell, 2001). The CM is usually abnormally increased in amplitude in ANSD subjects less than 10 years of age, although the functional significance of this finding remains unclear as no significant correlation has been found between CM amplitude and the pure tone audiogram, presence of neonatal risk factors, peripheral neuropathy, presence of a wave V, and family members with ANSD (Starr et al., 2001).

The SP represents the DC change produced in the cochlea in response to a sound. The source of the SP remains controversial, with some authors attributing it to the OHCs, some to IHCs, and others to both (Cheatham & Dallos, 1984; Durrant et al., 1998). The SP can be observed in some patients with ANSD (Santarelli et al., 2008, 2009; Starr et al., 2001) but it is not yet clear why it is present in some patients and not in others.

The CAP represents the synchronous depolarization/discharge of many single units of the auditory nerve. Presence of a CAP has been observed in several patients with ANSD (Santarelli & Arslan, 2002; Santarelli et al., 2008, 2009).

In a recent study, Santarelli et al. (2008) recorded transtympanic ECochG in 8 children and adults with ANSD and used an adaptation procedure that preferentially attenuates neural responses with minor changes in SP amplitude (Eggermont & Odenthal, 1974) to try to differentiate between ANSD of neural or hair cell origin. In normal subjects, this adaptation paradigm resulted in an amplitude reduction of the CAP that was twice that of SP without affecting their duration. In seven ANSD ears without CAP and with a prolonged negative potential, adaptation was accompanied by reduction of both the amplitude and duration of the negative potential to control values consistent with a neural generation site. In four ears without CAP and with normal-duration potentials, adaptation was without effect, consistent with receptor generation. In five ears with CAP, there was reduction in amplitude of CAP and SP similar to controls but with a significant decrease in response duration. These results reveal three patterns of cochlear potentials: (1) presence of receptor SP without CAP consistent with presynaptic disorder of IHC; (2) presence of both SP and CAP consistent with postsynaptic disorder of the proximal auditory nerve; and (3) presence of prolonged neural potentials without a CAP, consistent with postsynaptic or nerve terminal disorder. In their next study, ECochG responses obtained in 4 children with *OTOF* mutations was interpreted as a dendritic potential resulting from local depolarization of the distal portion of the afferent fibers without spike initiation. This would indicate decreased neurotransmitter release resulting in abnormal dendritic activation and impaired auditory nerve firing (Santarelli et al., 2009). McMahon et al. (2008) obtained the same type of results in transtympanic ECochG performed before cochlear implantation and also suggested that pre- and postsynaptic mechanisms of ANSD might be uncovered by ECochG. ECochG measurement has also been applied to two affected members of a family with an *OPA1* mutation (Huang et al., 2009). Again, ECochG testing showed prolonged low-amplitude negative potentials without auditory nerve CAPs. The latency of onset of the cochlear potentials was within the normal range found for IHC SP receptor potentials. The duration of the negative potential was reduced to normal during rapid stimulation, consistent with adaptation of neural sources generating prolonged potentials. Both subjects in this study had a cochlear implant placed with restoration of hearing thresholds, speech perception, and synchronous activity in auditory brainstem pathways. This suggests that deafness accompanying this *OPA1* mutation is due to altered function of terminal unmyelinated portions of auditory nerve.

Transtympanic ECochG testing seems to have great potential in refining the site of lesion in ANSD, understanding differences among some forms, and providing information that may be important in managing patients. The invasive nature of this technique and the requirement for anesthesia are limitations to its use in many clinical settings. Also, ECochG is more widely used in some practices and areas of the world than others. ECochG in some practices may be reserved for assessment prior to cochlear implantation. As more is learned about the value and utility of transtympanic ECochG in ANSD, it may be incorporated into more patient evaluations.

ANSD and Vestibular Neuropathies

True vestibular neuropathies appear to coexist with ANSD in some patients with concomitant peripheral neuropathies (Fujikawa & Starr, 2000). It is still unclear, however, if a presynaptic type of vestibular neuropathy might exist in cases of ANSD. There are few published reports regarding vestibular and balance disorders in general in the pediatric age group. This may be due to a lack of recognition of this pathology since children infrequently complain of vertigo, they may be considered "clumsy," and signs and symptoms of a balance disorder may be ignored. Children have also been noted to rapidly and readily accommodate for balance disorders (Balatsouras et al., 2007). Additionally, there are intrinsic difficulties in obtaining complete clinical histories and objective vestibular and balance testing in this age group. Although no balance defect has been observed as yet in children with *OTOF* mutations, Dulon et al. (2009) showed that OTOF is critical for a highly sensitive and linear calcium-dependent exocytosis at the vestibular hair cell ribbon synapses. This suggests that some type of balance dysfunction might appear in these children.

Although we do not know exactly what causes ANSD or the exact site of lesion in all instances, progress has been made. The use of a test battery that includes genetic testing, imaging studies and ECochG along with basic audiologic testing may sometimes delineate the problem and lead to more focused and accurate management. ANSD is a continuum in which a mosaic of present and functioning IHCs and OHCs and pre- and postganglionic single units of the auditory nerve may lead to various combinations of temporal disruption (Amatuzzi et al., 2001; Berlin et al., 1993; McMahon et al., 2008; Rance et al., 2004; Starr et al., 2000, 2008; Varga et al., 2003; Zeng et al., 1999, 2005). As described earlier in this chapter, the changes of nomenclature over the recent years reflect the evolution in understanding ANSD and its putative sites of lesion. New names (such as postsynaptic or type I ANSD; Starr et al., 2003 and presynaptic or type II ANSD; Rodriguez-Ballesteros et al., 2003; Starr et al., 2004) will certainly continue to emerge as we learn more about the details of ANSD.

UNDERSTANDING ANSD THROUGH ANIMAL MODELS

To increase understanding of ANSD, several animal models with hair cell/auditory nerve dysfunction have been proposed in recent years. The development of these experimental animal models has begun to provide insights into various mechanisms of the disorder and will hopefully lead to the development of treatment therapies.

Selective lesions to the IHCs have been obtained by intravenous administration of carboplatin in the chinchilla (Cowper-Smith et al., 2010 for a review of this model). IHC loss is not complete (from 54% to up to 95% depending on the studies) but OHCs seem to be mostly preserved and animals show relatively normal OAEs and CM in the presence of increased thresholds for CAP and ABR (Harrison, 1998; Wake et al., 1994; Wang et al., 1997). However, further studies reported that carboplatin also may induce a significant loss of auditory nerve fibers (El-Badry & McFadden, 2009). Although this model somewhat resembles ANSD, ABRs are still present in these chinchillas, only with elevated thresholds. In fact, surviving auditory nerve fibers retain normal thresholds and frequency tuning (Wang et al., 1997), but both spontaneous and driven spike rates of the fibers are significantly lower than normal.

Lesions to the spiral ganglion neurons have been achieved by injection of β-bungarotoxin to the round window in the rat (Palmgren et al., 2010). Such an injection decreases the number of spiral ganglion neurons by apoptosis, while keeping the hair cells intact. ABRs, however, still can be recorded in these animals, although their thresholds are elevated to levels consistent with severe to profound hearing loss. Application of ouabain to the round window of gerbils also results in a rapid loss of spiral ganglion neurons. There is a complete absence of the CAP, while the endocochlear potential and DPOAEs remain largely unaffected (Schmiedt et al., 2002; Wang et al., 2006). Pyridoxine intoxication induces auditory nerve fiber loss as well in mice in a dose-dependent manner. OAEs are preserved, while the ABR shows delayed latencies (Hong et al., 2009). Another method of lesion of the auditory nerve fibers has been achieved by compression of the auditory nerve. This technique induces a profound degeneration of the auditory nerve while preserving wave I in spite of significant depression of wave II and the following waves. IHCs and OHCs are almost completely preserved. A profound deterioration of the ABR is observed, while DPOAEs and CM are preserved (Matsumoto et al., 2008; Sekiya et al., 2000). Another animal model of ANSD is the sulfonamide-injected jj Gunn rat pup. Animals show abnormal spiral ganglion cells and selective loss of large, myelinated auditory nerve fibers with no abnormalities in cochlear hair cells (Shaia et al., 2005). Bilirubin neurotoxicity can specifically affect spiral ganglion neurons and their axons in the peripheral auditory nerve. Spiral ganglion neuron dendrites that innervate the cochlear hair cells might also be involved and the electrophysiology (ABR, CAP, and CM) is suggestive of ANSD.

Other animal models of ANSD now include mice that are genetically engineered to show defects affecting IHCs, synapses, or auditory nerve function. These models provide an opportunity to study how specific genes alter various aspects of auditory function (see Starr et al., 2008 for a review). The primary mechanisms result in defective IHC channelopathy, pre- and postsynaptic active zones, IHC vesicle fusion, IHC transmitter release, mislocalization of ion channels at initial axon segments and nodes of Ranvier, and axon/spiral ganglion neuron loss.

UNDERSTANDING ANSD THROUGH PHYSIOLOGIC AND PSYCHOACOUSTIC APPROACHES

Auditory Cortical Responses in ANSD

Cortical auditory evoked potentials (CAEPs) are inconsistently observed in patients with ANSD and are consistent with findings that, despite an absent ABR, some patients demonstrate some limited speech perception ability. Berlin et al. (1994) reported absent middle latency responses (MLR) and present N1-P2 CAEPs in a patient with ANSD related to Charcot-Marie-Tooth disease. Starr et al. (1996) found present MLRs in one of six patients but observed no MLRs on later evaluation of this patient. Long latency responses (LLRs) (N1-P2 and P300) were observed in one of six patients and abnormal N1-P2 responses in another patient in this group of primarily adult patients aged 15 to 49 years. However, responses were reported as small, and often slightly later than normal. Kraus et al. (2000) reported a case study of a 24-year-old female with ANSD who displayed P1/N1/P2 responses to synthetic syllables that were normal for one syllable and delayed for another stimulus syllable. Mismatch negativity (MMN) responses were normal when elicited to stimuli differing in formant duration but absent in response to stimuli differing in formant onset frequency. Results were consistent with behavioral perception on discrimination tasks.

We have recorded MLRs using click stimuli in 14 ANSD patients and found normal responses in one patient. In contrast, LLRs (N1-P2), obtained using long duration tonal stimuli, were present in 8 of 10 patients, although many of these patients demonstrated no speech recognition ability. This finding is generally consistent with Rance et al. (2002), who report present LLRs particularly in patients with residual speech recognition ability. LLRs, and perhaps particularly discriminatory responses such as P300 or MMN, may hold value in understanding speech processing ability in ANSD patients (Kraus et al., 2000; Rance et al., 2002). Given the wide variation in auditory perception ability observed in ANSD patients, evaluation is needed across a wide range of patients, across various well-controlled stimuli, and in the context of other functional measures.

CAEPs are valuable in characterizing detection as well as discrimination of speech signals and also as objective measures of processing of various dimensions of sound. Applications in ANSD should be useful in understanding some of the variants of ANSD, in management planning, and in basic understanding of the nature of various evoked potentials. Although CAEPs are not typically included in the audiologic test battery in clinical settings, their use may increase as we strive to understand the nature of various forms of ANSD, evaluate benefit from traditional amplification, determine candidacy for cochlear implantation in infants and young children, and define psychophysical discrimination where behavioral testing cannot be completed.

CAEPs have been used to assess performance with amplification and to make comparisons between children with ANSD and SNHL. Rance et al. (2002) measured aided and unaided performance on open-set word identification in quiet and compared those results to LLRs (P1, N1, P2) to tones and speech. Although all children in the SNHL group demonstrated a significant improvement in speech perception in the aided condition, only half of the ANSD subjects exhibited performance gains with amplification. The subjects who failed to show benefit from hearing aids also exhibited the poorest word recognition scores and absent LLRs. Contrary to Rance's finding, Kumar and Jayaram (2005) did not find any correlation between the parameters of the LLRs and the speech perception scores, but observed that many of their subjects who showed normal MMN could not discriminate the contrast of the stimuli behaviorally. In another study of older children and adults with ANSD, average N1-P2 amplitude of good performers was significantly higher than that of poor performers (Narne & Vanaja, 2008), whereas there was no relationship

between pure tone thresholds and speech identification scores. Variation is again expected, possibly related to etiology and underlying mechanisms, as patients with good LLRs but no word recognition ability also have been reported (Hood, 1999; Starr et al., 1996).

Auditory LLRs may also be helpful in characterizing psychophysical responses in individuals with ANSD. Measures of gap detection via LLRs provide neurophysiologic evidence of alterations in temporal processing in ANSD patients (Michalewski et al., 2005). In this study, N1 LLRs were significantly delayed in the majority of individuals in the ANSD group relative to controls and were absent at all gap durations tested in some ANSD subjects.

Insights from Psychoacoustic Studies

Studies utilizing psychophysical tasks to explore temporal, frequency and intensity processing provide insight into the aspects of auditory signals that are affected by ANSD and how speech understanding is impacted. Psychoacoustic studies from Zeng et al. (1999, 2001) indicate that ANSD patients have particular difficulty with the timing (temporal) characteristics of sound. Psychophysical studies of children and adults with ANSD have identified significant differences in temporal processing (gap detection, temporal modulation) and, to a lesser extent, frequency discrimination (for lower frequencies) for patients with ANSD versus SNHL (Rance et al., 2004; Zeng et al., 1999). Findings in patients with ANSD are generally different from patients with SNHL. For example, Rance et al. noted that children with SNHL have normal temporal modulation detection ability and less difficulty with frequency discrimination, but reduced frequency resolution abilities, which are normal in ANSD subjects. This timing deficit is consistent with a lack of neural synchrony and Kraus et al. (2000) present an interesting case discussion of evidence for neural asynchrony. This, coupled with a role of the nervous system in marking the onset of stimuli, following changes in signals, and preserving timing information, underscores the difficulties that patients with desynchronized neural responses may experience in understanding speech.

Rance and colleagues (2004) also reported a positive relationship between modulation detection thresholds and speech recognition ability. To further illustrate the link between temporal processing ability and speech understanding, Zeng and colleagues (1999) used temporal modulation functions derived from the responses of ANSD subjects to simulate ANSD-type hearing loss in normal hearing adults. Simulated hearing loss produced poorer speech recognition scores and elevated gap detection thresholds, which resembled those of ANSD subjects.

VARIATION AMONG PATIENTS WITH ANSD

As noted in previous sections, the classification of ANSD may include several different possible sites of abnormality, all of which result in the clinical observation of present cochlear OHC responses accompanied by poor neural responses. ANSD varies in a number of factors including age of onset, presence or absence of neurologic abnormalities, putative etiology, changes over time, and unilateral versus bilateral involvement. Furthermore, some patients, including infants, children and adults, have no known risk factors or associated neurologic disorders.

A Continuum of ANSD

Berlin et al. (2001, 2010) describe a continuum along which these patients distribute in relation to their functional communication ability. There are a few patients at one extreme who exhibit no overt delays or auditory complaints until adulthood, or until they are first evaluated with MEMRs or ABR. They are the patients who generally demonstrate the greatest residual speech recognition ability in quiet, though they report difficulty in noise. These patients would most likely be good candidates for FM technology as they generally report a considerable increase in listening difficulty in noisy situations.

At the other extreme are the ANSD patients who exhibit a total lack of sound awareness. Between these two groups is the largest group of patients we have seen. These patients demonstrate inconsistent auditory responses, and manage the best in quiet and the

poorest in noise. Their audiograms are in-consistent with other test results. The ABR is always desynchronized and MEMRs are absent. Visual phonetic language usually works best until cochlear implantation, unless the family prefers cultural Deafness.

Variation in Speech Recognition Characteristics

Speech recognition in ANSD patients is typically poorer than expected based on pure tone thresholds (Starr et al., 1996; Zeng et al, 1999), but performance varies widely across individuals. As noted earlier, some patients with normal or near-normal hearing thresholds for pure tone stimuli will exhibit reduced speech recognition ability in quiet and in noise. Others display some understanding of speech in quiet but considerable difficulty in noisy listening conditions. And yet another small group of patients are able to function quite well in quiet and, despite greater than expected difficulty in noise, are able to develop speech and language and good communication function.

Examination of specific word recognition scores shows that some ANSD patients demonstrate word recognition ability in quiet similar to subjects with SNHL while word recognition ability in noise for ANSD patients is below what is expected in SNHL (Berlin et al., 2010). These findings are consistent with other studies (e.g., Rance et al., 2007; Starr et al., 1996). This widely varying ability presents a particular challenge in both understanding ANSD and planning appropriate management.

Association with Other Neurologic Abnormalities

Patients with ANSD vary in demonstration of other peripheral neuropathies. Although some patients have no evidence of neurologic abnormalities, others have neurologic disorders affecting other nonauditory neural systems. Other patients have less apparent nonauditory neuropathies, which are only evident on clinical examination and still other patients demonstrate no signs of nonauditory neuropathy. In many cases, the primary complaint of patients in the latter two groups is difficulty in understanding speech, particularly in noise.

As noted in an earlier section, several neurological problems are identified in patients with ANSD, including HMSN, Charcot-Marie-Tooth disease, Friedreich ataxia, Mohr-Tranebjaerg syndrome, gait ataxia, loss of deep tendon reflexes, or motor system disturbances (Berlin et al., 2010; Butinar et al., 1999; Starr et al., 1996). Not all instances of these disorders include auditory problems; for example, it is possible to have HMSN or Friedreich ataxia affect the motor neural system without accompanying sensory problems involving the auditory system. When the auditory system is affected, characteristics such as absent or highly abnormal ABRs with preserved OAEs provide evidence consistent with ANSD. As with ANSD from other sources, broad variation in auditory characteristics such as speech understanding exist, perhaps related to underlying genetic characteristics as well as the stage of progress of the disease. HMSN generally has an onset in teenage and young adult years whereas Friedreich ataxia may have an earlier onset.

Onset of various characteristics may vary. For example, in a patient with Mohr-Tranebjaerg syndrome (deafness and dystonia), the hearing loss started at age 4 years, blindness and dystonia developed in his fifties and sixties, and the spiral ganglion fibers degenerated while the organ of Corti and presumably the OAEs and CMs remained normal (Merchant et al., 2001). Although ANSD may occur as part of or in conjunction with various neurological disorders, it is important to note that not all patients with such disorders have auditory problems.

Unilateral ANSD

Although most cases of ANSD identified to date are bilateral though often asymmetric, a few patients have unilateral ANSD where the pattern of test results is consistent with ANSD only in one ear. Auditory function in the other ear ranges from normal hearing to varying degrees of cochlear hearing losses with ABR, MEMR and OAE results consistent with behavioral results, patient complaint and history, and other aspects of auditory status. Functionally, patients with unilateral ANSD appear to have some of the same listening difficulties as patients with other types of unilateral hearing loss. The

increasing use of imaging is currently revealing that bilateral or unilateral absent or deficient auditory nerves is not uncommon among patients with ANSD (Buchman et al., 2006; Morlet, unpublished data).

Stability and Changes Over Time

Progressive worsening of hearing ability is observed in some patients, though it is not characteristic of all patients. This may involve factors such as loss of OAEs and CM over time in infants as well as progressive decreases in speech recognition and/or hearing sensitivity. Other patients demonstrate stable physiologic responses and behavioral audiometric thresholds over many years. In some cases ANSD is associated with fluctuating hearing. As described earlier, Starr et al. (1998) reported a patient with temperature-sensitive ANSD, where symptoms only occur with elevation of body temperature and auditory function is normal between periods of increased temperature. Gorga et al. (1995) reported another patient with fluctuations in hearing sensitivity that was felt to be related to an autoimmune disorder, where OAEs remained intact while the ABR was affected.

ANSD and Loss of OHC Function

Although ANSD is defined as a disorder of the IHC, their synapses and/or the auditory nerve in the presence of normal OHC function, there is now evidence that some types of ANSD may also involve loss of OHC function. First, although the preservation of OAEs and CM in cases of ANSD has been considered evidence that cochlear OHC function is normal in this disorder, CM in ANSD is especially prominent and persists several milliseconds after a transient click stimulus, may suggest some type of OHC dysfunction. Secondly, the disorder appears to be progressive in a significant number of patients, which is shown by abnormal OAEs, a loss of OAEs over time, a progression in the extent of hearing loss, or development of peripheral neuropathy (Deltenre et al., 1999; Kovach et al., 2002; Starr et al., 2000, 2001). The fact that a significant number of infants are diagnosed with ANSD in the absence of recordable OAEs does not naturally signify that OHC dysfunction is due to ANSD. Many risk factors independent of ANSD can impair OHC function.

Question 2

Why do you think some children with ANSD do well with cochlear implants?

Answer 2

As we have noted in our discussion, the vast majority of the children we have seen and who have obtained cochlear implants have done well with cochlear implants. Although persons with ANSD who have received cochlear implants likely have varying underlying mechanisms, those with conditions that affect the inner hair cells and/or synaptic junction, leaving the auditory neural connections intact, might be expected to perform the best. Future research will likely be able to tell us whether or not this is correct. Certainly, those whose imaging shows compromise of the eighth nerve, such as cochlear nerve agenesis, would be expected to be among the poorest performers with a CI, despite their clinical picture being consistent with ANSD (e.g., Teagle et al., 2010). Aside from the underlying anatomy, physiology, and mechanisms, there are a number of other factors that contribute to success with cochlear implants in individuals with various forms of hearing loss. We would anticipate that the same factors, such as parental support, educational setting, communication mode, etc. would contribute to success among ANSD patients.

ANSD AND NEWBORN HEARING SCREENING

Since the description of ANSD (Starr et al., 1996), and as a result of the rising number of universal newborn hearing screening programs being implemented around the globe, the number of newborns diagnosed with ANSD is continually increasing. The growing population of infants diagnosed with ANSD also has underscored the heterogeneity of this population. Numerous etiologies (hereditary, infectious, and metabolic) and potential risk factors (hypoxia, hyperbilirubinemia, among others) have been identified. Still, at least half of the patients cannot be assigned an etiology and do not seem to present any concomitant disorders. Despite progress in newborn hearing screening programs and techniques, many infants with ANSD remain undiagnosed when screened in an OAE-based screening program that does not include an ABR. OAE-based programs cannot specifically target ANSD and only infants with abnormal or absent OAEs may receive a proper diagnosis once an ABR recorded with both condensation and rarefaction polarities is performed after failing the OAE test.

Risk Factors in ANSD

As early as 2000, Starr et al. estimated that about 40% of cases of ANSD are due to genetic causes. Toxic-metabolic (anoxia, hyperbilirubinemia), immunological (drug reaction, demyelination), and infectious disease (postviral) account for about 10%, and the rest of the patients appear to have no defined etiology. Recent reports on larger samples of individuals diagnosed with ANSD have been increasing the number of risk factors and associated disorders, and are unraveling more varieties of ANSD (Berlin et al., 2010; Beutner et al., 2007; Xoinis et al., 2007).

Several groups of causes for ANSD can be defined.

Neonatal Causes

Several risk factors have been associated with ANSD, although a direct link between ANSD and a specific factor or a group of factors cannot always be established with certainty. The current list of risk factors includes: history of prematurity, low birth weight, hyperbilirubinemia, anoxia, hypoxia, previous meningitis, ototoxic drug exposure, cerebral palsy, intracranial hemorrhage, sepsis, traumatic brain injury, ischemia, central nervous system immaturity, and infection (mumps) alone or in combination (Amatuzzi et al., 2001; Attias & Raveh, 2007; Berlin et al., 2010; Beutner et al., 2007; Dowley et al., 2009; Madden et al., 2002; Rance et al., 1999; Raveh et al., 2007; Sheykholesami & Kaga, 2000;).

One of the main risk factors, hyperbilirubinemia, has been found to cause severe degeneration of spiral ganglion neurons and a paucity of myelinated axons in a jaundiced Gunn rat model compared with a nonjaundiced model (Conlee & Shapiro, 1991; Shaia et al., 2005). The anatomic changes observed in the auditory system, although small, were statistically significant, and their distribution corresponded to the location of generators of the ABR components shown to be abnormal in the same animals. In the Gunn rats, it is unlikely that gross alterations of CM occur in acute bilirubin toxicity, as ABR changes can appear without CM changes. In humans, bilirubin has been found to cause lesions in the CNS, including the brainstem auditory nuclei. These lesions often occur in the cochlear nucleus, trapezoid body, superior olive, lateral lemniscus, inferior colliculus, and medial geniculate (Shapiro & Teselle, 1994). As early as 1979, Chisin et al. found absent ABRs in 11 of 13 neonates presenting with hyperbilirubinemia, but a CM was observed in 9 out of 13, suggesting hearing loss with functioning hair cells and absent neural responses.

Another risk factor is hypoxia. The IHC/cochlear afferent system seems to be primarily affected in mild, chronic hypoxia whereas OHCs seem to be relatively unaffected (Sawada et al., 2001). It is clear that in certain types of cochlear insults (carboplatin treatment, for example, in chinchillas at least) the IHCs are more vulnerable than the OHCs.

Hereditary Causes

As described earlier, several genetic causes related to ANSD have been discovered in recent years (Bette et al., 2007; Ceranic & Luxon, 2004; Corley and Crabbe, 1999; Forli et al, 2006; Jutras et al., 2003; Merchant et al, 2001; Rodriguez-Ballesteros et al., 2003; Rodriguez-Ballesteros et al., 2008; Starr et al., 1996; Varga et al., 2003; Yasunaga et al., 1999). These include *OTOF* mutations, hereditary sensorimotor neuropathies (Charcot-Marie-Tooth disease; Waar-

denburg type 2 syndrome; Leber's hereditary optic neuropathy; autosomal dominant optic atrophy), and mitochondrial defects.

Inner Ear Abnormalities

Several cases of ANSD in children who present with enlarged vestibular aqueduct (EVA) have been reported (Ahmmed et al., 2008; Morlet et al., 2008). EVA is the most common radiological abnormality seen in children with SNHL. EVA can be associated with other congenital ear anomalies, such as a hypoplastic cochlea. Onset of SNHL may occur from birth to adolescence, usually during childhood, and may be precipitated by various factors such as head trauma. Hearing loss is often progressive and can fluctuate. Children with an EVA present with a wide variety of audiometric thresholds and physiologic measurement, and may present with the clinical characteristics of ANSD.

Immunologic Causes

Guillain-Barre syndrome is an inflammatory demyelinating polyneuropathy, an autoimmune disorder affecting the peripheral nervous system, usually triggered by an acute infectious process and can cause ANSD (Kowalski et al., 1991; Nelson et al., 1988; Wong, 2007).

Miscellaneous Causes

Other factors leading to ANSD have been mentioned in the literature, such as a case report of a newborn with ANSD presumably caused by a cerebellopontine angle arachnoid cyst (Boudewyns et al., 2008). Not all risk factors have been confirmed as a direct cause of ANSD. It is important to note that the risk factors discussed in this chapter may occur without leading to hearing loss and may occur in newborns with normal hearing as well as those diagnosed with SNHL rather than ANSD (Berg et al., 2005). In addition, not all children with ANSD have known associated pathologies or risk factors (Raveh et al., 2007). Clearly more research is needed in this area, as other risk factors leading to a diagnosis of ANSD have yet to be discovered.

Diagnosis of ANSD in Newborns

To detect ANSD as well as other hearing pathologies, the current consensus is that all newborns should be screened using both ABR and OAEs. A protocol of both OAE and ABR testing in a dual-testing paradigm is more specific than testing with either ABR or OAEs alone (Joint Committee on Infant Hearing, 2007). With the widespread implementation of newborn hearing screening programs using this dual-testing paradigm, early diagnosis of ANSD is becoming more and more frequent. A two-stage measurement of automated-ABR alone for newborn hearing screening is also a possibility as it has a lower referral rate and a lower false positive rate (Iwasaki, 2003). Some also support the use of conventional ABR for screening high-risk neonates, as it seems to provide more reliable results (Suppiej et al., 2007). Alternatively, a dual system combining wideband-MEMR/OAEs might prove to be useful, although further studies to assess its potential value are necessary (Keefe et al., 2010).

Outgrowing ANSD

Several reports indicate that some infants with an initial diagnosis of ANSD appear to resolve over time based on their follow-up ABR testing. They are effectively "outgrowing" the initial diagnosis. Psarommatis et al. (2006) found that 13 (65%) out of 20 of children suffering from ANSD demonstrated ABR recovery on re-examination. In 12 cases, a complete ABR recovery was observed with a clear and reproducible waveform at 40 dB nHL bilaterally, whereas one infant showed ABR threshold restoration to 50 dB nHL bilaterally. Madden et al. (2002) observed improvement over time as well in 9 out of 18 pediatric patients. Interestingly, the behavioral thresholds in these cases improved, but not the ABR.

Children with jaundice were more likely to improve with time. Four cases of newborns/infants initially diagnosed with ANSD that later resolved were reported by Attias and Raveh (2007) and two other similar cases were reported by Dowley et al. (2009). Raveh et al. (2007) reported four patients who showed spontaneous improvement by age 8 months, including two with a history of hyper-

bilirubinemia, three born prematurely, and one conceived by in vitro fertilization. In Dowley et al. (2009), two patients with ANSD showed evidence of auditory maturation, one at 10 months (who was born at 37 weeks and later developed kernicterus and cerebral palsy) and the other at seven months, born at 29 weeks (who later developed hypoxia, intraventricular hemorrhage, sepsis, and chronic lung disease). The prevalence of children outgrowing ANSD is not yet precisely known. Aside from children with hyperbilirubinemia who seemed to have a better chance of showing some improvement during the first year of life, it remains unclear when and if recovery from ANSD might occur.

An ANSD diagnosis in newborns, including those with and without risk factors, is likely to increase in the future. As mortality rates for low birth weight and premature infants declines, it will likely lead to an enhancement in the adverse neurological consequences in the surviving neonates. The goal of Universal Newborn Hearing Screening is to begin rehabilitation as soon as possible. However, the developmental consequences of ANSD cannot be predicted on the basis of test results obtained in infants. The known variation of ANSD raises important issues related to management in infants, such as use of amplification, as discussed below.

DISTINGUISHING ANSD FROM CENTRAL AUDITORY PROCESSING DISORDER

Similarities in Presentation

About 5% of children diagnosed with ANSD will be able to develop language normally and will start speaking within 12 to 18 months (Berlin et al., 2010), despite their abnormal ABR results. Many will show normal hearing in quiet environments but will have difficulty understanding speech in the presence of background noise. These children can often be misdiagnosed as having a (central) auditory processing disorder (APD).

A hallmark of an APD is a child who exhibits the ability to detect a pure tone in a soundproof booth, but fails to hear well in the presence of competing speech or background noise (e.g., Bamiou et al., 2001; Bellis, 1996; Chermak et al., 1999, 2002; Muchnik et al., 2004). Interestingly, some children with ANSD exhibit hearing behavior similar to children with APD, in that there is somewhat appropriate development of speech and language, normal understanding of speech in quiet, but difficulty understanding speech in noisy environments. Therefore, both categories of children will present with a normal pure tone audiogram, normal OAEs and similar speech discrimination scores in quiet and in noise.

As stated earlier, the MMN, auditory LLPs (P1/N1, P2/N2) and LLP components evoked with speech stimuli can be recorded in numerous patients with ANSD (Kumar & Jayaram, 2005; Michalewski et al., 2005; Narne & Vanaja, 2008; Rance et al., 2002;). Interestingly, when present, these evoked potentials show latencies and amplitudes that can be prolonged and smaller, respectively (Narne & Vanaja, 2008). They can also even be similar to those of normal-hearing children (Kumar & Jayaram, 2005; Rance et al., 2002). Hence, when present, these LLPs might not significantly differ between ANSD and APD.

As some children with APD present with deficits related to auditory percepts dependent on temporal cues, it is likely that some of them will share the same abnormally low scores as children with ANSD for tasks assessing temporal resolution, temporal masking, temporal integration, temporal ordering gap detection, backward and forward masking, as well as for auditory performance with competing acoustic signals and detection of degraded acoustic signals.

Overall psychoacoustic testing revealed that in ANSD the auditory cortex might be able to adjust to the faulty signal representations present at earlier stages along the auditory pathway which can mimic APD in some instances.

Differences Between ANSD and APD

An APD may be broadly defined as a deficit in the processing of information that is specific to the auditory modality, despite normal pure tone hearing sensitivity (Jerger & Musiek, 2000). APDs may manifest as a deficit in sound localization, discrimination, pattern recognition, temporal processing, and poor per-formance in the presence of competing or degraded acoustic signals (ASHA, 1996). Approximately 5% of school-age children have some type of APD (Musiek et al., 1990). APDs are often associated with other listening and learning deficits, such as specific language impairment and dyslexia. APDs may also be associated with the presence of neurological conditions in a few cases (such as tumors), delayed maturation of the central auditory pathways, and developmental abnormalities (Bamiou et al., 2001).

Although the two disorders share the above-mentioned characteristics, there are differences that can be determined through audiologic testing. Children with ANSD will present with absent MEMRs (in rare cases, MEMRs can be present but elevated) and absent or abnormal ABR waveforms, whereas children with an APD typically have normal MEMR thresholds and normal ABRs to a click stimulus. It is therefore important initially to include MEMR testing for all children suspected of having an APD. If MEMRs are absent or elevated, an ABR recorded with both click polarities to rule out ANSD will then be necessary to determine which type of hearing disorder the child has.

Most children diagnosed with ANSD are not able to develop speech and language without specific intervention. It is important that this diagnosis made as early as possible. However, numerous newborn screening programs continue to be strictly OAE-based (this is mostly the case in well-baby units). This means that such children who actually have ANSD will not be flagged for follow-up by newborn screening because they still have present OAE function and will pass the OAE testing. Their hearing disorder may not be discovered until much later, when parental concern about the lack or delay in speech development surfaces.

These children will at least be referred for further testing once it has become apparent to the parents and/or pediatrician that there is a hearing problem. However, children who do not show major delays in the first few years of life may be completely missed. Some of them will later be inappropriately diagnosed with an APD (or other type of learning disability) if a hearing evaluation includes only the pure tone audiogram, word recognition in quiet, tympanometry, and OAE measures. This is why a preaudiometric triage including tympanometry,

MEMRs, and OAEs is strongly recommended for all children seen in consultation for the first time (Berlin et al., 2003a).

IMPLICATIONS FOR MANAGEMENT OF PERSONS WITH ANSD

Variation in clinical presentation across individuals with ANSD impacts the effectiveness of various management approaches. Individual management approaches are needed along with the ability to tailor and refine these approaches based on changes in an individual's characteristics and needs. Although some patients demonstrate benefit from amplification, the majority of patients with ANSD have not shown benefit sufficient to support speech and language development or auditory communication through the use of amplification alone.

Audibility varies widely among ANSD patients and this translates to broad variation in the need for and utility of amplification. Challenges exist in determining audibility in young infants since reliable behavioral testing is difficult and clinicians typically rely on ABR data, which is not obtainable in infants with characteristics consistent with ANSD. In infants with ANSD, management may be based on behavioral responses and parental reports of functional abilities. A hearing aid trial is often recommended and the child's responsiveness to sound and speech is closely monitored to estimate benefit from the amplification. A dilemma exists in that the use of amplification may damage functioning OHCs and result in additional changes in function that were not present at the time of the original diagnosis. The broad benefits of hearing aids to develop proper speech and language are unclear for children with ANSD, since not only are they providing amplification to a system that may not require it, they may be amplifying sounds that remain unclear and meaningless to the child. Despite the lack of clear information or guidelines, the general practices at present attempt to provide audible signals in those with ANSD who display poor sound awareness or reduced audibility. Benefit in the form and communication development in children is regularly assessed.

Use of an FM system (alone or with other devices) can be helpful to persons with ANSD in noisy settings such as a classroom, car, restaurant, and so forth. Providing a clearer signal to an auditory system that cannot cope with interference, as in ANSD, can be particularly helpful in those patients with some residual word recognition in quiet (Hood et al., 2004). Visual information through communication systems, such as cued speech or sign language, facilitate language development in infants and children, and captioning and other visual cues are useful in children and adults (Berlin et al., 2002). Other techniques such as clear speech (Zeng & Liu, 2006) and envelope enhancement (Narne & Vanaja, 2009) show some promise in improving word recognition.

Both children and adults with ANSD demonstrate improved speech perception and significant benefit from cochlear implants (Peterson et al., 2003; Shallop et al., 2001; Trautwein et al., 2000; Zeng & Liu, 2006). Improvement is observed related to sensitivity, speech perception in quiet and in noise, as well as evidence of synchronous neural responses in EABRs and neural response telemetry. As might be expected, more favorable speech perception scores post cochlear implantation are reported for ANSD subjects with normal cochlear nerves as compared to those with cochlear nerve anomalies (Buchman et al., 2006; Walton et al., 2008).

Also, as described earlier, some infants may show maturational changes and/or complete or partial recovery from ANSD during the first months of life. Based on this, amplification in high-risk infants, especially those with low birth weight, may be carefully considered with fitting only after at least 6 months of age, as any maturation that may occur is still in progress. After that time period, amplification may be useful but should be monitored closely since many infants with ANSD do not benefit from the use of hearing aids as the sole method to support speech and language development.

Collaboration with speech-language pathologists, otolaryngologists, neurologists, other physicians and health care professionals, as well as early interventionists and teachers of the deaf, is of great value to the patients and their families. Although the audiologist is likely to be one of the first professionals to encounter a patient with ANSD, management should focus on the global communication skills and abilities of the patient necessary to acquire language, become literate and be self-sufficient.

Some Challenges

The observed variation among patients underscores the importance of developing information and methods that will allow clinicians to accurately distinguish among the various forms of ANSD. Progress in this area will likely include additional discoveries in genetics, improved sensitivity of physiologic responses, further exploration of psychophysical tasks, particularly those related to temporal resolution, and auditory LLRs may provide insight into underlying mechanisms and functional abilities. One hopes that future research and clinical assessment will see greater utilization of novel stimuli and paradigms, more sensitive approaches, and development of clinically feasible methods that include these advances. Even within various forms of ANSD, we expect that variation will exist and we will need to understand the range of variation and contributing factors.

Advances in understanding various forms of ANSD should guide us toward a better understanding of those characteristics that may derive benefit from amplification, versus cochlear implants, versus those in need of little intervention. Guidelines and protocols for determination of need for and success with hearing aids, FM systems, and cochlear implants are needed, as well as the ability to predict who will develop speech/language with minimal intervention despite poor neural synchrony. Patient and parent education is critical as we learn more about ANSD and use our knowledge to guide our patients and their families in making informed decisions.

Acknowledgments. Research at Kresge Hearing Research Laboratory in New Orleans was supported by the NIH National Institute on Deafness and Other Communication Disorders (NIDCD), Oberkotter Foundation, Deafness Research Foundation, American Hearing Research Foundation, National Organization for Hearing Research, Marriott Foundation, Kam's Fund for Hearing Research, and the Louisiana Lions Eye Foundation.

The following colleagues at Kresge Hearing Research Laboratory and the Audiology Clinic, Department of Otolaryngology, Louisiana State University Health Sciences Center, New Orleans, have contributed to our research on auditory neuropathy/dys-synchrony: Charles I. Berlin, PhD, Harriet Berlin, MA, Jill Bordelon, MCD, Shanda Brashears Morlet, AuD, Leah Goforth-Barter, MS, Annette Hurley-Larmeau, PhD, Jennifer Jeanfreau-Taylor, MCD, Bronya Keats, PhD, Elizabeth Montgomery, MS, Kelly Rose-Mattingly, MA, Patti St. John, MCD, Sonya Tedesco, MCD, Melanie Thibodeaux, MCD, Han Wen, MSBE, and Diane Wilensky, MA.

FURTHER READINGS

Berlin, C. I., Hood, L. J., Morlet, T., Wilensky, D., Li, L., Rose-Mattingly, K., . . . Frisch, S.A. (2010). Multi-site diagnosis and management of 260 patients with Auditory Neuropathy/Dys-synchrony (Auditory Neuropathy Spectrum Disorder). *International Journal of Audiology, 49*, 30–43.

Rance, G., McKay, C., & Grayden, D. (2004). Perceptual characterization of children with auditory neuropathy. *Ear Hearing, 25*, 34–46.

Santarelli, R., Starr, A., Michalewski, H. J., & Arslan, E. (2008). Neural and receptor cochlear potentials obtained by transtympanic electrocochleography in auditory neuropathy. *Clinical Neurophysiology, 119*, 1028–1041.

Starr, A., Zeng, F. G., Michalewski, H. J., & Moser, T. (2008). Perspectives on auditory neuropathy: Disorders of inner hair cell, auditory nerve, and their synapse. In A. I. Basbaum, A. Kaneko, G. M. Shepherd, & G. Westheimer (Eds.), *The senses: A comprehensive reference, Vol 3, Audition* (pp. 397–412). P. Dallos & D. Oertel (Eds.). San Diego, CA: Academic Press.

Zeng, F. G., Kong, Y. Y., Michalewski, H. J., & Starr, A. (2005). Perceptual consequences of disrupted auditory nerve activity. *Journal of Neurophysiology, 93*, 3060–3063.

REFERENCES

Abdala, C., Sininger, Y. S., & Starr, A. (2000). Distortion product otoacoustic emission suppression in subjects with auditory neuropathy. *Ear and Hearing, 21*, 542–553.

Ahmmed A., Brockbank C., & Adshead J. (2008). Cochlear microphonics in sensorineural hearing loss: Lesson from newborn hearing screening. *International Journal of Pediatric Otorhinolaryngology, 72*, 1281–1285.

Amantini A., Rossi L., De Scisciolo G., Bindi A., Pagnini P., & Zappoli R. (1984). Auditory evoked potentials (early, middle, late components) and audiological tests in Friedreich's ataxia. *Electroencephalography and Clinical Neurophysiology, 58*, 37–47.

Amati-Bonneau P., Guichet A., Olichon A., Chevrollier A., Viala F., Miot S., . . . Reynier P. (2005). OPA1 R445H mutation in optic atrophy associated with sernsorineural deafness. *Annals of Neurology, 58*, 958–963.

Amatuzzi, M. G., Northrop, C., Liberman, M. C., Thornton, A., Halpin, C., Herrmann, B., . . . Eavey, R. D. (2001). Selective inner hair cell loss in premature infants and cochlea pathological patterns from neonatal intensive care unit autopsies. *Archives of Otolaryngology-Head and Neck Surgery, 127*, 629–636.

American Speech and Language Hearing Association. (1996). Central auditory processing: Current status of research and implications for clinical practice. *American Journal of Audiology, 5*, 41–54.

Aran, J.-M., & de Sauvage, R. C. (1976). Clinical value of cochlear microphonic recordings. In R. J. Ruben, C. Elberlin, & G. Salomon (Eds.), *Electrocochleography* (pp. 55–65). Baltimore, MD: University Park Press.

Attias, J., Buller, N., Rubel, Y., & Raveh, E. (2006). Multiple auditory steady-state responses in children and adults with normal hearing, sensorineural hearing loss, or auditory neuropathy. *Annals of Otology, Rhinology, and Laryngology, 115*, 268–276.

Attias, J., & Raveh, E. (2007). Transient deafness in young candidates for cochlear implants. *Audiology and Neurotology, 12*, 325–333.

Bahmad, F., Merchant, S. N., Nado, J. B., & Tranebjærg, L. (2007). Otopathology in Mohr-Tranebjærg syndrome. *Laryngoscope, 117*, 1202–1208.

Bahr, M., Andres, F., Timmerman, V., Nelis, M. E., Van Brockhoven, C., & Dichgans, J. (1999). Central visual, acoustic, and motor pathway involvement in a Charcot-Marie-Tooth family with an Asn205Ser mutation in the connexin 32 gene. *Journal of Neurology, Neurosurgery, and Psychiatry, 66*, 202–206.

Balatsouras, D. G., Kaberos, A., Assimakopoulos, D., Katotomichelakis, M., Economou, N. C., & Korress, S. G. (2007). Etiology of vertigo in children. *International Journal of Pediatric Otorhinolaryngology, 71*, 487–494.

Bamiou, D. E., Musiek, F. E., & Luxon, L. M. (2001). Aetiology and clinical presentations of auditory processing disorders—a review. *Archives of Disease in Childhood, 85*, 361–365.

Bellis, T. R. (1996). *Assessment and management of central auditory processing disorders in the educational settings.* San Diego, CA: Singular.

Berg, A. L., Spitzer, S. B., Towers, H. M., Bartosiewicz, C., & Diamond, B. E. (2005). Newborn hearing screening in the NICU: Profile of failed auditory brainstem response/passed otoacoustic emission. *Pediatrics, 116*, 933–938.

Berlin, C. I., Bordelon, J., St. John, P., Wilensky, D., Hurley, A., Kluka, E., & Hood, L. J. (1998). Reversing click polarity may uncover auditory neuropathy in infants. *Ear and Hearing, 19*, 37–47.

Berlin, C. I., Hood, L. J., Cecola, R. P., Jackson, D. F., & Szabo P. (1993). Does Type I afferent neuron dysfunction reveal itself through lack of efferent suppression? *Hearing Research, 65*, 40–50.

Berlin, C. I., Hood, L. J., Hurley, A., & Wen, H. (1994). Contralateral suppression of otoacoustic emissions: An index of the function of the medial olivocochlear system. *Otolaryngology-Head and Neck Surgery, 100*, 3–21.

Berlin, C. I., Hood, L. J., Hurley, A., Wen, H., & Kemp, D. T. (1995). Bilateral noise suppresses click-evoked otoacoustic emissions more than ipsilateral or contralateral noise. *Hearing Research, 87*, 96–103.

Berlin, C. I., Hood, L. J., Morlet, T., Den, Z., Goforth, L., Tedesco, S., . . . Keats, B. (2000). The search for auditory neuropathy patients and connexin 26 patients in schools for the Deaf. *ARO Abstracts, 23*, 23.

Berlin, C. I., Hood, L. J., Morlet, T., Li, L., Brashears, S., Tedesco, S., Rose, K., . . . Keats, B. J. B. (2003a). Auditory neuropathy/dys-synchrony (AN/AD): Management and results in 193 patients. *ARO Abstracts, 26*, 191.

Berlin, C. I., Hood, L. J., Morlet, T., Wilensky, D., Li, L., Rose-Mattingly, K., . . . Frisch, S. A. (2010). Multi-site diagnosis and management of 260 patients with Auditory Neuropathy/Dys-synchrony (Auditory Neuropathy Spectrum Disorder). *International Journal of Audiology, 49*, 30–43.

Berlin, C. I., Hood, L. J., Morlet, T., Wilensky, D., St. John, P., Montgomery, E., & Thibodeaux, M. (2005). Absent or elevated middle ear muscle reflexes in the presence of normal otoacoustic emissions: A universal finding in 136 cases of auditory neuropathy/dys-synchrony. *Journal of the American Academy of Audiology, 16*, 546–553.

Berlin, C., Hood, L., & Rose, K. (2001). On renaming auditory neuropathy as auditory dys-synchrony: Implications for a clearer understanding of the underlying mechanisms and management options. *Audiology Today, 13*, 15–17.

Berlin, C. I., Li, L., Hood, L. J., Morlet, T., Rose, K., & Brashears, S. (2002). Auditory neuropathy/dys-synchrony: After the diagnosis, then what? *Seminars in Hearing, 23*, 209–214.

Berlin, C. I., Morlet, T., & Hood, L. J. (2003). Auditory Neuropathy/Dys-Synchrony: Its diagnosis and management. *Pediatric Clinics of North America, 50*, 331–340.

Bette, S., Zimmermann, U., Wissinger, B., & Knipper, M. (2007). *OPA1*, the disease gene for optic atrophy type Kjer, is expressed in the inner ear. *Histochemistry and Cell Biology, 128*, 421–430.

Beutner, D., Foerst, A., Lang-Roth, R., von Wedel, H., & Walger, M. (2007). Risk factors for auditory neuropathy/auditory synaptopathy. *ORL Journal of Oto-rhino-laryngology and Its Related Specialties, 69*, 239–244.

Boerkoel, C. F., Takashima, H., Garcia, C. A., Olney, R. K., Johnson, J., Berry, K., . . . Lupski, J. R. (2002). Charcot-Marie-Tooth disease and related neuropathies: Mutation distribution and genotype-phenotype correlation. *Annals of Neurology, 51*, 190–201.

Boudewyns, A. N., Declau, F., De Ridder, D., Parizel, P. M., van den Ende, J., & Van de Heyning, P. H. (2008). Case report: "Auditory neuropathy" in a newborn caused by a cerebellopontine angle arachnoid cyst. *International Journal of Pediatric Otorhinolaryngology, 72*, 905–909.

Buchman, C. A., Roush, P. A., Teagle, H. F., Brown, C. J., Zdanski, C. J., & Grose, J. H. (2006). Auditory neuropathy characteristics in children with cochlear nerve deficiency. *Ear and Hearing, 27*, 399–408.

Butinar, D., Starr, A., Zidar, J., Koutsou, P., & Christodoulou, K. (2008). Auditory nerve is affected in one of two different point mutations of the neurofilament light gene. *Clinical Neurophysiology, 119*, 367–375.

Butinar, D., Zidar, J., Leonardis, L., Popovic, M., Kalaydjieva, L., Angelicheva, D., . . . Starr, A. (1999). Hereditary auditory, vestibular, motor, and sensory neuropathy in a slovenian roma (Gypsy) kindred. *Annals of Neurology, 46*, 36–44.

Campuzano, V., Montermini, L., Molto, M.D., Pianese, L., Cossée, M., Cavalcanti, F., . . . Pandolfo, M. (1996). Friedreich's ataxia: Autosomal recessive disease caused by an intronic GAA triplet repeat expansion. *Science, 271*, 1423–1427.

Cassandro, E., Mosca, F., Sequino, L., De Falco, F. A., & Campanella, G. (1986). *Audiology, 25*, 84–91.

Ceranic, B., & Luxon, L. M. (2004). Progressive auditory neuropathy in patients with Leber's hereditary optic neuropathy. *Journal of Neurology, Neurosurgery and Psychiatry, 75*, 626–630.

Chapon, F., Latour, P., Diraison, P., Schaeffer, S., & Vandenberghe, A. (1999). Axonal phenotype of Charcot-Marie-Tooth disease associated with a mutation in the myelin protein zero gene. *Journal of Neurology, Neurosurgery and Psychiatry, 66*, 779–782.

Cheatham, M. A., & Dallos, P. (1984). Summating potential (SP) tuning curves. *Hearing Research, 16*, 189–200.

Chermak, G. D. (2002). Deciphering auditory processing disorders in children. *Otolaryngology Clinics of North America, 35*, 733–749.

Chermak, G. D., Hall, J. W., & Musiek, F. E. (1999). Differential diagnosis and management of central auditory processing disorder and attention deficit hyperactivity disorder. *Journal of the American Academy of Audiology, 10*, 289–303.

Chisin, R., Perlman, M., & Sohmer, H. (1979). Cochlear and brain stem responses in hearing loss following neonatal hyperbilirubinemia. *Annals of Otology, 88*, 352–357.

Collet, L., Kemp, D. T., Veuillet, E., Duclaux, R., Moulin, A., & Morgon, A. (1990). Effect of contralateral auditory stimuli on active cochlear micro-mechanical properties in human subjects. *Hearing Research, 43*, 251–262.

Conlee, J. W., & Shapiro, S. M. (1991). Morphological changes in the cochlear nucleus and nucleus of the trapezoid body in Gunn rat pups. *Hearing Research, 57*, 23–30.

Corley, V. M., & Crabbe, L. S. (1999). Auditory neuropathy and a mitochondrial disorder in a child: Case study. *Journal of the American Academy of Audiology, 10*, 484–488.

Cossée, M., Schmitt, M., Campuzano, V., Reutenauer, L., Moutou, C., Mandel, J. L., & Koenig, M. (1997). Evolution of the Friedreich's ataxia trinucleotide repeat expansion: Founder effect and premutations. *Proceedings of the National Academy of Sciences of the United States of America, 94*, 7452–7457.

Cowper-Smith, C. D., Dingle, R. N., Guo, Y., Burkard, R., & Phillips, D. P. (2010). Synchronous auditory nerve activity in the carboplatin-chinchilla model of auditory neuropathy. *Journal of the Acoustical Society of America, 128*(1), EL56–62.

Cullen, J. K. Jr, Ellis, M. S. Berlin, C. I., & Lousteau, R. J. (1972). Human acoustic nerve action potential recordings from the tympanic membrane without anesthesia. *Acta Otolaryngologica, 74*, 15–22.

Dallos, P. (1983). Some electrical circuit properties of the organ of Corti. I. Analysis without reactive elements. *Hearing Research, 12*, 89–120.

Dallos, P. (1993). *The auditory periphery*. New York, NY: Academic Press.

De Jonghe, P., Timmerman, V., Nelis, E., De Vriendt, E., Löfgren, A., Ceuterick, C., . . . Van Broeckhoven, C. (1999). A novel type of hereditary motor and sensory neuropathy characterized by a mild phenotype. *Archives of Neurology, 56*, 1283–1288.

Delmaghani, S., del Castillo, F. J., Michel, V., Leibovici, M., Aghaie, A., Ron, U., . . . Petit, C. (2006). Mutations in the gene encoding pejvakin, a newly identified protein of the afferent auditory pathway, cause DFNB59 auditory neuropathy. *Nature Genetics, 38*, 770–778.

Deltenre, P., Mansbach, A. L., Bozet, C., Christiaens, F., Barthelemy, P., Paulissen, D., & Renglet, T. (1999). Auditory neuropathy with preserved cochlear microphonics and secondary loss of otoacoustic emissions. *Audiology, 38*, 187–195.

De Michele, G., Perrone, F., Filla, A., Mirante, E., Giordano, M., De Placido, S., & Campanella, G. (1996). Age of onset, sex, and cardiomyopathy as predictors of disability and survival in Friedreich's disease: A retrospective study on 119 patients. *Neurology, 47*, 1260–1264.

Dowley, A. C., Whitehouse, W. P., Mason, S. M., Cope, Y., Grant, J., & Gibbin, K. P. (2009). Auditory neuropathy: Unexpectedly common in a screening newborn population. *Developmental Medicine and Child Neurology, 51*, 642–646.

Dulon, D., Safieddine, S., Jones, S. M., & Petit, C. (2009). Otoferlin is critical for a highly sensitive and linear calcium-dependent exocytosis at vestibular hair cell ribbon synapses. *Journal of Neuroscience, 29*, 10474–10487.

Dürr, A., Cossee, M., Agid, Y., Campuzano, V., Mignard, C., Penet, C., . . . Koenig, M. (1996). Clinical and genetic abnormalities in patients with Friedreich's ataxia. *New England Journal of Medicine, 335*, 1169–1175.

Durrant, J. D., Wang, J., Ding, D. L., & Salvi, R. J. (1998). Are inner or outer hair cells the source of summating potentials recorded from the round window? *Journal of the Acoustical Society of America, 104*, 370–377.

Eggermont, J. J., & Odenthal, D. W. (1974). Action potentials and summating potentials in the normal human cochlea. *Acta Otolaryngology, 316*(Suppl.), 39–61.

El-Badry, M. M., & McFadden, S. L. (2009). Evaluation of inner hair cell and nerve fiber loss as sufficient pathologies underlying auditory neuropathy. *Hearing Research, 255*, 84–90.

Finocchiaro, G., Formenti, A., Baiocco, F., & Di Donato, S. (1985). Brainstem auditory-evoked responses and clinical picture in a one year follow-up of 18 patients with Friedreich ataxia. *Italian Journal of Neurological Sciences, 6*, 47–52.

Forli, F., Mancuso, M., Santoro, A., Dotti, M.T., Siciliano, G., & Berrettini, S. (2006). Auditory neuropathy in a patient with mitochondrial myopathy and multiple mtDNA deletions. *Journal of Laryngology and Otology, 120*, 888–891.

Fujikawa, S., & Starr, A. (2000). Vestibular neuropathy accompanying auditory and peripheral neuropathies. *Archives of Otolaryngology-Head and Neck Surgery, 126*, 1453–1456.

Gibson, W. P. R., & Sanli, H. (2007). Auditory neuropathy: An update. *Ear and Hearing, 28*, 102S–106S.

Gorga, M. P., Stelmachowicz, P. G., Barlow, S. M., & Brookhouser, P. E. (1995). Case of recurrent, reversible, sudden sensorineural hearing loss in a child. *Journal of the American Academy of Audiology, 6*, 163–172.

Gravel, J. S. (2008). Keynote address, NHS meeting. Como, Italy. June 19–21, 2008.

Gravel, J. S., & Stapells, D. R. (1993). Behavioral, electrophysiologic and otoacoustic measures for a child with auditory processing dysfunction: Case report. *Journal of the American Academy of Audiology, 4*, 412–419.

Hallpike, C. S., Harriman, D. G., & Wells, C. E. (1980). A case of afferent neuropathy and deafness. *Journal of Laryngology and Otology, 94*, 945–964.

Harding, A. E. (1981). Friedreich's ataxia: A clinical and genetic study of 90 families with an analysis of early diagnostic criteria and intrafamilial clustering of clinical features. *Brain, 104*, 589–620.

Harrisson, R. V. (1998). An animal model of auditory neuropathy. *Ear and Hearing, 19*, 355–361.

Hattori, N., Yamamoto, M., Yoshihara, T., Koike, H., Nakagawa, M., Yoshikawa, H., . . . Sobue, G. (2003). Study Group for Hereditary Neuropathy in Japan. Demyelinating and axonal features of Charcot-Marie-Tooth disease with mutations of myelin-related proteins (PMP22, MPZ and Cx32): A clinicopathological study of 205 Japanese patients. *Brain, 126*, 134–151.

Hirsh, I. J. (1948). The influence of interaural phase on interaural summation and inhibition. *Journal of the Acoustical Society of America, 20*, 536–544.

Hood, L. J. (1999). A review of objective methods of evaluating auditory neural pathways. *Laryngoscope, 109*, 1475–1478.

Hood, L. J., Berlin, C. I., Bordelon, J., & Rose, K. (2003). Patients with auditory neuropathy/dys-synchrony lack efferent suppression of transient evoked otoacoustic emissions. *Journal of the American Academy of Audiology, 14*, 302–313.

Hood, L. J., Berlin, C. I., Hurley, A., Cecola, R. P., & Bell, B. (1996). Contralateral suppression of click-evoked otoacoustic emissions: Intensity effects. *Hearing Research, 101*, 113–118.

Hood, L. J., Wilensky, D., Li, L., & Berlin, C. I. (2004). The role of FM technology in the management of patients with auditory neuropathy/dys-synchrony. *Proceedings of the International Conference on FM Technology*, Chicago, Illinois, November, 2003.

Hong, B. N., Yi, T. H., Kim, S. Y., & Kang, T. H. (2009). High-dosage pyridoxine-induced auditory neuropathy and protection with coffee in mice. *Biological Pharmaceutical Bulletin, 32*, 597–603.

Huang, T., Santarelli, R., & Starr, A. (2009). Mutation of OPA1 gene causes deafness by affecting function of auditory nerve terminals. *Brain Research, 1300*, 97–104.

Iwasaki, S., Hayashi, Y., Seki, A., Nagura, M., Hashimoto, Y., Oshima, G., & Hoshino, T. (2003). A model of two-stage newborn hearing screening with automated auditory brainstem response. *International Journal of Pediatric Otorhinolaryngology, 67*, 1099–1104.

Jerger, J., & Musiek, F. (2000). Report of the consensus conference on the diagnosis of auditory processing disorders in school aged children. *Journal of the American Academy of Audiology, 11*, 467–474.

Joint Committee on Infant Hearing. (2007). Year 2007 position statement: Principles and guidelines for early hearing detection and intervention programs. *American Academy of Pediatrics, 120*, 898–921.

Joo, I. S., Ki, C. S., Joo, S. Y., Huh, K., & Kim, J. W. (2004). A novel point mutation in PMP22 gene associated Scandinavian Audiology, 25,with a familial case of Charcot-Marie-Tooth disease type 1A with sensorineural deafness. *Neuromuscular Disorders, 14*, 325–328.

Jutras, B., Russell, L. J., Hurteau, A. M., & Chapdelaine, M. (2003). Auditory neuropathy in siblings with Waardenburg's syndrome. *International Journal of Pediatric Otorhinolaryngology, 67*, 1133–1142.

Kaga, K., Nakamura, M., Shinogami, M., Tsuzuku, T., Yamada, K., & Shindo, M. (1996). Auditory nerve disease of both ears revealed by auditory brainstem responses, electrocochleography and otoacoustic emissions. *Scandinavian Audiology, 25*(4), 233–238.

Kalaydjieva, L., Gresham, D., Gooding, R., Heather, L., Baas, F., de Jonge, R., . . . Thomas, P. K. (2000). N-myc downstream-regulated gene 1 is mutated in hereditary motor and sensory neuropathy—Lom. *American Journal of Human Genetics, 67*, 47–58.

Kalaydjieva, L., Nikolova, A., Turnev, I., Petrova, J., Hristova, A., Ishpekova, B., . . . Thomas, P. K. (1998). Hereditary motor and sensory neuropathy—Lom, a novel demyelinating neuropathy associated with deafness in gypsies. Clinical, electrophysiological and nerve biopsy findings. *Brain, 121*, 399–408.

Keefe, D. H., Fitzpatrick, D., Liu, Y. W., Sanford, C. A., & Gorga, M. P. (2010). Wideband acoustic-reflex test in a test battery to predict middle ear dysfunction. *Hearing Research, 263*, 52–65.

Kim, T. B., Isaacson, B., Sivakumaran, T. A., Starr, A., Keats, B. J., & Lesperance, M. M. (2004). A gene responsible for autosomal dominant auditory neuropathy (AUNA1) maps to 13q14-21. *Journal of Medical Genetics, 41,* 872–876.

Kirkim, G., Serbetcioglu, B., Erdag, T. K., & Ceryan, K. (2008). The frequency of auditory neuropathy detected by universal newborn hearing screening program. *International Journal of Pediatric Otorhinolaryngology, 72,* 1461–1469.

Kovach, M. J., Campbell, K. C. M., Herman, K., Waggoner, B., Gelber, D., Hughes, L. F., & Kimonis, V. E. (2002). Anticipation in a unique family with Charcot-Marie-Tooth syndrome and deafness: Delineation of the clinical features and review of the literature. *American Journal of Medical Genetics, 108,* 295–303.

Kowalski, J. W., Rasheva, M., & Zakrzewska, B. (1991). Visual and brainstem auditory evoked potentials in hereditary motor-sensory neuropathy. *Electromyography and Clinical Neurophysiology, 31,* 167–172.

Kraus, N., Bradlow, A. R., Cheatham, M. A., Cunningham, J., King, C. D., Koch, D. B., . . . Wright, B. A. (2000). Consequences of neural asynchrony: A case of auditory neuropathy. *Journal of the Association for Research in Otolaryngology, 1,* 33–45.

Kraus, N., Özdamar, Ö., Stein, L., & Reed, N. (1984). Absent auditory brainstem response: Peripheral hearing loss or brain stem dysfunction? *Laryngoscope, 94,* 400–406.

Kumar, A. U., & Jayaram, M. (2005). Auditory processing in individuals with auditory neuropathy. *Behavioral and Brain Functions, 1,* 1–21.

Lee, J. S. M., McPherson, B., Yuen, K. C. P., & Wong, L. L. N. (2001). Screening for auditory neuropathy in a school for hearing impaired children. *International Journal of Pediatric Otolaryngology, 61,* 39–46.

Licklider, J. C. R. (1948). The influence of interaural phase relations upon the masking of speech by white noise. *Journal of the Acoustical Society of America, 20,* 150–159.

López-Bigas, N., Olivé, M., Rabionet, R., Ben-David, O., Martínez-Matos, J.A., Bravo, O., . . . Estivill, X. (2001). Connexin 31 (GJB3) is expressed in the peripheral and auditory nerves and causes neuropathy and hearing impairment. *Human Molecular Genetics, 10,* 947–952.

Madden, C., Rutter, M., Hilbert, L., Greinwald, J., & Choo, D. (2002). Clinical and audiological features in auditory neuropathy. *Archives of Otolaryngology-Head and Neck Surgery, 128,* 1026–1030.

Marlin, S., Feldmann, D., Nguyen, Y., Rouillon, I., Loundon, N., Jonard, L., . . . Denoyelle, F. (2010). Temperature-sensitive auditory neuropathy associated with an otoferlin mutation: Deafening fever! *Biochemical and Biophysical Research Communications 394,* 737–742.

Matsumoto, M., Sekiya, T., Kojima, K., & Ito, J. (2008). An animal experimental model of auditory neuropathy induced in rats by auditory nerve compression. *Experimental Neurology, 210,* 248–256.

McDonald, W. I. (1980). Physiological consequences of demyelination. In A. J. Sumner (Ed.), *The physiology of peripheral nerve disease* (pp. 265–286). Philadelphia, PA: W. B. Saunders.

McMahon, C. M., Patuzzi, R. B., Gibson, W. P. R., & Sanli, H. (2008). Frequency-specific electrocochleography indicates that presynaptic and postsynaptic mechanisms of auditory neuropathy exist. *Ear and Hearing, 29,* 314–325.

Merchant, S. N., McKenna, M. J., Nadol, J. B. Jr., Kristiansen, A. G., Tropitzsch, A., Lindal, S., & Tranebjaeizrg, L. (2001). Temporal bone histopathologic and genetic studies in Mohr-Tranebjaerg syndrome (DFN-1). *Otology and Neurotology, 22,* 506–511.

Michalewski, H. J., Starr, A., Nguyen, T. T., Kong, Y. Y., & Zeng, F. G. (2005). Auditory temporal processes in normal-hearing individuals and in patients with auditory neuropathy. *Clinical Neurophysiology, 116,* 669–680.

Misu, K., Yoshihara, T., Shikama, Y., Awaki, E., Yamamoto, M., Hattori, N., . . . Sobue, G. (2000). An axonal form of Charcot-Marie-Tooth disease showing distinctive features in association with mutations in the peripheral myelin protein zero gene (Thr124Met or Asp75Val). *Journal of Neurology, Neurosurgery and Psychiatry, 69,* 806–811.

Miyamoto, R. T., Kirk, K. I., Renshaw, J., & Hussain, D. (1999). Cochlear implantation in auditory neuropathy. *Laryngoscope, 109,* 181–185.

Morlet, T., O'Reilly, R., & Morlet, S. (2008). *Enlarged vestibular aqueduct in infants and children: What is the appropriate test battery?* NHS meeting. Como, Italy. June 19–21, 2008.

Muchnik, C., Ari-Even Roth, D., Othman-Jebara, R., Putter-Katz, H., Shabtai, E., & Hildesheimer, M. (2004). Reduced medial olivocochlear bundle system function in children with auditory processing disorders. *Audiology and Neurotology, 9,* 107–114.

Musiek, F. E., Gollegly, K. M., Lamb, L. E., & Lamb, P. (1990). Select issues in screening for central auditory processing dysfunction. *Seminars in Hearing, 11,* 372–383.

Narne, V. K., & Vanaja, C. S. (2008). Speech identification and cortical potentials in individuals with auditory neuropathy. *Behavioral and Brain Functions, 31,* 4–15.

Narne, V. K., & Vanaja, C. S. (2009). Perception of envelope-enhanced speech in the presence of noise by individuals with auditory neuropathy. *Ear and Hearing, 30,* 136–142.

Nelson, K. R., Gilmore, R. L., & Massey, A. (1988). Acoustic nerve conduction abnormalities in Guillain-Barre syndrome. *Neurology, 38,* 1263–1266.

Ngo, R. Y. S., Tan, H. K. K., Balakrishnan, A., Bee Lim, S., & Lazaroo, D. T. (2006). Auditory neuropathy/auditory dys-synchrony detected by universal newborn hearing screening. *International Journal of Pediatric Otorhinolaryngology, 70,* 1299–1306.

Palmgren, B., Jin, Z., Ma, H., Jiao, Y., & Olivius, P. (2010). ß-Bungarotoxin application to the round window: An in vivo deafferentation model of the inner ear. *Hearing Research, 265,* 70–76.

Peterson, A., Shallop, J., Driscoll, C., Breneman, A., Babb, J., Stoeckel, R., & Fabry, L. (2003). Outcomes of cochlear implantation in children with auditory neuropathy. *Journal of the American Academy of Audiology, 14,* 188–201.

Picton, T. W., John, M. S., Dimitrijevic, A., & Purcell, D. (2003). Human auditory steady-state responses. *International Journal of Audiology, 42*, 177–219.

Psarommatis, I., Riga, M., Douros, K., Koltsidopoulos, P., Douniadakis, D., Kapetanakis, I., & Apostolopoulos, N. (2006). Transient infantile auditory neuropathy and its clinical implications. *International Journal of Pediatric Otorhinolaryngology, 70*, 1629–1637.

Rance, G., Barker, E., Mok, M., Dowell, R., Rincon, A., & Garratt, R. (2007). Speech perception in noise for children with auditory neuropathy/dys-synchrony type hearing loss. *Ear and Hearing, 28*, 351–360.

Rance, G., Beer, D. E., Cone-Wesson, B., Shepherd, R. K., Dowell, R. C., King, A. M., . . . Clark, G. M. (1999). Clinical findings for a group of infants and young children with auditory neuropathy. *Ear and Hearing, 20*, 238–252.

Rance, G., Cone-Wesson, B., Wunderlich, J., & Dowell, R. (2002). Speech perception and cortical event related potentials in children with auditory neuropathy. *Ear and Hearing, 23*, 239–253.

Rance, G., Corben, L., Barker, E., Carew, P., Chisari, D., Rogers, M., . . . Delatycki, M. B. (2010). Auditory perception in individuals with Friedreich's ataxia. *Audiology and Neurotology, 15*, 229–240.

Rance, G., Fava, R., Baldock, H., Chong, A., Barker, E., Corben, L., & Delatycki, M. B. (2008). Speech perception ability in individuals with Friedreich ataxia. *Brain, 131*, 2002–2012.

Rance, G., McKay, C., & Grayden, D. (2004). Perceptual characterization of children with auditory neuropathy. *Ear and Hearing, 25*, 34–46.

Rance, G., Roper, R., Symons, L., Moody, L. J., Poulis, C., Dourlay, M., & Kelly, T. (2005). Hearing threshold estimation in infants using auditory steady-state responses. *Journal of the Amererican Academy of Audiology, 16*, 291–300.

Rapin, I., & Gravel, J. (2003). Auditory neuropathy: Physiologic and pathologic evidence calls for more diagnostic specificity. *International Journal of Pediatric Otorhinolaryngology, 67*, 707–728.

Raveh, E., Buller, N., Badrana, O., & Attias, J. (2007). Auditory neuropathy: Clinical characteristics and therapeutic approach. *American Journal of Otolaryngology, 28*, 302–308.

Rea, P. A., & Gibson, W. P. R. (2003). Evidence for surviving outer hair cell function in congenitally deaf ears. *Laryngoscope, 113*, 2030–2034.

Rodríguez-Ballesteros, M., del Castillo, F. J., Martín, Y., Moreno-Pelayo, M. A., Morera, C., Prieto, F., . . . del Castillo, I. (2003). Auditory neuropathy in patients carrying mutations in the otoferlin gene (OTOF). *Human Mutation, 22*, 451–456.

Rodríguez-Ballesteros, M., Reynoso, R., Olarte, M., Villamar, M., Morera, C., Santarelli, R., . . . del Castillo, I. (2008). A multicenter study on the prevalence and spectrum of mutations in the otoferlin gene (OTOF) in subjects with nonsyndromic hearing impairment and auditory neuropathy. *Human Mutation, 29*, 823–831.

Ryu, E. J., Wang, J. Y. T., Le, N., Baloch, R. H., Gustin, J. A., Schmidt, R. E., & Mildbrand, J. (2007). Misexpression of Pou3f1 results in peripheral nerve hypomelination and axonal loss. *Journal of Neuroscience, 27*, 11552–11559.

Santarelli, R., & Arslan, E. (2002). Electrocochleography in auditory neuropathy. *Hearing Research, 170*, 32–47.

Santarelli, R., del Castillo, I., Rodriguez-Ballesteros, M., Scimeni, P., Cama, E., Arslan, E., & Starr, A. (2009). Abnormal cochlear potentials from deaf patients with mutations in the Otoferlin gene. *Journal of the Association for Research in Otolaryngology, 10*, 545–556.

Santarelli, R., Starr, A., Michalewski, H. J., & Arslan, E. (2008). Neural and receptor cochlear potentials obtained by transtympanic electrocochleography in auditory neuropathy. *Clinical Neurophysiology, 119*, 1028–1041.

Satya-Murti, S., Cacace, A., & Hanson, P. (1980). Auditory dysfunction in Friedreich ataxia: Result of spiral ganglion degeneration. *Neurology, 30*, 1047–1053.

Sawada, S., Mori, N., Mount, R. J., & Harrison, R. V. (2001). Differential vulnerability of inner and outer hair cell systems to chronic mild hypoxia and glutamate ototoxicity insights into the cause of auditory neuropathy. *Journal of Otolaryngology, 30*, 106–114.

Schmiedt, R. A., Okamura, H., Lang, H., & Schute, B. A. (2002). Ouabain application to the round window of the gerbil cochlea: A model of auditory neuropathy and apoptosis. *Journal of the Association for Research in Otolaryngology, 3*, 223–233.

Sekiya, T., Hatayama, T., Shimamura, N., & Suzuki, S. (2000). An in vivo quantifiable model of cochlear neuronal degeneration induced by central process injury. *Experimental Neurology, 161*, 490–502.

Shaia, W. T., Shapiro, W. M., & Spencer, R. F. (2005). The jaundiced Gunn rate model of auditory neuropathy/dyssynchrony. *Laryngoscope, 115*, 2167–2173.

Shallop, J. K., Peterson, A., Facer, G. W., Fabry, L. B., & Driscoll, C. L. W. (2001). Cochlear implants in five cases of auditory neuropathy: Postoperative findings and progress. *Laryngoscope, 111*, 555–562.

Shapiro, S. M., & Teselle, M. E. (1994). Cochlear microphonics in the jaundiced Gunn rat. *American Journal of Otolaryngology, 15*, 129–137.

Sheykholesami, K., & Kaga, K. (2000). Otoacoustic emissions and auditory brainstem responses after neonatal hyperbilirubinemia. *International Journal of Pediatric Otothinolaryngology, 52*, 65–73.

Shirane, M., & Harrison, R. V. (1987). The effects of hypoxia on sensory cells of the cochlea in the chinchilla. *Scanning Microscopy, 1*, 1175–1183.

Sininger, Y. S. (2002). Auditory neuropathy in infants and children: Implications for early hearing detection and intervention programs. *Audiology Today, 14*, 16–21.

Spoendlin, H. (1974). Optic cochleovestibular degenerations in hereditary ataxias. II. Temporal bone pathology in two cases of Friedreich's ataxia with vestibulo-cochlear disorders. *Brain, 97*, 41–48.

Starr, A. (2001). The neurology of auditory neuropathy. In Y. S. Sininger & A. Starr (Eds.), *Auditory neuropathy: A new perspective on hearing disorders* (pp. 37–49). San Diego, CA: Singular Thomson Learning.

Starr, A., Isaacson, B., Michalewski, H. J., Zeng, F. G., Kong, Y. Y., Beale, P., . . . Lesperance, M. M. (2004). A dominantly inherited progressive deafness affecting distal auditory nerve and hair cells. *Journal of the Association for Research in Otolaryngology, 5,* 411–426.

Starr, A., McPherson, D., Patterson, J., Don, M., Luxford, W., Shannon, R., . . . Waring, M. (1991). Absence of both auditory evoked potentials and auditory percepts depending on timing cues. *Brain, 114,* 1157–1180.

Starr, A., Michalewski, H. J., Zeng, F. G., Fujikawa-Brooks, S., Linthicum, F., Kim, C. S., . . . Keats, B. (2003). Pathology and physiology of auditory neuropathy with a novel mutation in the MPZ gene (Tyr145→Ser). *Brain, 126,* 1604–1619.

Starr, A., Picton, T. W., Sininger, Y., Hood, L. J., & Berlin, C. I. (1996). Auditory neuropathy. *Brain, 119,* 741–753.

Starr, A., Sininger, Y., Nguyen, T., Michalewski, H. J., Oba, S., & Abdala, C. (2001). Cochlear receptor (microphonic and summating potentials, otoacoustic emissions) and auditory pathway (auditory brain stem potentials) activity in auditory neuropathy. *Ear and Hearing, 22,* 91–99.

Starr, A., Sininger, Y. S., & Pratt, H. (2000). The varieties of auditory neuropathy. *Journal of Basic and Clinical Physiology and Pharmacology, 11,* 215–230.

Starr, A., Sininger, Y., Winter, M., Derebery, M. J., Oba, S., & Michalewski, H. J. (1998). Transient deafness due to temperature-sensitive auditory neuropathy. *Ear and Hearing, 19,* 169–179.

Starr, A., Zeng, F. G., Michalewski, H. J., & Moser, T. (2008). Perspectives on auditory neuropathy: Disorders of inner hair cell, auditory nerve, and their synapse. In A. I. Basbaum, A. Kaneko, G. M. Shepherd, & G. Westheimer (Eds.), *The senses: A comprehensive reference, Vol 3, Audition* (pp. 397–412). P. Dallos & D. Oertel (Eds.). San Diego, CA: Academic Press.

Stein, L. K., Tremblay, K., Pasternak, J., Banerjee, S., & Lindemann, K. (1996). Auditory brainstem neuropathy and elevated bilirubin levels. *Seminars in Hearing, 17,* 197–213.

Suppiej, A., Rizzardi, E., Zanardo, V., Franzoi, M., Ermani, M., & Orzan, E. (2007). Reliability of hearing screening in high-risk neonates: Comparative study of otoacoustic emission, automated and conventional auditory brainstem response. *Clinical Neurophysiology, 118,* 869–876.

Takeno, S., Harrison, R. V., Mount, R. J., Wake, M., & Harada, Y. (1994). Induction of selective inner hair cell damage by carboplatin. *Scanning Microscopy, 8,* 97–106.

Tang, W., Zhang, Y., Chang, Q., Ahmad, S., Dahlke, I., Yi, H., . . . Lin, X. (2006). Connexin29 is highly expressed in cochlear Schwann cells, and it is required for the normal development and function of the auditory nerve in mice. *Journal of Neuroscience, 26,* 1991–1999.

Teagle, H. F, Roush, P. A., Woodard, J. S., Hatch, D. R., Zdanski, C. J., Buss, E., & Buchman, C.A. (2010). Cochlear implantation in children with auditory neuropathy spectrum disorder. *Ear and Hearing, 31,* 325–335.

Trautwein, P., Sininger, Y., & Nelson, R. (2000). Cochlear implantation of auditory neuropathy. *Journal of the American Academy of Audiology, 11,* 309–315.

Varga, R., Kelley, P. M., Keats, B. J., Starr, A., Leal, S. M., Cohn, E., & Kimberling, W. J. (2003). Non-syndromic recessive auditory neuropathy is the results of mutations in the otoferlin (OTOF) gene. *Journal of Medical Genetics, 40,* 45–50.

Wake, M., Takeno, S., Ibrahim, D., & Harrison, R. (1994). Selective inner hair cell ototoxicity induced by carboplatin. *Laryngoscope, 104,* 488–493.

Walton, J., Gibson, W. P., Sanli, H., & Prelog, K. (2008). Predicting cochlear implant outcomes in children with auditory neuropathy. *Otology and Neurotology, 29,* 302–309.

Wang, L., Cao, K., Wang, Z., & Chen, Z. (2006). Cochlear function after selective spiral ganglion cells degeneration induced by ouabain. *Chinese Medicine Journal, 119,* 974–979.

Wang, J., Powers, N. L., Hofstetter, P., Trautwein, P., Ding, D., & Salvi, R. (1997). Effects of selective inner hair cell loss on auditory nerve fiber threshold, tuning and spontaneous and driven discharge rate. *Hearing Research, 107,* 67–82.

Withnell, R. H. (2001). Brief report:The cochlear microphonic as an indication of outer hair cell function. *Ear and Hearing, 22,* 75–77.

Wong, V. (1997). A neurophysiological study in children with Miller Fisher syndrome and Guillain-Barré syndrome. *Brain and Development, 19,* 197–204.

Worthington, D. W., & Peters, J. F. (1980). Quantifiable hearing and no ABR: Paradox or error? *Ear and Hearing, 1,* 281–285.

Xoinis, K., Weirather, Y., Mavoori, H., Shaha, S. H., & Iwamoto, L. M. (2007). Extremely low birth weight infants are at high risk for auditory neuropathy. *Journal of Perinatology, 11,* 718–723.

Yasunaga, S., Grati, M., Cohen-Salmon, M., El-Amraoui, A., Mustapha, M., Salem, N., . . . Petit C. (1999). A mutation in *OTOF*, encoding otoferlin, A FER-1-like protein, causes DFNB9, a nonsyndromic form of deafness. *Nature Genetics, 21,* 362–369.

Yellin, M. W., Jerger, J., & Fifer, R. C. (1989). Norms for disproportionate loss in speech intelligibility. *Ear and Hearing, 10,* 231–234.

Zeng, F. G., & Liu, S. (2006). Speech perception in individuals with auditory neuropathy. *Journal of Speech, Language and Hearing Research, 49,* 367–380.

Zeng, F.G., Oba, S., Garde, S., Sininger, Y., & Starr, A. (1999). Temporal and speech processing deficits in auditory neuropathy. *NeuroReport, 10,* 3429–3435.

Zeng, F. G., Oba, S., Garde, S., Sininger, Y., & Starr, A. (2001). Psychoacoustics and speech perception in auditory neuropathy. In Y. S. Sininger & A. Starr (Eds.), *Auditory neuropathy: A new perspective on hearing disorders* (pp. 141–164). San Diego, CA: Singular Thomson Learning.

Zeng, F. G., Kong, Y. Y., Michalewski, H. J., & Starr, A. (2005). Perceptual consequences of disrupted auditory nerve activity. *Journal of Neurophysiology, 93,* 3060–3063.

3

Time and Timing in Audition: Some Current Issues in Auditory Temporal Processing

Dennis P. Phillips

Key Words. Auditory perception, auditory neuroscience, temporal processing, temporal acuity, temporal gap detection, temporal asymmetries, auditory saltation, temporal windows

LEARNING OBJECTIVES

- What do we mean by "temporal processing"? What kinds of sensory-perceptual processes are embraced by that term? In this chapter, you will encounter three, quite different, ways of approaching how the auditory system confronts the task of dealing with a stimulus which, by its very nature, unfolds over time.
- First, what is auditory temporal gap-detection? How do the perceptual processes engaged by that task change according to whether the sounds that bound the gap are the same or different? In what way might gap detection paradigms help us understand the formation of phonetic categories in speech?
- Second, in what way(s) have studies using temporally asymmetric sounds informed us about the sensory-perceptual processing of the stream of sound with which we are continuously presented? Why is it that the auditory system seems to extract more information from sound onsets than from sound offsets?
- Third, what is "auditory saltation"? How have studies of auditory saltation helped us to understand the time course of, and the processing that goes into, the generation of a conscious perceptual event?

INTRODUCTION

Auditory perception is confronted with a substantial, multilevel temporal processing problem. In the first place, any auditory event is, by definition, a mechanical disturbance whose acoustical identity resides in the fashion in which the disturbance is distributed in time. This means that the nervous system must contain mechanisms for representing or encoding that temporal pattern of energy. Second, the acoustic world, often composed of many sound sources, arrives at each ear as a single waveform, so the auditory system faces the further task of executing a spectrotemporal decomposition of that single *physical* waveform and then building a *perceptual* auditory scene composed of separate objects. It can do this in part based on the temporal coherence of energy fluctuations in different frequency ranges; that is, spectral regions that undergo near-synchronous, correlated variations in energy may be grouped as belonging to a single object (after Bregman, 1990). The auditory system can also use the spatial locations of energy fluctuations to define the sound sources. In this regard, note that determining the spatial location of a sound source is itself in part

69

based on an interaural correlation of acoustic event *times*. Third, auditory events that make up our proximal stimulus (i.e., the acoustical signal at the ears) are themselves often closely spaced in time. Spoken language is a fine example: it reminds us that phonetically important auditory events can have a temporal "grain" in the ms to tens-of-ms range, so it behooves the auditory processor to have a temporal acuity capable of resolving those events. Finally, the act of generating any percept in response to the physical stimulus itself takes neural processing *time*.

The purpose of this chapter is to provide an overview of some recent research that provides insights into the role of time and timing in auditory perception, or that has exploited auditory perceptual timing tasks to reveal new information about auditory perceptual architecture. "Temporal processing," perhaps somewhat like binaural hearing, has always had a special place in the endeavors of hearing scientists. In recent years, there has been a number of new advances, or revisitations to older ones, that have alerted us to the multiplicity of levels at which time and timing are core to the auditory perceptual process. If there is a general theme in what follows, then, it is that "temporal processing" in audition is simply not a unitary process; it is an umbrella term with a wide capture (see also Divenyi, 2004; Hirsh, 1959; Rosen, 1992). This point takes on special significance from the fact that there is currently much focus on the existence of auditory temporal processing deficits in persons with developmental language disorders; viewed in the present sense, attributions of normal or impaired behavioral performance simply to impoverished "temporal processing" might actually provide relatively little specification of the processing problem. The brain is a temporal correlator par excellence (Eggermont, 1990), and auditory perception is inherently a temporal- processing problem (after Bregman, 1990) executed by the brain (Phillips, 1995, 2002). It should thus come as no surprise that any disturbance in brain function mediating auditory perception might receive behavioral expression in impaired "temporal processing." It is the specification of particular temporal mechanism(s) that is informative about the architecture of auditory perceptual processing, and disorders of it.

We begin with a description of auditory temporal gap detection, which has been a popular measure of auditory temporal acuity. This will lead naturally into a description of the monaural "temporal window," and into an exploration of the roles of perceptual channels in auditory temporal processing. Next, we examine the importance of stimulus onsets in auditory perception. Finally, we consider some recent experiments on auditory saltation, which have exploited a merger of challenges to spatial hearing and challenges to temporal processing, in order to provide an independent reminder of the time required for the generation of auditory percepts. This chapter is also colored by an interest in exploring the relation between neural processing architecture, and the perceptual architecture it supports. To be sure, in many domains, attempts to specify that relation may be premature; nevertheless, there is no doubt that knowledge of one can usefully inform inquiry into the other. We further hope that referencing of the arguments that follow is sufficiently liberal that readers can elect to pursue their own enquiries into temporal aspects of audition not covered here. What follows is far from exhaustive in its coverage of temporal processes in hearing, and it necessarily assumes a modest knowledge of basic auditory psychophysics and auditory neuroscience. Readers who are less well versed in these topics might wish to consult Moore (2003) or Plack (2005) on psychophysics, and Ruggero (1992) and Phillips (2001) for overviews of peripheral auditory nerve and central auditory function, respectively.

AUDITORY TEMPORAL ACUITY STUDIED WITH TEMPORAL GAP DETECTION PARADIGMS

"Within-Channel" Gap Detection

A primary dimension in sensory systems is temporal acuity or temporal resolution. There are many paradigms that one might employ to measure the temporal "grain" of the auditory perceptual process. These include temporal gap detection, click fusion, and the temporal ordering of clicks with different amplitudes or of sound pulses that differ in some dimension (frequency, amplitude, location, etc.). One of the most popular methodologies is gap detection, in which the general task is to detect a brief period of silence in an otherwise ongoing stream of sound; the measure of interest is the shortest detectable gap ("gap threshold"). In its now classical formulation, temporal gap detection provides a measure with relatively little cognitive "overhead" in a task that is close to being purely temporal, that is, with little possibility of subjects' use of unintended spectral cues as a means to perform the task. Typically, the gap detection task offers the listener a 2-interval, 2-alternative, forced-choice design (Figure 3–1, upper). A (carrier) sound occurs in each interval (the "standard" and the "signal"), but in one of them (the "signal"), the carrier has a silent period (gap)

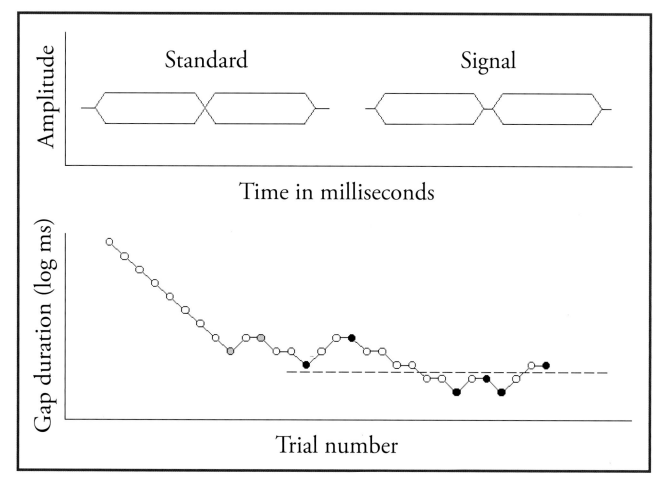

Figure 3–1. An auditory temporal gap detection paradigm. Upper panel is a schematic illustration of a single trial. The subject is presented, in randomized order, with a "standard," which contains no silent period, and a "signal," which contains the gap to be detected. The task of the listener is to specify whether the first or second sound contained the gap. Typically, this trial structure is embedded in an adaptive tracking paradigm. Lower panel shows the time course of responses in one such paradigm. The first trial contains a signal with a long silent period, which, if correctly identified by the listener, is reduced in duration (by a fixed factor, e.g., 1.2) for the next trial. This strategy is repeated until the listener commits the first error. At that point, the gap duration is increased (by the same factor) until the listener correctly identifies the signal in two successive trials; at that point, the direction of the adaptive step is reversed until the listener makes another error. This "two-down/one-up" adaptive tracking of the shortest detectable gap continues until there has been some predetermined number of reversals of the adaptive step. Gap detection threshold is then defined as the mean of the gap durations associated with the last six (or more) reversals in the sign of the adaptive step (dashed line). For detailed analysis of adaptive tracking procedures, see Levitt (1971).

inserted at some point during its time course. The task of the listener is to specify the interval containing the gap. The gap detection threshold is then usually measured using some form of adaptive tracking methodology (see Figure 3–1, lower).

Many stimulus considerations are important in designing "clean" measures of temporal gap detection thresholds. We do not dwell on them at length here, but mention a few of them simply to alert the reader to the range of stimulus control issues to check for when reading this literature. The bandwidth of the carrier is an issue, because the salience of spectral splatter introduced by the gating of the carrier to produce gap onset and gap offset is minimized when the carrier bandwidth is large. When gap detection thresholds are sought for narrowband noises (or tones), one can use carefully chosen fall-rise times to shape the carrier envelope, or the target bandwidth can be embedded in a (spectrally complementary) notched-noise masker. The durations of the "markers" (i.e., the carriers that precede and follow the silent period) are also important. This is because one wishes to avoid the possibility of listeners using the overall stimulus duration (leading marker + gap + trailing marker) as a cue to the interval containing the gap. Nor, in the case of short stimuli in which the gap is inserted destructively into a carrier of otherwise constant overall length, does one want to permit the overall energy in the stimulus to be used as such a cue. Solutions to these problems include the deliberate introduction of jitter to the length of the markers bounding the gap, the use of markers which are very long in relation to the duration of the inserted gap, or manipulations (roving) of marker amplitudes.

Using wideband noises, human auditory temporal gap detection thresholds can be as short as about 2 to 3 ms or less, depending on measurement methodology (Eddins et al., 1992; Penner 1977: Phillips et al., 1997; Plomp, 1964; Shailer & Moore, 1983). This is comparable to the shortest gap that is represented in the averaged spike trains recorded from single cochlear neurons in animals (Zhang et al., 1990). There is thus a correspondence between perceptual performance and that of the encoding mechanisms of the auditory periphery. This correspondence is important for two reasons. One is that it points to strictly *peripheral* limitations on behav-

ioral gap-detection performance. The second reason emerges from how we conceptualize the auditory periphery. We can construe cochlear output as a bank of narrowly tuned filters, each responsible for transmitting information about the presence, amplitude and timing of energy within its passband (Phillips et al., 2002; Ruggero, 1992). That being said, the detection of a gap between identical markers reduces to a process of "within-channel discontinuity detection" (after Phillips et al., 1997). That is, the perceptual operation itself is simply the detection of a discontinuity or interruption in the stream of activity aroused in the neural/perceptual channel activated by the stimulus (Figure 3–2, lower left). There is no need to postulate that the listener separately resolves the leading marker offset, the presence of a silent period, and the subsequent trailing marker onset, particularly at threshold gap durations (Moore, 1993).

Gap-detection thresholds vary inversely with the bandwidth of the carrier sounds (Eddins et al., 1992). At least one reason for this is probably the number of peripheral channels carrying information about the presence of the temporal gap. In this regard, when very narrowband noises are used as carriers, gap-detection performance is better with two bands than with one, even with spectral separations of up to five octaves (Grose, 1991; Hall et al., 1996; Phillips & Hall, 2000). This may be because the narrowband noises have waveforms characterized by random amplitude-envelope fluctuations; those fluctuations might be confused with the gap to be detected (e.g., Moore & Glasberg, 1988), and so a disambiguation may be afforded by the temporal coherence of the (intended) gap's representation in activity carried by more than one channel. In this regard, the benefit of having two noises over one is largely independent of the spectral separation of the noise carriers (Hall et al., 1996). It is likely that recovery of the gap can be aided by "central" processes operating across frequency channels (after Viemeister; 1979: "central," because there is no peripheral neural infrastructure for sampling across cochlear output channels).

If the output of the auditory periphery is construed as a bank of frequency-specific channels describing the energy of the stimulus within its respective passband, then gap detection can use-

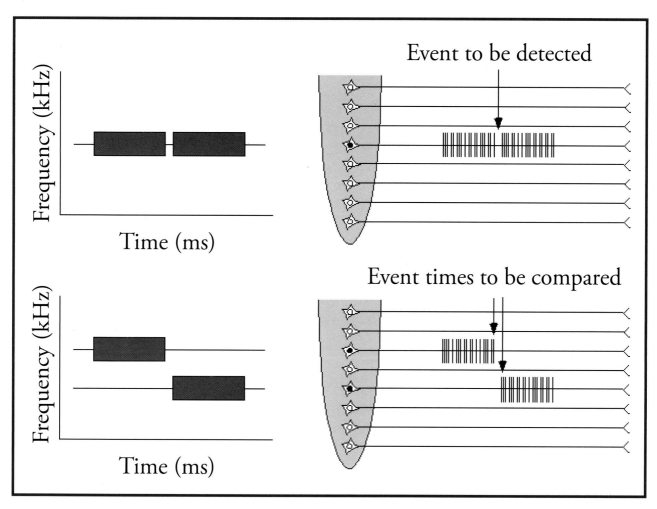

Figure 3–2. The distinction between within-channel and between-channel gap detection. In within-channel gap detection, the leading and trailing markers that bound the gap are spectrally identical (*upper left*), and so activate the same population of cochlear neurons (*lower left*). The perceptual process required to detect the silent period is the detection of a discontinuity in the activity of that population of cochlear neurons. The case for between-channel gap detection is quite different. In this instance, the spectral content of the leading and trailing markers can be quite different (*upper right*), so that the two markers activate different populations of cochlear neurons (*lower right*). Successful detection of the silent period may now require the relative timing of the offset of the leading marker and the onset of the trailing marker. For further discussion, see Phillips et al. (1997) and Formby et al. (1998).

fully be thought of as an extreme case of decrement detection, that is, the case of detecting a transient, 100% amplitude decrement. This raises the question of the existence of any trade-off between depth and duration of the decrement. In practice, at threshold levels of decrement detectability, there is such a trade-off because the listener is typically unable to distinguish a brief, deep energy decrement from a longer, more shallow one. One way of thinking about this acknowledges that the decision about the presence

of a temporal gap depends on a temporally sliding, running average of the output of peripheral filters. A "smearing" of the output occurs because the output of the temporal window at any given moment is a weighted average of the input across time. This smearing is shaped by at least two factors: the width (duration in time) and the shape (weighting across time) of the temporal window within which activity is averaged. It is this windowing that has the consequence of the perceptual ambiguity of gap duration/depth at threshold levels of detectability. Indeed, one can use psychophysical data to calculate the properties of the temporal window, and there is agreement that its width can be as narrow as about 8 ms, although this depends on the shape of the window assumed (e.g., rounded exponential versus Gaussian: Moore et al., 1988; Plack & Moore, 1990). Note that this does not mean that the temporal acuity of the auditory system is of that order; only that the sliding temporal window within which the representation of stimulus energy shows significant smearing has that duration. Parenthetically, one should perhaps not construe such a temporal window as a selected-for feature in neural evolution; it might simply be an emergent property of the neural hardware and/or perceptual-sampling mechanisms.

Something of a modification of the decrement-detection view of gap detection has been offered by Oxenham (1997; see also Florentine et al., 1999). Oxenham provided modeling evidence that while one might construe decrement (and therefore gap) detection as some kind of discontinuity detection in the channel activated by the sound, the discontinuity being detected is the onset of the trailing marker, rather than reduction of energy at the offset of the leading marker. In this regard, Oxenham pointed out that the detectability of the rise in energy after a stimulus decrement would be sensitive to the duration of the decrement if "masking" of the decrement by the prior pedestal were significant. By this view, it is the slope of output of the temporal window that plays significantly into the decision about the presence of the gap. As will be seen below, this shift in emphasis from detection of the energy decrement at gap onset, towards detection of energy increment at gap offset, is paralleled in neurophysiological studies (Barsz et al., 1998; Eggermont 1999, 2000), and in animal behavioral studies (Ison et al., 2002). This account is not without question, however. Allen et al. (2002) showed (using noise stimuli) that human listeners are sensitive to marker-ramp configuration only to the extent that changes in the ramp also change the effective gap duration. That observation favors a model of gap detection based on detection of loudness or energy level changes. This finding is thus in contrast to conclusions drawn from modeling efforts that suggest that the detectability of the onset of the trailing marker may play a significant role in

determining gap-detection thresholds (Florentine et al., 1999; Oxenham, 1997). Allen et al.'s (2002) conclusion has recently been supported by Plack et al. (2006), who studied ramp shape for its effects on increment and decrement detection. Plack et al. (2006) found that rapid envelope changes contributed little to the detection for threshold-magnitude increments and decrements.

It is difficult to know exactly what to conclude from these disparate findings. Detection of threshold-level gaps based on sensitivity to trailing marker onset is attractive because of the fact that stimuli with abrupt onsets best synchronize neural responses and thus provide a salient neural substrate for event detection. It is possible, however, that the simple detection of a threshold-level gap is based on response-rate decrement among sustained-firing neurons that are common in the auditory brainstem, while discrimination responses may be based on representations in higher centers where transient responses are often dominant.

A further question for within-channel gap detection concerns the importance of the temporal proximity of the silent period to the onset of the leading marker or the offset of the trailing marker, that is, the temporal location of the silent period within the signal. Studies with highly practiced listeners often show that gap-detection thresholds are independent of the temporal location of the gap (Forrest & Green, 1987; Phillips et al., 1997). Other authors have found that gap thresholds are elevated when the leading or trailing marker is very short, particularly in relatively unpractised listeners (Phillips et al., 1998; Snell et al., 1999) or in older ones (Schneider & Hamstra, 1999). The reasons for the existence of marker-duration effects are unclear. One might be tempted to account for the marker-duration effects in terms of non-simultaneous, energetic-masking phenomena, that is, sensitivity reductions for very short leading or trailing markers based on adaptive or other responses to the temporally proximate, more energetic marker (backward and forward masking, respectively). Certainly, the auditory system is replete with examples of such sensitivity adjustments at behavioral and neurophysiological levels (Phillips, 1990; Phillips et al., 2002; Schneider & Hamstra, 1999; Smith, 1977). Having said that, why this particular behavioral expression of such adjustments might be susceptible to practice effects is unclear. It is perhaps possible that some listeners learn to deliberately employ the detectability of the shorter marker as a cue to the signal.

"Between-Channel" Gap Detection

The perceptual operations involved in gap detection become more complicated when the temporal gap is bounded by dissimilar markers (Divenyi & Danner, 1977; Formby & Forrest, 1991; Formby et al., 1996, 1998; Grose et al., 1999, 2001; Oxenham, 2000; Phillips & Hall, 2000;Phillips et al., 1997, 1998, 1999; see Figure 3–2, right). If the markers have non-overlapping spectra, or are presented to different ears, then the perceptual process used to detect the silent period must be central in origin and between-channel in nature. It must be central because there is no peripheral machinery available to sample activity in both of the channels activated by the stimulus. It is between-channel in the sense that detection of the silent period may require a relative timing of the offset of activity in the channel driven by the leading marker, and the onset of activity in the channel representing the trailing marker. Note also that both the signal and standard in these between-channel paradigms necessarily contain a perceptible discontinuity, as the stimulus switches from the leading to trailing marker; only the signal contains a non-zero duration silent period. Subjects find the between-channel task more difficult, and the adaptive-tracking functions that emerge from gap-threshold determinations are more variable in shape (Heinz et al., 1996). All of these data suggest that the perceptual operation required to detect the silent period between the markers is more complex than that involved in the classical within-channel paradigm.

Between-channel gap thresholds, whether studied with acoustic stimuli in normal listeners, or with electrical stimuli in cochlear implantees (Chatterjee et al., 1998; Van Wieringen & Wouters, 1999), are almost always longer than within-channel thresholds in the same listeners. Between-channel paradigms have most often employed tonal markers of different frequencies, or bandpass noise markers that differ in spectral content (e.g., Formby & Forrest, 1991; Formby et al., 1996, 1998; Phillips et al., 1997;

Williams & Perrott, 1972). Gap thresholds increase with increasing spectral distance between the markers, with the caveat that in some listeners there is a plateau effect, with gap thresholds at asymptotic maxima for trailing markers significantly higher in frequency than leading ones (Formby et al., 1996, Phillips et al., 1997). The absolute value of the threshold difference between within- and between-channel conditions can be as great as an order of magnitude; thus listeners with within-channel thresholds for bandpass noises on the order of 5 ms may have between-channel thresholds closer to 40 to 50 ms.

For example, Phillips and Smith (2004) used 0.25-octave bandpass noises centered on 4.0 kHz and 1.0 kHz to obtain within- and between-channel gap thresholds from 95 normal-hearing listeners, ranging in age from 18 to 57 years. Leading and trailing markers were of 10 and 300 ms duration respectively, and stimuli were presented at 30 to 40 dB sensation level. Thresholds were obtained using a two-down/one-up adaptive-tracking method. The distributions of gap thresholds for the within-channel conditions were highly peaked and centered on quite small values (means ± standard deviations were 5.06 ± 2.19 ms and 8.43 ± 3.66 ms, for 4.0 and 1.0 kHz noise, respectively). These values were comparable to those reported for practised listeners in psychophysical studies (see Eddins et al., 1992). In contrast, the between-channel thresholds for the same listeners, obtained using 4 kHz leading markers and 1.0 kHz trailing markers were very broadly distributed (mean ± s.d. = 28.68 ± 18.87 ms) and only very rarely were in the range of within-channel thresholds. The between-channel thresholds were, however, in keeping with values from the same (Phillips et al., 1997, 1998, Phillips & Hall, 2000) and other laboratories using other between-channel stimulus designs (Formby et al., 1998; Grose et al., 1999, 2001; Oxenham, 2000).

The long gap thresholds seen when the gap's markers differ significantly in frequency are also seen for spectrally identical markers that differ in ear of presentation (Phillips et al., 1997; see also Penner, 1977 for an earlier demonstration that this might be the case). Using 4-kHz narrowband noises, Phillips et al. showed that "within-ear" gap thresholds were typically on the order of 4 to 5 ms, but that "between-ear" thresholds were, on average, closer to 20 ms, and even longer if the leading marker was very short. Interestingly, if the leading marker was presented to one ear, while the trailing marker was presented diotically (i.e., with zero interaural level difference), then gap thresholds were comparable to the "within-ear" cases. The diotic task, of course, offers the listener a special opportunity to attend selectively to the stimulus at either ear alone, and so it is possible that the similarity in the monotic and dichotic conditions reflects the use of that strategy.

Between-channel gap thresholds appear to be more prone to significant individual differences than are within-channel thresholds, and it is often the case that there are longer learning curves in between-channel paradigms, that is, more experience is required for listeners to reach best performance (minimum thresholds; Phillips et al., 1997). Furthermore, gap thresholds in between-channel tasks are often sensitive to the duration of the leading marker, with gap thresholds increasing for leading markers shorter than about 30 ms. This effect is not seen in all listeners, but in listeners showing the effect, it is robust in the face of amplitude adjustments that equate leading and trailing markers for sensation level, and in the case of markers presented to different ears (Phillips et al., 1997). These two stimulus configurations make it highly unlikely that the leading marker duration effect has its genesis in peripheral masking or adaptation phenomena. Again, these phenomena illustrate that between-channel gap detection likely involves higher-level perceptual-cognitive operations. The existence of marked individual differences in absolute between-channel gap-detection thresholds, and in the vulnerability of those thresholds to stimulus manipulations, suggests that different listeners might employ different perceptual strategies to execute the task. It should be noted, however, that not all authors have seen systematic evidence of leading-marker duration effects in between-channel gap detection (Grose et al., 2001; Oxenham, 2000).

Following the work of Fitzgibbons et al. (1974), one hypothesis is that the mechanisms involved in between-channel gap detection are highly cognitive (Phillips et al., 1997). It proposes that detection of leading marker offset requires attention allocation to the perceptual channel representing that marker, that there is then a time-consuming attentional shift to the channel activated by the trailing marker, and it is only after that shift has occurred that the onset of the trailing marker can be timed relative to attentional allocation to that channel. The shortest detectable gap thus must exceed any attentional dwell time on the leading marker channel (if the leading marker is shorter in duration than that dwell time), plus the mandatory switch time. Neither of these is required in within-channel gap detection, and it is for this reason that between-channel thresholds are so much longer than within-channel thresholds. Note that this hypothesis predicts longer gap thresholds for stimuli with short leading marker durations, though the predicted relationship is not exactly of the form seen empirically (Phillips et al., 1997). A related, but lower level hypothesis is simply that allocation of attention to the channel activated by the leading marker reduces resources available for the time-stamping of events in any other channel (Phillips et al., 1997). This suggestion is a minor elaboration of the fact that selective attention to one frequency channel can reduce the detection rate of threshold-level events in unattended channels (Scharf et al., 1987).

Forrest and Formby (1996) provided a different explanation of why gap-detection thresholds are elevated for sinusoidal markers that differ in frequency. Their model is based on the hypothesis that the temporal gap detection is mediated by the peripheral frequency channel lying between those centered on the frequencies of the two markers. For small marker-frequency separations, the single-channel model does a good job of approximating human gap thresholds. Once the frequency separation is beyond about an octave, the two markers no longer activate a single peripheral channel, and gap detection must rely on some other, perhaps relative-timing, operation on the activity in different channels. For these large frequency separations, gap-detection thresholds may become asymptotic both in modeling efforts (Forrest & Formby, 1996) and in human behavior (Formby et al., 1998).

Grose et al. (1999) offered a novel experiment that helps to clarify the nature of the processes involved in between-channel gap detection. Their stimuli were pairs of tones, each present throughout each (signal and standard) interval. The "gap" to be detected existed only in the envelope of a modulating 8-Hz sinusoid imposed on one carrier in the leading marker, and in the other carrier tone for the trailing marker. The "gap" itself was an interruption in the continuity of the modulating waveform. In this "modulation gap detection," the temporal event to be recovered was one that traversed frequency, but with the twist that both frequencies were continuously present. The authors reported that when the temporal event existed in a single frequency, gap thresholds were in the range from about 12 to 20 ms; in the between-channel cases studied, gap thresholds were 80 to 150 ms, or were above the authors' 250-ms measurement limit. When the modulation gap-detection paradigm was extended to the case of an isofrequency carrier, but presented "across ears" (following Phillips et al., 1997), then gap thresholds were again high. The absolute values of gap thresholds in Grose et al. (1999)'s study were higher than those in the Phillips and Smith (1999) data set, but this is unsurprising given the differences in stimulus design. What matters is that between-channel gap detection thresholds were poorer than within-channel thresholds in the same listeners, that the effect size was dramatic, and extended to include both "across frequency" and "across ear" paradigms.

It is thus likely that between-channel temporal gap detection relies not simply on a discontinuity detection, but on some form of relative timing of activity in the channels activated by the two markers. Two further, independent lines of empirical evidence support the general hypothesis that the mechanisms mediating the two forms of gap detection are separable. First, Lister, et al. (2000) showed, using quite long gap markers, that between-channel thresholds appear to be more susceptible to deleterious effects of aging than are within-channel gap thresholds in the same listeners. Second, Phillips and Smith (2004; see above) showed that in a given set of listeners, gap thresholds for different within-channel stimuli tend to be highly correlated with each other, whereas within-channel and between-channel gap thresholds tend to be poorly correlated with each other. Within-channel gap thresholds for 1.0 kHz noise and those for 4.0 kHz noise in the same listeners were highly correlated ($r = 0.74$, $p < 0.0001$), and the relationship accounted for 54.1% of the variance in the data. By comparison, gap thresholds for the between-channel task were more weakly correlated

with those for either the 1.0 kHz ($r = 0.29$, $p < 0.01$) or the 4.0 kHz noise within-channel conditions ($r = 0.43$, $p < 0.001$). These correlations accounted for only 8.4% and 18.9%, respectively, of the variance in the two data sets. Because of the within-subjects design, one would expect all of the measures to show some degree of correlation. It is the fact that the correlation between the two within-channel gap thresholds is greater than that for either of the other data sets (*t*-test, $p < 0.001$ in both cases) that argues for the separability of the processes mediating the two kinds of gap-detection performance.

Finally, there is a question as to whether strictly central effects in between-channel gap detection are larger or smaller than peripheral ones. This is a difficult question to ask (e.g., because we need to be very clear about what constitutes a "peripheral" or "central" effect), and a very difficult one to answer, because it requires that the stimulus manipulations used to compare peripheral and central effect sizes on gap thresholds produce markers of equivalent perceptual dissimilarity (Grose et al., 2001; Phillips & Hall, 2000). One recent study (Phillips & Hall, 2002) used low- and high-pass noises as markers in a between-channel paradigm, and systematically varied the amount of overlap and separation of the marker spectra. That study found that in stimuli with sufficient within-channel marker energy to support very low gap thresholds, the presence of irrelevant stimulus energy (which altered the pitch of the markers) was sufficient to elevate gap thresholds. Grose et al. (2001) have presented comparable data: they showed that gap detection thresholds often deteriorated if the bandwidths of the markers differed, even when the spectral content of a narrowband marker was subsumed within that of a wideband marker with which it was paired. These data suggest that the perceptual dissimilarity of the markers can override the availability of within-channel information that would otherwise support very low gap thresholds. Oxenham (2000) measured gap detection thresholds using unresolved harmonic tone complexes as markers bounding the gap. In one set of conditions, the markers had the same spectral envelopes but different fundamental frequencies (and therefore different pitches); in other conditions, the fundamental frequencies of the leading and trailing markers were the same, but the markers had different spectral envelopes. By comparison with within-channel "control" stimuli, both of the between-channel paradigms resulted in longer gap thresholds. This effect was greater in the case of markers differing in spectral envelope. This was taken to suggest that gap detection thresholds are more sensitive to marker differences in peripheral input patterns than to differences in central processing of shared peripheral inputs. It is possible, however, that the *perceptual* dissimilarity of the markers was not equivalent in the two designs.

Neurophysiology of Gap Detection

We mentioned above that, for within-channel designs, direct recordings from the cochlear nerve in chinchillas reveal that averaged spike trains are capable of encoding silent periods located late in a noise stimulus almost as short as those detectable behaviorally (Zhang et al., 1990). The same may be true for the mouse auditory midbrain (Walton et al., 1997). As one ascends the auditory neuraxis, however, sustained discharges become less common, and responses to acoustic stimulation become increasingly dominated by an onset transient (Phillips et al., 2002). This has the consequence that the central neural representation of the temporal gap resides more in the presence of a response to the onset of the trailing marker than it does in a quiescent period following the offset of the leading marker (e.g., Barsz et al., 1998; Eggermont, 1999). Insofar as the neural representation or correlate of gap-detection threshold is concerned, this has resulted in a shift in emphasis from analyzing spike activity during the energy decrement (e.g., Zhang et al., 1990) to the detectability of a response to trailing-marker onset. This shift parallels that suggested independently in human psychophysics (Oxenham, 1997), although it is at variance with the more recent psychophysical efforts that show gap-detection thresholds to be uninfluenced by envelope shape *per se* (Allen et al., 2002; Plack et al., 2006). This is surprising, because one would have expected rapid envelope changes (viz., onset of the trailing marker) to best synchronize neural responses and so optimize the possibility of a salient response to serve as a substrate for gap detection.

Eggermont (1999, 2000) has studied the cortical coding of gap stimuli in cats. In one study, he compared the encoding of gaps placed 5 ms (early) or 500 ms (late) after the onset of a wideband noise stimulus. Cortical neural responses are dominated by brief responses to onset transients (Phillips et al., 2002), and Eggermont used the presence of such a response to the onset of the trailing marker as evidence of the neural detection of the stimulus gap. For late gaps, minimal gap "thresholds" clustered around 5 and 10 ms or less, although the tail of the distribution of thresholds extended to 60 ms. For early gaps, minimum encodable gaps were broadly distributed, with only a small minority of neurons responding to gaps less than 5 to 10 ms in duration. Some of those neurons responded *selectively* to short gaps, suggesting the operation of some form of synaptic facilitation or perhaps a delay in a postonset after-hyperpolarization (see Eggermont, 1999; Phillips et al., 2002) which would otherwise terminate the response to noise onset and prevent a response to trailing marker onset at longer durations. Eggermont suggested that human behavioral gap-detection performance across various temporal-gap locations likely follows the envelope of the thresholds of the neurons with the greatest gap sensitivities for those locations.

In a subsequent study of cat cortical cells, Eggermont (2000) argued that the neural encoding of between-channel gap stimuli might be based on the onset responses to the leading and trailing markers. He showed, using *within*-channel stimuli, that minimally detectable gaps decreased in exponential fashion with increases in leading-marker duration, with an asymptote near 50 or 100 ms, and that this behavior was well modeled by properties of synaptic depression and after-hyperpolarization driven by the leading marker. The pattern of minimally detectable gaps showed a striking similarity to that seen in behavioral studies of *between*-channel gap detection (Phillips et al., 1997). Eggermont argued that to link the two bodies of data, one simply needed to postulate the existence of single cells receiving input with these temporal properties, but from separate frequency channels, or the existence of neural assemblies representing the activity of the two channels. This issue needs further study, perhaps in the form of experiments directly examining the cortical coding of between-channel gap stimuli. Note, though, that this account of the neurophysiology of between-channel gap detection does smack of "grandmother cells," that is, the notion that a strictly single-unit account of the perception of complex sounds is required at all. It is, arguably, just as likely that the relative timing operation does not exploit a single-unit representation of the combined stimulus.

Human Perceptual Channels for Auditory Azimuth

Following traditional cognitive science (Broadbent, 1958; Moray, 1969), channels need not be restricted to those defined by peripheral wiring. "Information enters the system through a number of parallel sensory channels. In addition to obvious channels such as the left and right auditory nerves, the visual pathways, and so forth, a channel may also be a position in auditory space or a wave envelope of a particular fundamental frequency or similar functional channels. These are presumed to have a distinct neural representation somewhere in the brain, which allows messages to be selected on the basis of their pitch, loudness, and spatial location characteristics" (Moray, 1969, p. 28). In this regard, between-channel gap thresholds in normal listeners for markers distinguished by pitch but not by spectral disposition are also high (Oxenham, 2000), and in cochlear implantees, gap thresholds are higher for markers that differ in pulse rate or amplitude than for those that don't (Chatterjee et al., 1998). The pitch examples in particular constitute elegant evidence on the purely central contribution to gap detection.

Following the demonstration of between-channel effects on gap thresholds through the "ear" dimension (Phillips et al. 1997), Phillips et al (1998) reported that free-field markers on opposite (left or right) sides of the head, but not free-field markers at the same locus on either side, also produced between-channel effects on gap thresholds for wideband noise stimuli, namely elevated thresholds and an effect of leading-marker duration in most listeners. Later, Boehnke and Phillips (1999) used the free-field gap-detection paradigm to explore the tuning of perceptual channels for azimuth in man. For leading wideband noise markers positioned at

each of a number of azimuths, they measured gap thresholds for stimuli in which the trailing marker was located elsewhere in azimuth. They reasoned that for leading and trailing markers in the same perceptual channel, gap thresholds would be low, and that longer gap thresholds would reflect the extent to which leading and trailing markers were located in different perceptual channels. Their main finding was that azimuthal channels had (left and right) hemifield tuning, with medial borders straddling the midline. These psychophysical "channels" displayed the same azimuthal tuning as do the free-field spatial receptive fields of cortical neurons in animals (see Stecker et al., 2005; Phillips, 2008). Neural receptive fields are generated by the conjunction of binaural interactions (sensitivity to interaural time and intensity disparities—which likely contribute to receptive field boundaries) and pinna directionality and head-shadow effects (which likely shape response strength within the receptive field: see Phillips and Brugge, 1985, for review). In this regard, neurophysiologic data suggest that each auditory forebrain processes spatial information only for the contralateral acoustic hemifield (Phillips & Brugge, 1985; Phillips & Irvine, 1981), and behavioral data indicate that unilateral auditory forebrain lesions create sound localization deficits only for sources in the contralateral hemifield (Jenkins & Masterton, 1982; Jenkins & Merzenich, 1984; Kavanagh & Kelly, 1987). The behavior-lesion data do not speak to the spatial tuning of individual elements in the cerebral representation, but only to the range of azimuths encoded in the ablated structure. In this sense, the behavior-lesion data are certainly compatible with the hemifield spatial receptive fields seen in single-unit studies. The hemifield tuning of human psychophysical channels for space thus appeared congruent with independent neurophysiological evidence on spatial coding in animals.

Oxenham (2000), however, quite correctly pointed out that markers located at different eccentricities not only produce different *interaural* disparities (thus available for binaural coding) but also different proximal stimuli at *either ear alone*, notably through the effects of the head shadow. Accordingly, if the proximal stimuli for the markers differ at one ear, then that difference might limit the peripheral encoding of the gap available for central elaboration (notably through masking effects). In turn, this means that the psychophysical tuning of spatial channels described by Boehnke and Phillips might reflect monaural mechanisms in addition to binaural ones. Thus, without disputing the spatial tuning itself, there is some debate about the balance of mechanisms in which that tuning has its genesis. Interestingly, highly similar patterns of dependence on spatial location to those in Boehnke and Phillips (1999) can be seen in the free-field release from masking data provided by Saberi et al (1991) and Phillips et al. (2003). This issue is somewhat difficult to resolve in a satisfying manner, because changes in the locations of free-field markers generate changes in interaural stimulus parameters and changes in monaural marker levels that are perfectly correlated with each other.

Whatever the origins of the spatial channels, the channel architecture itself offers new insights into a variety of spatial phenomena in hearing. Cocktail party effects (e.g., Cherry, 1953; Yost et al., 1996) and spatial release from masking effects (Kidd et al., 1998) all should exploit the two-channel architecture such that the perceptual elaboration of a target signal in the presence of a spatially separate distractor will be more efficient when the signal and distractor occupy different spatial channels. Note that it should be the location of signal and distractor relative to the perceptual channels that matters, as much as the absolute spatial separation of the stimuli. Empirically, this is the case: a 90-degree separation of source and distractor results in a greater access to the signal if the two stimuli are in different spatial channels than if they occupy the same channel (Phillips et al., 2003). There is some effort at developing clinical tools for measuring speech intelligibility in the presence of noise in the free-field (Nilsson et al., 1994; Soli & Nilsson, 1994). Such efforts might benefit by being informed by the spatial-channel hypothesis, so that it would be possible to probe spatial release from masking within auditory hemifields separately.

Gap Detection and Voice Onset Time Phonetic Boundaries

When the leading marker is short in a between-channel gap-detection paradigm, the stimulus begins

to have spectrotemporal properties that resemble a stop-consonant-vowel (CV) syllable, that is, one spectral event (consonantal burst, with most energy at high frequencies) followed by a period of relative quiet, followed by the resumption of sound (vowel, with most energy at low frequencies). What makes this interesting is that CV syllables for the same place of articulation are distinguished by voice onset time (VOT; e.g., /ba/ and /pa/), and the VOT continuum has the unusual property of supporting distinctly "categorical" perception. That is, presented with CV exemplars differing only in VOT, subjects label exemplars from short VOT range exclusively as the voiced member of the CV pair (e.g., /ba/), and those from the long VOT end of the continuum as the unvoiced member of the pair (/pa/). The VOT associated with the switch in phonetic identity of the stimulus is known as the phonetic boundary. It takes the form of an abrupt shift in label selection, reflecting an abrupt switch from one percept to the other. The general finding ultimately led to the proposal of "linguistic feature detectors" in spoken language processing (Eimas & Corbit, 1973). Somewhat later, Kuhl and Miller (1978) showed that chinchillas also displayed categorical perception of VOTs. In the face of nonlinguistic animals showing categorical perception of VOTs, Kuhl and Miller made the important discussion point that the speech system might exploit natural psychophysical discontinuities, that is, that some phonetic boundaries in speech might be built on some sort of psychophysical boundaries.

At that time, the identities of the relevant psychophysical discontinuities were unclear, but evidence from studies of between-channel gap detection has offered one possibility. Recall that when markers bounding a gap differ significantly in spectrum, gap-detection thresholds are not uncommonly in the range from 20 to 40 ms, that is, in the same range as VOT phonetic boundaries. This finding extends to the case of stimuli with spectrotemporal configurations specifically designed as analogs of CV syllables (Phillips et al., 1997), and has been used as circumstantial evidence that between-channel gap threshold may be one determinant of VOT phonetic boundaries (Phillips et al., 1997; Phillips & Smith, 2004). The account has some viability, first, because mean between-channel gap thresholds have values in the same range as VOT boundaries, and second, because the distinction between detectable and undetectable gaps is arguably a categorical one.

Elangovan and Stuart (2008) took this line of argument a step further. They measured within- and between-channel gap thresholds, and perceptual VOT boundaries, in the same listeners. They showed that between-channel gap thresholds were highly correlated with perceptual VOT boundaries, while within-channel gap thresholds were not. This is not to say that between-channel gap thresholds were equal in value to VOT boundaries in the Elangovan and Stuart study, only that they were correlated. In natural speech, exemplars of voiced and unvoiced consonants for the same articulatory place likely also differ in factors other than VOT (e.g., Soli, 1983). The covariation of multiple stimulus features might help explain the difference in absolute values of gap thresholds and VOT boundaries in that study, and the steepness of the phonetic boundary.

Evidence on the further relevance of these findings is available. Children with specific language impairment display less obvious categorical perception and production of CV syllables distinguished by VOT than do unimpaired children. Thus, the measured VOTs from voiced and unvoiced stop consonants have overlapping distributions in language-impaired children, but not in controls (Stark & Tallal, 1979), and differential responses to consonant-vowel syllables differing only in VOT are also impaired (Tallal & Stark, 1980). These data in themselves do not mean that between-channel gap detection processes are at fault in developmental language delay. Interestingly, however, adults with acquired aphasia display more severe deficits in between-channel gap processing than in within-channel gap processing (Stefanatos et al., 2007; Sidiropoulos et al., 2010). In this general regard, Walker et al. (2006) showed that phonological reading performance in normally developing, unselected readers was correlated with between-channel gap detection performance, but not with within-channel performance; in contrast, orthographic reading performance was more highly correlated with within-channel gap detection performance. Highly proficient adult readers tend to have low (good) within-channel gap thresholds (Au & Lovegrove, 2001a,b). These observations, drawn from all parts of the language/reading performance continuum, serve to reinforce the general hypothesis of an association between "temporal processing" performance on the one hand, and language performance on the other.

This raises the question of whether the dominance of language in the left cerebral hemisphere reflects a greater temporal acuity on that side (e.g., Creese, 1999). Studies of gap-detection thresholds have provided conflicting data on this point. Detailed studies of normal listeners have failed to find ear, and therefore hemispheric, asymmetries in within-channel (Baker et al., 2008; Carmichael et al., 2008) or between-channel gap thresholds (Carmichael et al., 2008) even when contralateral masking is employed. Other recent studies have found a significant right-ear superiority in within-channel gap-detection thresholds or gap processing (Brown & Nicholls, 1997; Nicholls et al., 1999; Sininger & deBode, 2008), although the effect appears to be highly stimulus dependent (e.g., Sininger & deBode, 2008; Sulakhe et al., 2003).

Question 1

Does gap detection show any relation to speech perception? If so, what types of errors (problems) do people with impaired temporal processing show?

Answer 1

One of the most explicit studies on the relation between gap detection and speech perception is that by Elangovan and Stuart (2008). They studied within- and between-channel gap thresholds and perceptual phonetic boundaries for a /ba/-/pa/ continuum in the same listeners. They found that between-channel gap thresholds were highly correlated with the voice onset time boundary (VOT, in ms), whereas within-channel gap thresholds were not. Although these data are correlational, they do suggest that there may be a contribution of the between-channel timing process(es) to the formation of phonetic (VOT) boundaries. That view is consistent with a history of earlier evidence (Kuhl & Miller, 1978; Phillips & Smith, 2004).

The applied question is more awkward to address in a satisfying way. First, most studies of the relation between speech perception errors and temporal processing performance begin with a clinically defined population and seek to determine if there are temporal processing correlates of the disorder (e.g., Stefanatos et al., 1989, 2007), rather than the other way around. Second, "temporal processing" is an umbrella term, and so the spectrum of perceptual/cognitive difficulties to be expected of patients with impaired temporal processing is likely as diverse and subtle as the processes caught in "temporal processing's" umbrella. Third, although this chapter has been about some temporal processes in hearing, temporal factors are inherently involved in all brain information processing. Thus, it is not at all difficult to imagine that a temporal processing deficit could find expression in multiple sensory, cognitive and/or motor systems. This is not a new conclusion. Tallal et al. (1981) saw multimodal temporal processing deficits in young children with language-learning impairments, and it continues to be an issue in how best to conceptualize central "auditory" processing disorders (Cacace & McFarland, 1998). Finally, it is good to remember that temporal processing deficits present early in childhood might impair language acquisition or reading or cognition, but then resolve. By that point, however, some children may well have learned to avoid the tasks at which they are poor and thus be somewhat isolated from situations which might promote their skills. This leaves the older child with no overt auditory or temporal processing disorder at a time at which they do have poor language or cognitive skills. If we have only one measurement point, and it is from later childhood, then the relationship between basic perceptual processing performance and concurrent language or cognitive performance may be seen as weak. This is one of the reasons for the importance of longitudinal developmental studies.

DOMINANCE OF STIMULUS ONSETS

Psychophysics

One of the interesting areas of study to emerge in the modern auditory psychophysical literature is that of temporal asymmetries in hearing (Phillips et al, 2002). By this we mean that the percepts evoked by a brief, temporally asymmetric sound and its temporally reversed analog are unexpectedly different, particularly given that the two sounds are spectrally identical. Most often, this asymmetry has been demonstrated using asymmetrically modulated carriers. Thus, periodically damped sinusoids (i.e., those with an abrupt onset and a slower decay) are described as sounding like a tapping on a hollow wooden block, while their temporally reversed analogs, ramped sinusoids, sound more like a thumping on a nonresonant surface, but in the presence of a continuous tone at the carrier frequency (Irino & Patterson, 1996; Patterson, 1994a,1994b). The fact that a temporally asymmetric sound and its temporally reversed analog are perceptually different is unsurprising: what is important here is the unexpected nature of the perceptual differences, for example, the distinction between the percussive quality of damped sinusoids and the presence of the continuous tone in ramped ones.

This kind of asymmetry extends to modulations of noise carriers: the percept evoked by ramped noise has a continuous hiss whereas that evoked by damped noise does not (Akeroyd & Patterson, 1995). This is important, because it suggests that the reasons for the perceptual asymmetry do not reside in a strictly temporal (phase-locking) neural code of the stimuli. Consider the following. When the carrier is a sinusoid, a damped tone begins with an abrupt onset which likely activates a broad array of low-frequency cochlear channels which will "ring" at their own preferred frequencies. In contrast, the ramped sinusoid is likely to drive phase-locked carrier responses in a narrow range of cochlear neurons tuned near the carrier frequency. This distinction in the auditory encoding process appears plausibly to account for the percussive quality of damped sinusoids and the presence of the continuous tone in the percept of the ramped one. However, when noise is the carrier signal, there is little or no such opportunity for differential phase-locked responses, yet the perceptual asymmetry exists nonetheless.

Patterson and his colleagues have generated an "auditory image model" that provides an understanding of this behavior. The model begins with conceptualizing the cochlea as a filter bank whose output is a neural activation pattern constituted by the array of cochlear nerve fibers. It assumes that each cochlear frequency channel has a decaying output, and that this output is subject to a "strobelike integrator" mechanism. The output of the integrator is then supplied to a static image buffer, and the complete array of those strobe-integrated signals constitutes the model's representation of the auditory image of the sound. The model emphasizes that the strobe integrator has an adaptive threshold, so that the threshold for the next "snapshot" is set in part by the stimulus level of the preceding snapshot. This has the consequence that more strobe snapshots are obtained on the rising slope of an auditory amplitude envelope than on the falling slope, and it is for this reason that more information is extracted from sound onsets, and/or that sound onsets are perceptually more heavily weighted (after Irino & Patterson, 1996; Akeroyd & Patterson, 1995; Phillips et al., 2002).

As discussed in more detail elsewhere (Phillips et al., 2002), there are now many documented examples and correlates of this perceptual asymmetry. Listeners are more sensitive to gating transients at sound onsets than to those at sound offsets (Miyaska & Sakai, 1982). Sounds with slow onsets and abrupt decays are judged as louder than their temporally reversed counterparts (Stecker & Hafter, 2000). Akeroyd and Patterson (1997) tested listeners' abilities to detect and to discriminate noise modulated by temporally symmetric and temporally asymmetric waveforms. *Detection* of symmetric and asymmetric modulations were comparable up to quite high rates, but *discrimination* of the stimuli was most difficult when the modulating waveforms differed only in their falling shapes.

The perceptual dominance of sound onsets is expressed in other ways as well. First, as mentioned above, one account of within-channel gap-detection mechanisms suggests that gap thresholds may be determined by the slope of the monaural temporal window output, that is, by the detectability of the trailing marker's onset, rather than by the detectability of the energy decrement per se. Second, it is possible to construct sounds whose interaural-onset delay is different from the interaural delay of the ongoing sound. When the ongoing delay provides weak or ambiguous laterality information, the interaural onset delay dominates the percept (Freyman et al., 1997; Kunov & Abel, 1981). Aoki and Houtgast (1992; Houtgast & Aoki,1994) studied responses to brief noise bursts in which the first half of the sound had an interaural disparity lateralizing the source to one side, whereas the second half of the stimulus had an equivalent disparity favoring the opposite ear. When listeners were required to judge the "overall sensation," the temporal location of the switchpoint had to be shifted significantly toward sound onset in order for the perceptual dominance of the sound onset to be overcome. Third, in speech, the onsets of acoustic events across the frequency domain are important cues to phonetic identity (Howell & Rosen 1983; Rosen, 1992). Fourth, in music, the rate of sound onset contributes significantly to the determination of perceptual attack time and timbre (Gordon, 1987; Rosen & Howell, 1981; Saldanha & Corso, 1964). Finally, the temporal coherence of sound onsets is one of the most important stimulus parameters that promotes the perceptual grouping of energy in different frequency bands into single events (Bregman 1990; Turgeon et al., 2002). This factor may be significant in temporal gap-detection processes for those instances in which the disposition of spectral energy on the two edges of the gap is asymmetric (Formby et al., 1998; Phillips & Hall, 2002).

Neurophysiology

There has been a long-standing interest in the fashion and fidelity with which the auditory nervous system can encode or "represent" the time structure of sounds. For our immediate purposes, there are two general kinds of time structure that we need to address. One is periodicities, and the other is singular or isolated auditory event times. In the paragraphs that follow, our goal is to describe some of the basic phenomenology of the two types of temporal neural coding, and to emphasize the extent to which the auditory forebrain has preserved the temporal precision of coding developed in the auditory periphery.

Perhaps the most basic form of periodicity coding is phase-locking of auditory nerve fiber action potentials to a tonal stimulus. Phase-locking arises from the fact that cochlear hair cell neurotransmitter release is proportional to membrane depolarization, which in turn is driven by upward motion of the basilar membrane (toward scala vestibuli). For frequencies that do not exceed the low-pass filtering of the transduction process, this has the consequence that periodic upward motions of the basilar membrane are preserved in the spike times of cochlear nerve cells. In turn, the central nervous system can recover the frequency content of the sound, either by sampling the interspike intervals of spike trains within individual neurons across time, or by sampling across neurons for a short time.

There are a number of ways to quantify the temporal fidelity of this encoding, and these are based on the degree to which spike times are synchronized with the phase of the stimulus waveform. In the cochlear nerve, phase-locking for single tones is strongest at low frequencies, but remains detectable at frequencies up to about 3000 Hz. If phase-locking to the sinusoidal amplitude modulation of high-frequency carrier is studied, then phase locking to the modulating waveform is a little poorer, again being best at low frequencies, but detectable as high as about 1500 Hz (Joris & Yin, 1992). The temporal fidelity of this coding, expressed as the cutoff frequency in the lowpass function, declines with each ascending station along the auditory neuraxis. By the level of the cortex, phase-locked responses to single tones or to modulated carriers rarely are seen for modulating frequencies above about 40 to 60 Hz, at least in anesthetized animals (Eggermont, 1994). The reasons for this are unclear, although synaptic depression is a likely candidate mechanism (Eggermont, 2002). In unanesthetized animals, phase-locking to simple or complex sounds sometimes extends to modestly higher frequencies (Creutzfeldt

et al., 1980; Steinschneider et al., 1982). In awake primates studied with amplitude- and frequency-modulated tones, best modulation frequencies for cortical cells may extend into the hundreds of Hz range, but the responses at those modulation frequencies are rarely phase-locked ones (Liang et al., 2002). This suggests a shift in coding principle from a temporal code to a rate-based one.

The temporal precision of responses to auditory event onsets is usually measured as the standard deviation of the mean latency to the first spike. These standard deviations vary with a host of stimulus parameters, but in the cat's cochlear nerve, their minima tend to be less than a millisecond (Rhode & Smith, 1986). In the cat's auditory cortex, minimal standard deviations of first spike latencies are also generally less than a millisecond (Phillips & Hall, 1990). Thus, in stark contrast to the case for periodicity coding, the afferent auditory nervous system has preserved the precision of event onset timing. These onset responses, though short in duration, are sensitive to a wealth of stimulus parameters, including stimulus envelope shape at sound onset (Heil, 1997a,1997b), stimulus spectral content and amplitude (Phillips et al., 1994) and binaural properties (Semple & Kitzes, 1993; Kitzes, 2008). Because all of those stimulus parameters affect the spike rate of any given cortical neuron, the spike output of any given single-unit is an inherently ambiguous indicator of the set of stimulus parameters evoking the response. A disambiguation lies in the pattern of activity evoked by the stimulus across the tonotopic cortical neural array, because different neurons across the array will have different patterns of sensitivity to those parameters.

Stimulus onsets likely evoke these responses widely across the cortex, and so there will be a stimulus-dependent synchrony or correlation in the timing of responses to the same stimulus event across cortical neurons. Eggermont (1997) has shown that the combination of the intercortical synchrony of spike discharges and the absolute firing rates, distinguish the responses to stimulus onsets, stimulus amplitude changes, responses to steady-state stimuli, and spontaneous activity. Specifically, high intercortical synchrony and high spike rates differentiate responses to stimulus onsets from the other responses studied. This temporal coherence may be a contributor to the importance of stimulus onsets in perceptual binding.

The further question concerns the reasons for the prevalence of onset responses in the auditory forebrain. This topic has been discussed elsewhere in some detail (Phillips et al., 2002), and so will be mentioned only briefly here. The sustained response to acoustic stimulation seen in the cochlear nerve appears to be prone both to adaptation and to the development of post-onset hyperpolarization responses in central neurons, especially in the cortex (Eggermont, 1991, 1996; Phillips, 1985; Phillips & Sark, 1991). The adaptation component of the response is particularly interesting in the present context. First, it develops over a time course of milliseconds or tens of milliseconds (Phillips, 1985), and is likely built on short-term adaptation already present at the level of the cochlear nerve (Smith 1977). Second, it is a mechanism by which the tone threshold sensitivity of cortical neurons tracks the level of ongoing stimulation. Thus, the tone thresholds of cortical auditory cells adaptively track the level of background noise stimulation, and the threshold adjustments match background stimulus-level adjustments with a slope very close to unity (Phillips, 1990). Very similar behavior is seen psychophysically (Hawkins & Stevens, 1950). The fact that a single-unit's tone threshold tracks the level of a continuous noise background has the further effect that the cell's whole tone input-output function (dynamic range) is similarly adjusted. Figure 3–3 shows stylized impressions of one cell's tone input-output functions in the absence (tone alone, TA) and presence of a continuous wideband noise masker;

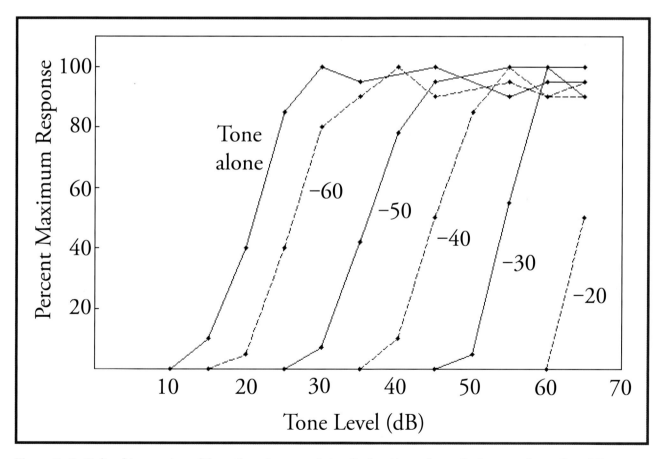

Figure 3–3. Stylized impression of the spike rate-versus-intensity functions of a cortical neuron for preferred-frequency tones presented in the absence (tone alone, TA) and presence of a continuous wideband noise masker. The parameter is the masker level, arbitrarily expressed in dB attenuation. Note that the tone threshold tracks the level of background noise, resulting in a displacement of the tone intensity function toward higher tone levels as masker level increases.

the parameter is the noise level, expressed arbitrarily in dB attenuation. The important point to be gleaned from Figure 3–3 is that once the noise level is sufficient to elevate tone thresholds, the whole tone intensity profile is shifted toward higher tone levels, and the magnitude of the shifts roughly match the increases in masker level. This has the interesting implication that the cell's tone intensity responses are driven by signal to noise ratio rather than by absolute stimulus level (Phillips, 1990), that is, the relevant intensity parameter for cortical cells is auditory "contrast" (Phillips et al., 1991). Recent data from event-related potential studies suggest that the human auditory cortex may behave in the same way (Billings et al., 2009).

To this point in the discussion, we have assumed that the mechanism mediating the responses to masked tones has been adaptation, and we should at least briefly examine the evidence for that assumption (see also Plack, 2005). We have already seen (above) that inhibitory responses are very common in cortical circuits, so it behooves us to try to disentangle at least those two. One circumstantial line of evidence derives from the fact that cortical cells differ in whether they are excited or inhibited by the presentation of noise *burst* stimuli; both cell types, however, show the dynamic range shifts seen for tones presented against *continuous* noise backgrounds. A second line of evidence comes from Phillips and Cynader (1985). They described studies of cortical cells' tone responses both against continuous noise maskers and against simultaneously gated ones. For cells that are inhibited by noise-burst stimuli, simultaneous gating of tones and noise results in a noise-level dependent suppression of the tone response, as might be expected. The latencies of the weakened tone responses are the same as those seen in the absence of the gated masker. In this paradigm, then, the level of the masker determines the level of the inhibitory response available to summate with the excitatory tone response; the response timing is that of the tone response itself. In contrast, when the same cells are studied with continuous noise backgrounds, the tone intensity function undergoes the now-familiar dynamic range shift, and so too do the cells' tone latency-intensity functions. The coupling of these spike rate and spike timing responses constitute a sensitivity shift for the tone when continu-

ous noise is present. It is this difference in the latency behavior of the responses seen in the two paradigms that suggests that adaptation is a significant mechanism mediating the sensitivity adjustments driven by continuous maskers.

The adaptation behavior is seen in other stimulus paradigms. When amplitude modulations of a carrier tone are presented as increments or decrements on a background, only increments are effective in evoking spikes (Phillips & Hall, 1987). When cortical neurons are studied with narrow frequency modulations presented in the form of a ramp of an ongoing tone, then only those frequency changes toward the center of a cell's effective frequency range are successful in evoking spikes; indeed, the strength of the cell's direction preference for frequency modulation is strikingly correlated with the slope of the cell's spike count versus frequency function over the excursion covered by the modulation (Phillips et al., 1985). The latter finding is easily interpreted as the neuron treating the frequency change as if it were an effective amplitude modulation of the excitatory drive on the neuron (Phillips & Hall, 1987). Still, more generally, the adaptation response may be one factor that makes the responses of cortical cells to a given stimulus so sensitive to the stimulus-response history that immediately preceded the stimulus (Phillips, 2001).

Note that this kind of adaptive behavior seen in the neurophysiology bears a strong resemblance to the adaptive threshold tracking proposed in Patterson's auditory image model (Phillips et al., 2002). This is not necessarily meant to imply that the former is the neurological instantiation of the latter; only that when two completely independent lines of research converge on a common hypothesis, there is likely some merit to it. What the congruence offers us here is a partial explanation for the perceptual dominance of auditory onsets: there is a more fully developed representation of auditory onsets in the nervous system, and this affords a greater information extraction from them. Lu et al. (2001) have recorded the responses of cortical neurons to periodically ramped and damped sinusoids (preferred- or characteristic-frequency tones) in unanesthetized primates (marmosets). Of the cells that showed systematic preferences for one over the other, preference was more common for ramped than damped carriers. Of some interest was the fact that responses to the periodic signals (i.e., the envelope shapes) were not themselves periodic, that is, the representation was in the form of a rate code rather then a temporal one.

Question 2

How does this information relate to spectral processing since speech contains both temporal and spectral cues?

Answer 2

This is a good question, but one that is not easy to answer. One approach to it might be based on patients with so-called "pure word deafness" (see Phillips, 1995, 1998; Stefanatos et al., 2005). This is a rare disorder, usually following bilateral damage to the auditory cortex, or damage to the left cortex and isolation of the right cortex from cerebral language processors. Because the condition is rare, there are relatively few detailed data on affected patients' psychophysical performance. Interestingly, however, the patients often describe speech as sounding like "noise" or a "buzz," suggesting that the percepts aroused by successive spectral elements in the stream of speech are not well differentiated. In this regard, a failure to be able to temporally segregate sounds might result in some kind of integration or smearing of the perceptual responses to spectral events that should in fact be segregated. In this way, an impaired temporal process might give rise to impaired spectral processing.

AUDITORY SALTATION

Phenomenology

"Saltation" is an orderly misperception of the spatial location of repetitive, transient stimuli. It was originally described in the somatosensory modality (Geldard & Sherrick, 1972), but it is also seen in vision (Geldard, 1976) and in hearing (Bremer et al., 1977; Hari, 1995; Shore et al., 1998). In the original cutaneous demonstration, the stimulus was a series of taps delivered to the wrist, and then to the midpoint of the forearm, and then to a point near the elbow. At appropriately short intertap intervals, the resulting percept was of a stimulus not only at the points of contact, but also at points between them. In the auditory modality, the stimulus is usually a train of 3 to 4 dichotic clicks favoring one laterality (usually through the imposition of an interaural time disparity on each click: Hari, 1995; Shore et al., 1998), followed in perfect temporal cadence by a second sequence of 3 to 4 dichotic clicks of the opposite laterality. A priori, one would expect the resulting percept to be of a brief train of clicks lateralized to one side, followed by an identical train of clicks lateralized to the other side. When long interclick intervals (ICIs; ≥120 ms) are used, this is, indeed, often the percept reported (Figure 3–4, left side). At shorter ICIs (usually less than about 120 ms), however, the percept is of a single train of clicks more evenly distributed around the intracranial azimuth, as if there were a single auditory object moving between the stimulus anchor points, emitting clicks as it moves (Figure 3–4, right side).

In recent years, the most common way of quantifying the perceptual response has been to ask listeners to rate the "continuity" of motion evoked by the click train (Shore et al., 1998; Phillips & Hall, 2001; Phillips et al., 2002), that is, the extent to which the perceived locations of the clicks are evenly spaced through the intracranial azimuth. Such ratings are high for short ICIs, and steadily fall for longer ICIs (Phillips & Hall, 2001; Shore et al., 1998). As a control condition, some authors include monaural click trains, in which the first clicks are delivered to one ear, and the remainder are delivered to the other ear; these stimuli evoke much poorer percepts of motion. Still another control condition is the "veridical motion" click train, in which each click in the train has a new interaural time difference designed to result in their perceived locations (genuinely) shifting smoothly in azimuth (Phillips et al., 2002). These latter click trains are given high ratings for continuity of motion, irrespective of ICI, and it

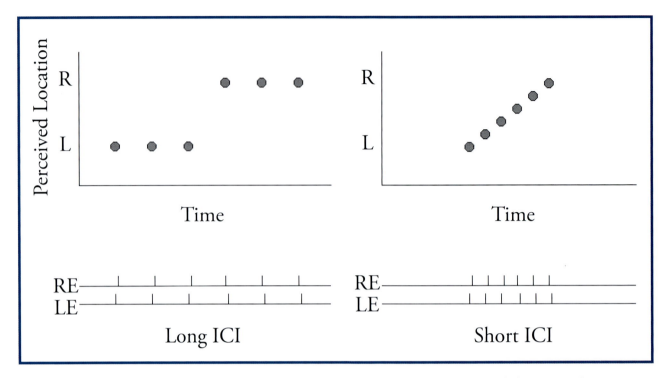

Figure 3–4. Auditory saltation. The auditory saltation stimulus is usually a train of dichotic clicks presented at a constant interclick interval (ICI). The first half of the clicks contain an interaural time difference favoring one ear, and the second half of the train contains clicks with an equivalent ITD favoring the opposite ear. When the ICI is long, the intracranial locations of the clicks are perceived veridically (*upper left*). When the ICI is short, the same dichotic clicks are perceived as originating not only at the anchor points, but along a path between them (*upper right*). Other abbreviations: R, right; L, left; RE, right ear; LE, left ear.

is this independence from ICI that distinguishes the veridical stimulus from the saltation one.

There are three reasons for our interest in auditory saltation. The first is that it is a remarkable instance in which the perceptual processing of one event in a sequence *appears* to influence the processing of *earlier* events in the sequence. Second, saltation appears to be a general property of spatiotemporal processing, yet there has been relatively little study of it, so the mechanisms that mediate it are of interest in their own right. Third, the ICIs which support the illusion appear to extend to significantly longer values in persons with dyslexia (Hari & Kiesilä, 1996), although this finding is not without significant dispute (Kidd & Hogben, 2007). Nevertheless, auditory saltation might offer a new probe of temporal-perceptual mechanisms lying at the root of some developmental disorders.

As mentioned, the dichotic clicks used to generate the illusion typically are lateralized using interaural time differences (Hari, 1995; Hari & Kiesilä, 1996; Shore et al. 1998). Clicks lateralized using interaural intensity disparities work equally well (Phillips & Hall, 2001), suggesting that it is not the presence of a specifically temporal disparity in the proximal stimulus which is required for the illusion. Indeed, at the switchpoint in the click train, one can shift the lateralization cue from being an interaural time disparity to an interaural intensity disparity without effect on the illusion (Phillips et al., 2002). This suggests that the illusion is operating on a spatial representation sufficiently "high" that it has not preserved the stimulus information in which the representation has its origins. In this regard, the illusion also works for free-field stimuli. Thus, clicks emitted from speakers in the free field will, given appropriate ICIs, generate a percept of clicks taking a trajectory between the actual sources. What makes this finding of special interest is that the illusion is quite robust for free-field sources at eccentricities deep in the lateral hemifields (i.e., opposite one or other ear) where cues to source location are dominated by *monaural* stimulus information (Ishigami & Phillips, 2008; Phillips et al., 2002). This confirms that the illusion exploits the properties of a spatial representation irrespective of the stimulus cues in which the representation has its origins (see above), but extends the generality of that to include predominantly monaural cases. The illusion also works in the elevation dimension at the frontal midline where the only cues to source location are monaural in nature (Boehnke & Phillips, 2005), providing a further confirmation of this point.

Temporal Window and Mechanisms

The interpretation of the saltation effect, that is, that it apparently reflects an effect of the perceptual processing of late elements in the train on the processing of earlier ones, raises the intriguing question of the time course over which this effect operates. Phillips and Hall (2001) conducted an experiment to explore this question. In general, the click trains used to elicit the illusion contain relatively few elements (6 to 8), and so the temporal window for processing of the percept might be at least as wide as the duration of those click trains (ICI × number of clicks). Phillips and Hall reasoned that one could increase the number of clicks in the train preceding the laterality reversal and ask subjects not to rate the continuity of any perceived motion, but simply to detect the presence of any *stationarity* of the clicks at the beginning of the stimulus. By doing this for various conditions of click numbers and ICIs in the leading train, they were able to measure the probability of detecting that stationarity as a function of the duration of the leading click train and for click trains differing in ICI (Figure 3–5). These functions usually were sigmoidal and independent of the ICIs of which the leading train was composed, with near-zero probability of detecting stationarity when the leading click train was short, but near-unity proba-

bility of detecting stationarity when the leading click train was long—meaning that the leading click train was long enough that its beginning section was now outside the window for contamination by the later laterality reversal. The midpoint of the sigmoidal function constitutes a measurement of the distance in time backward from the laterality reversal over which the effect operated. Such measurements must be regarded as preliminary, since there were a number of arbitrary decisions made in the measurement process, and the measurement process itself is naïve with regard to the shape of the temporal window. In the analysis of data from nine listeners, window widths varied from 250 to 500 ms, with most listeners having a window width near 300 to 400 ms. This "window" is, of course, not to be confused with the simple, energy-monitoring, monaural temporal window we discussed earlier in reference to gap detection.

These values derive some special interest from their correspondence with measures of other expressions of auditory processing or integration times. Thus, attempts to measure auditory integration times electrophysiologically report values on the order of 200 ms (Nagarajan et al., 1999; Winkler et al., 1998; Yabe et al., 1998). The extent to which spectral slices of speech sounds can be temporally offset without significant consequence to word discrimination performance is on the order of 140 ms, and 50%-correct word recognition can be seen with asynchronies of more than 200 ms (Arai & Greenberg, 1998). In this regard, a case can be made that the functional unit of speech is the syllable (as opposed to the phoneme), and the mean duration of syllables is again on the order of 200 ms (Greenberg, 1999; Massaro, 1972). In quite a different domain, Akeroyd and Summerfield (1999) have examined the duration of the "binaural temporal window," i.e., a binaural analog of the monaural temporal window discussed above. It can be thought of as the duration of the sampling window for interaural correlation change detection, within which there can be significant smearing of the neural representation of the interaural correlation. Estimates of this window width vary widely between listeners and may be quite long (50 to 300 ms: Akeroyd & Summerfield, 1999; 85 ms, Boehnke et al., 2002, giving rise to the notion of "binaural

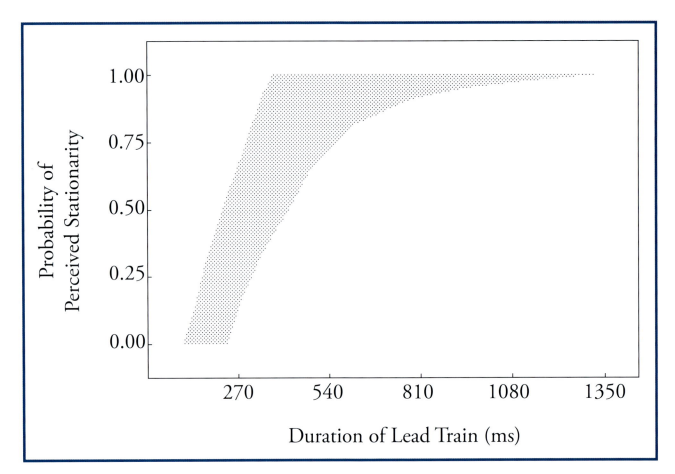

Figure 3–5. Schematic depiction of data from an auditory saltation study. In this experiment, the independent variable was the duration of the click train that preceded the laterality reversal. Note that in separate trials, the leading train could be composed of clicks with different ICIs. The dependent variable was the (yes/no) report of any perceived stationarity of the click train at the beginning of the stimulus. The responses are distributed as a relatively narrow swath. When the leading train was short in duration, there were few or no reports of stationarity, indicating that the leading train was wholly within the window through which information about subsequent clicks (i.e., those after the laterality reversal) could contaminate its perceptual processing. In contrast, when the leading train was lengthened, the probability of a perceived stationarity increased to unity, indicating that at least some part of the leading train was now outside the window for contamination by the processing of the clicks following the laterality reversal. Based on Phillips and Hall (2001).

sluggishness," after Grantham & Wightman, 1979). On the other hand, there is some evidence that the width and of the binaural temporal window may be task dependent, and, construed as a symmetric, double exponential one, the time constants could be as low as 16 ms (Bernstein et al 2001). Because auditory saltation is effective in free-field domains in which spatial processing is dominated by monaural cues, it is not necessarily clear how the binaural temporal window plays into the mechanisms mediating the

effect. The general point to emerge from this listing is that there appears to be a host of perceptual processes, operating over a time scale of a few hundred milliseconds, which significantly shapes the resulting percept, but access to which we have only at the output level. The width of this window is reminiscent of what Massaro (1972) much earlier called "perceptual processing time."

This raises the question of exactly what "processing" is going on during this time. An appeal can be made to quite low-level mechanisms to explain auditory saltation (Phillips & Hall 2001). One of them is "binaural adaptation," the phenomenon in which, during click trains at very short ICIs, the usefulness of the interaural information extracted from the successive elements in the train declines, until the system is "reset" by the introduction of some form of a change in the stimulus train (Buell & Hafter, 1988; Hafter & Buell, 1990). In this regard, however, binaural adaptation might provide a partial explanation for the malleability of the percepts evoked by clicks preceding the switchpoint, but it does not explain why the click marking the switch is also misperceived in its location (Phillips et al., 2002). A higher level explanation for the saltation effect is based on perceptual grouping phenomena. The illusion is strongest for ICIs at which it becomes difficult to individuate elements of the train (after Shore et al., 1998), raising the possibility that the clicks at short ICIs are grouped as a single event (i.e., a "buzz"). Now, the proximal stimulus for saltation is actually ambiguous. One interpretation is of a brief train of clicks in one location followed in perfect temporal cadence by a second train at the second location. A second interpretation is that all of the clicks arise from a single distal stimulus (i.e., the clicks are grouped on the basis of ICI), namely one which initially resided at one anchor point and then moved to the second, emitting clicks as it went. If the perceptual system defaults to the "single object" interpretation, then illusory motion is the result (Ishigami & Phillips, 2008). Note that at longer ICIs, the clicks in the train are more readily individuated, and so can be assigned their own (veridical) spatial location and thus be less susceptible to the illusion. The "default" to a single object interpretation might thus be driven by the inability to individuate the clicks in the train.

For readers new to this material, a rather counterintuitive conceptualization of the act of auditory perception (and likely perception in general) emerges from these considerations. We normally take for granted that the physical world unfolds on a seamless, continuous, ms-by-ms basis, that this leads to the (equally continuous), ms-by-ms updating of the neurophysiologic representations of the proximal stimulus, and in turn to the event-by-event, veridical mental elaboration of the stimulus. In fact, the conscious percept is a time-delayed, highly edited weaving together of the outcomes of a wide array of representational and interpretative processes of the physical events executed in parallel, and probably subject to attentional filtering (the "multiple drafts model" of Dennett, 1991). In this kind of model, the representation of time in the perceptual process need not have a simple relationship with the unfolding of time in neural events, any more than the representation of space in the brain necessarily is spatial in form. The perceptual elaboration of the early clicks in the train, indeed of any event, is continuously subject to an updating and editing (perhaps on the basis of perceptual grouping mechanisms), and the window for that perceptual editing is a few hundreds of ms wide, which is long enough for the writing of the percepts of clicks early in the train to have been influenced by the occurrence of subsequent clicks in the train. This means that the "content" of the percept depends on when in the processing stream it is sampled. Auditory saltation has provided one measure of the time occupied by the processes that lead to the writing of the percept, and a reminder of some of the levels of processing that go into the editing of the percept that is written.

We still have much to learn about the relation between the cortical sensory representation of the stimulus and the percepts it supports. On the one hand, it is clear that the properties of those neurophysiological representations of the stimulus set limits on the properties of the percepts that ultimately arise from them (e.g., Phillips, 1987, 1998; Phillips & Brugge, 1985; Phillips & Hall, 1990). On the other hand, the response latencies of the neurophysiologic representations can be as short as 15 to 30 ms, and the short-latency activity in those representations themselves is clearly active in animals under general anesthesia. It follows that the direct, short-latency activation of those sensory representations is not itself the basis of the generation of a conscious percept.

Question 3

What kind of therapies can be aimed at impaired temporal processing?

Answer 3

There is now fairly wide support for auditory training regimes, in the sense that intense practice can improve performance on some auditory tasks (see Chapter 6; Agnew et al., 2004; Merzenich et al., 1996; Moore & Amitay, 2007). Plasticity of central auditory responses expressed in the effects of behavioral training has a quite long history in animal neurophysiologic studies. In the early days, the form taken by the plasticity was often described in terms of the simple enhancement or weakening of responses to attended stimuli by comparison with responses to the same stimuli when unattended. Perhaps more interesting from the applied point of view is the history of research showing that behavioral training can change the stimulus selectivity of central neurons—most commonly demonstrated in the auditory cortex. Thus, neurons which receive a highly convergent input across the frequency domain can have a frequency specificity imposed on them through behavioral training in which the target frequency takes on a special significance (e.g., Diamond & Weinberger, 1986). In narrowly tuned neurons, behavioral training can shift the strength of responses within the tuning curve (Weinberger, 1997). In part, both of these responses may reflect a "selection" process exerted on the range of available inputs by the training (after Suga et al., 1997; Phillips & Hall, 1992). They may be mediated by the forebrain cholinergic neural systems, because pairing of nucleus basalis stimulation with acoustic stimuli can bring about comparable effects in the absence of behavioral training (Weinberger, 1997).

From the standpoint of remediation in human listeners, a host of questions remain, and these echo some of the concerns already raised by Moore and Amitay (2007). One question concerns the range of auditory perceptual dimensions that are susceptible to this kind of training. Does it extend to temporal processing, and if so, which forms of it? A second question concerns whether attention needs explicitly to be assigned to the auditory stimuli in the training program, or whether engagement in another task with correlated (e.g., visual) stimuli is sufficient to provoke improved auditory discrimination along the dimension of interest. A third question concerns listeners with a language-learning impairment presumed to have a root cause in auditory temporal processing deficits. Is auditory training with nonverbal stimuli that target auditory temporal processing skills sufficient to help remediate the language-learning problem (for example, through a cascade mechanism), or is training specifically with speech and language materials also required? Relatedly, what are the relative merits of the various training programs available (e.g., Cohen et al., 2005)?

CONCLUSIONS AND IMPLICATIONS

The purpose of this chapter has been to survey some recent advances in auditory perception and their neurophysiologic underpinnings, and to use the descriptions of that research to explore issues of time and timing. In the context of auditory temporal gap detection, we saw a host of temporal processes, and these varied with stimulus marker content. Thus, we saw a distinction between discontinuity detection and relative timing, and even within relative timing, we saw reason to consider the relative timing of marker offset and onset (Phillips et al., 1997) and the relative timing of marker onsets alone (Eggermont, 2000). We saw the emergence of the concept of a "temporal window," a weighted-averaging process executed on the amplitude envelope of peripheral output, not necessarily as a design feature of the nervous system, but perhaps as an emergent property of the hardware and higher level sampling mechanisms. We turned then to consider the perceptual salience of event onsets, and the origins of that salience as seen in Patterson's auditory image model and in the quite rapid, short-term adaptation of neurons in the auditory nervous system (Phillips et al., 2002). Finally, we considered auditory saltation, an illusion which itself depends on the temporal intervals of the elements making up the stimulus, but which also provided a reminder of the extent of sensory processing executed before the percept is written, and of the width of the temporal window for that more high-level processing. Note that there are still more temporal coding issues we have not discussed, such as the temporal cross-correlation of information from the two ears used in sound localization, the temporal asymmetries that emerge from relative timing operations on events in different perceptual streams, the detection of periodic modulations in a carrier's amplitude or frequency, periodicity pitch phenomena, masking phenomena, the perhaps more cognitively loaded temporal order judgments, and so on.

Auditory perception engages any or all of these mechanisms according to circumstance, and does so in a way which weaves together parallel lines of processing in a continuous updating and editing of the information entering conscious perception. It is because of the wealth of temporal processes ascribed to the brain in the act of perception that "temporal processing" or even "rapid temporal processing" have become ambiguous umbrella terms. It is an empirical question as to whether any of the foregoing temporal processes can be impaired in isolation, that is, whether a pathology affecting perception can be expected to respect processing or structural boundaries in any simple way. There have been some precedents in this regard, mostly at the level of analysis of particular stimulus features. We have thus seen reports of relatively focal auditory processing deficits, including those of auditory motion perception (Griffiths et al., 1996), sound localization (Sanchez-Longo & Forster, 1958), and periodic frequency modulations (Stefanatos et al., 1989); but see also the higher level effects of brain damage on melody processing (Peretz et al., 1994). The selective impairment of between-channel gap detection in the aphasias (Sidiropoulos et al., 2010; Stefanatos et al.,

2007) and in other pathologies is another promising line of enquiry, both from the standpoint of isolating temporal processes in within- and between-channel gap detection, and from the standpoint of showing their relations to speech perception.

The highly diverse ways in which time and timing play into the process of auditory perception have important implications for how we should address the possibility that some form of auditory temporal processing problem may be at the root of developmental language disorders in some children. First, it is now obvious that one must be very clear about the process(es) to which one alludes in such a claim because "auditory temporal processing" is an umbrella term with a wide capture. The same applies more generally to "temporal processing" (Farmer & Klein, 1995; Klein 2002) and to categories of language disorder (Phillips, 2002). Second, one needs to know if the demonstrable presence of a specifiable auditory processing problem is correlated with (i.e., a marker for), or causally related to, the language/reading performance deficit. One therefore needs to have a theoretical framework that connects the nature of the processing problem with the nature of the language-performance deficit. In this regard, a causal relation between a nonverbal auditory temporal-processing problem and language performance might be most important or evident during language *acquisition* or while *learning* to read, and not necessarily after language and/or reading performance has reached any adult plateau.

There is much debate about the concurrent existence of nonverbal auditory processing problems in persons with developmental language disorders, with some authors finding a systematic relationship (Hari & Renvall, 2001; Helenius et al., 1999; McAnally & Stein, 1996; Tallal, 1980; Tallal & Piercy, 1974; Tallal et al., 1993; Witton et al., 1998; Wright et al., 1997) and others not (Bishop et al., 1999; McArthur & Bishop, 2001; Rosen, 1999; Schulte-Korne et al., 1998; Watson & Kidd, 2002). Much of the dispute likely has its origins in the foregoing issues. One of the more interesting hypotheses on the role of auditory processing in dyslexia has come from Hari and her colleagues (Hari & Renvall, 2001). They have shown the existence of a variety of "temporal" auditory processing abnormalities in dyslexics (Hari & Kiesilä, 1996; Helenius et al., 1999), and have sought to integrate these into a hypothesis with plausible causal links to language/reading performance. At the core of the hypothesis is the general notion that the temporal chunking of information available to the perceptual processor is more coarse than normal (i.e., dyslexics have a "prolonged cognitive integration window" [Hari & Renvall, 2001]). One result of this is that in the perceptual processing stream, acoustic events which are relatively closely spaced in time are able to interfere with each other over greater than normal temporal distances (see above discussion of auditory saltation). In principle, such a mechanism could give rise to ambiguous representations of sounds that, for the purposes of phonology, need to be tempo-

rally differentiated (see also Phillips, 1995, 1998). In this regard, persons with reading disabilities appear not to have impaired within-channel gap-detection thresholds (Schulte-Korne et al., 1998), suggesting that some percepts based on low-level temporal analyses may be intact in persons with reading disabilities. These findings all need to be confirmed, not the least because the basic empirical finding of prolonged temporal windows in dyslexics has been significantly challenged (Kidd & Hogben, 2007). Longitudinal studies capable of revealing the time course of auditory-perceptual and language/reading-performance development are particularly important.

Question 4

The section on saltation describes mechanisms or processes that could lead our perceptual experience not to be a truthful representation of the acoustic world. Is that right?

Answer 4

Yes. Saltation may be a special case, but this author's suspicion is that a purely data-driven (bottom-up) and complete, veridical perceptual representation of the world on a moment-by-moment basis would require neural processing machinery that exceeds the brain's resources. Nørretranders (1991) characterizes the problem as one of processing "bandwidth." He argues that the information transmission rate from the sense organs is on the order of millions of bits per second, whereas the bandwidth of conscious perception is orders of magnitude below that. As a strategy to cope with this, the perceptual processor chunks stimulus elements into objects, or hypotheses about objects. We have evidence of this at the perceptual level. One obvious auditory demonstration is phonemic restoration, in which the physical speech stimulus at the ear contains a phonetically ambiguous, substituted sound, and the perceptual system resolves the ambiguity by replacing the ambiguous element with a context-driven choice of phoneme

(Warren, 1970). In vision, each eye contains a blindspot: the portion of the retina devoid of photoreceptors because it is occupied by departing ganglion cell axons and by blood vessels entering and leaving the eye. With one eye open at a time, therefore, there is a patch of retina not sending information centrally, yet we are not aware of any visual field defect associated with that blindspot; indeed we have to contrive an experiment to demonstrate its existence. Again, the perceptual system has "filled in" (disambiguated) a local region of impoverished retinal output based on context, in this instance, prior experience with that portion of the visual scene. Both of these are examples of the fact that much of our perceptual world is "constructed." This is true first in the sense that it contains a binding or stitching together of independently represented components of the sensory scene. It is also true in the sense that we have mechanisms to increase processing efficiency by use of top-down resources, with the result that parts of the subjective perceptual scene can almost be thought of as hypotheses about the state of the sensory scene rather than direct mental representations of it. The part of the stimulus scene which receives the most elaborate conscious processing is presumably the fraction of the scene to which we specifically allocate our attention.

In this regard, there has been recent interest in the phenomena of "change blindness" and "change deafness." In the former case, subjects alternately view images (usually separated by a visual mask) that differ in the presence or absence of some object. The viewer is typically blind to the change through many alternations of the scenes, although once the change is detected, it remains very obvious. Change blindness suggests that the visual perceptual world is not based directly on a highly detailed representation of the scene; rather, it is built in large part on hypotheses about what is there. When attention is captured by some element in the scene, then it may be subject to detailed processing. In studies of change deafness, the listener is presented with two successive naturalistic auditory scenes containing a number of auditory objects or sources; the auditory scenes differ in the presence, absence or identity of one of the objects (e.g., Pavani & Turatto, 2008). Listeners often do not detect the change unless they are cued to it (Eramudugolla et al., 2005). There are probably some differences between the processes at work in change detection in hearing and vision (Pavani & Turatto, 2008). Nevertheless, in both sensory modalities, failure to detect the change means that at any given moment, we don't have conscious access to any complete internal representation of the sensory world. The effects of cueing on sensitivity to change tell us that access to a detailed perceptual representation of the world, or part of it, is subject to an attentional filter.

On the one hand, these lines of evidence suggest that the richness and continuity of the subjective perceptual world is something of an illusion. On the other hand, it may be that the constructed nature of our perceptual world is a corollary of a computationally efficient means of interacting with the physical world, and one which works quite well in the vast majority of circumstances.

Acknowledgments. Thanks are due to Drs. Kelly Tremblay and Robert Burkard for inviting this contribution, and to them, and their students, for helpful feedback on previous versions of this chapter. Some of the research described in this chapter, and the preparation of the chapter itself, was supported by grants from the Natural Sciences and Engineering Research Council (NSERC) of Canada, the Canadian Language and Literacy Research Network (CLLR-Net), and the Killam Trust to DPP. Special thanks go to Susan E. Hall and Susan E. Boehnke, who were active contributors to much of the work described herein, and to Rachel N. Dingle for outstanding commentary on an earlier draft.

FURTHER READINGS

Readers seeking more comprehensive accounts of basic auditory psychophysics are referred to Moore (2003) and Plack (2005). Readers wishing to "stretch" into cognitive aspects of hearing, or, indeed, into neurophilosophy, are referred to the following books:

Blackmore, S. (2004). *Consciousness. An introduction.* Oxford, UK: Oxford University Press.
Handel, S. (1989). *Listening. An introduction to the perception of auditory events.* Cambridge, MA: MIT Press.
McAdams, S., & Bigand, E. (1993). *Thinking in sound. The cognitive psychology of human audition.* New York, NY: Oxford University Press.

REFERENCES

Agnew, J. A., Dorn, C., & Eden, G. F. (2004). Effect of intensive training on auditory processing and reading skills. *Brain and Language, 88,* 21–25.
Akeroyd, M. A., & Patterson, R. D. (1995). Discrimination of wideband noises modulated by a temporally asymmetric function. *Journal of the Acoustical Society of America, 98,* 2466–2474.
Akeroyd, M. A., & Patterson, R. D. (1997). A comparison of detection and discrimination of temporal asymmetry in amplitude modulation. *Journal of the Acoustical Society of America, 101,* 430–439.

Akeroyd, M. A., & Summerfield, A. Q. (1999). A binaural analog of gap detection. *Journal of the Acoustical Society of America, 105,* 2807–2820.

Allen, P. D., Virag, T. M., & Ison, J. R. (2002). Humans detect gaps in broadband noise according to effective gap duration without additional cues from abrupt envelope changes. *Journal of the Acoustical Society of America, 112,* 2967–2974.

Aoki, S., & Houtgast, T. (1992). A precedence effect in the perception of inter-aural cross correlation. *Hearing Research, 59,* 25–30.

Arai, T., & Greenberg, S. (1998). Speech intelligibility in the presence of cross-channel spectral asynchrony. *Proceedings of the IEEE Conference on Acoustics, Speech, and Signal Processing* (pp. 933–936). Seattle, WA.

Au, A., & Lovegrove, B., (2001a). Temporal processing ability in above average and average readers. *Perception and Psychophysics, 63,* 148–155.

Au, A., & Lovegrove, B., (2001b). The role of visual and auditory temporal processing in reading irregular and nonsense words. *Perception, 30,* 1127–1142.

Baker, R. J., Jayewardene, D., Sayle, C., & Saeed, S. (2008). Failure to find asymmetry in auditory gap detection. *Laterality, 13,* 1–21.

Barsz, K., Benson, P. K., & Walton, J. P. (1998). Gap encoding by inferior collicular neurons is altered by minimal changes in signal envelope. *Hearing Research, 115,* 13–26.

Bernstein, L. R., Trahiotis, C., Akeroyd, M. A., & Hartung, K. (2001). Sensitivity to brief changes of interaural time and interaural intensity. *Journal of the Acoustical Society of America, 109,* 1604–1615.

Billings, C. J., Tremblay, K. L., Stecker, G. C., & Tolin, W. M. (2009). Human cortical activity to signal-to-noise ratio rather than absolute signal level. *Hearing Research, 254,* 15–24.

Bishop, D. V. M., Carlyon, R. P., Deeks, J. M., & Bishop, S. J. (1999). Auditory temporal processing impairment: Neither necessary nor sufficient for causing language impairment in children. *Journal of Speech, Language and Hearing Research, 42,* 1295–1310.

Boehnke, S. E., Hall, S. E., & Marquardt, T. (2002). Detection of static and dynamic changes in interaural correlation. *Journal of the Acoustical Society of America, 112,* 1617–1626.

Boehnke, S. E., & Phillips, D. P. (1999). Azimuthal tuning of human perceptual channels for sound location. *Journal of the Acoustical Society of America, 106,* 1948–1955.

Boehnke, S. E., & Phillips, D. P. (2005). Auditory saltation in the vertical, midsagittal plane. *Perception, 34,* 371–377.

Bregman, A. S. (1990). *Auditory scene analysis: The perceptual organization of sound.* Cambridge, MA: MIT Press.

Bremer, C. D., Pittenger, J. B., Warren, R., & Jenkins, J. J. (1977). An illusion of auditory saltation similar to the cutaneous "rabbit." *American Journal of Psychology, 90,* 645–654.

Broadbent, D. (1958). *Perception and communication.* London, UK: Pergamon.

Brown, S., & Nicholls, M. E. R. (1997). Hemispheric asymmetries for the temporal resolution of brief auditory stimuli. *Perception and Psychophysics, 59,* 442–447.

Buell, T. N., & Hafter, E. R. (1988). Discrimination of interaural differences of time in the envelopes of high-frequency signals: Integration times. *Journal of the Acoustical Society of America, 84,* 2063–2066.

Cacace, A. T., & McFarland, D. J. (1998). Central auditory processing disorder in school-aged-aged children: A critical review. *Journal of Speech, Language, and Hearing Research, 41,* 355–373.

Carmichael, M. E., Hall, S. E., & Phillips, D. P. (2008). Ear and contralateral masking effects on auditory temporal gap detection thresholds. *Hearing Research, 245,* 18–23.

Chatterjee, M., Fu, Q-L., & Shannon, R. V. (1998). Within-channel gap detection using dissimilar markers in cochlear implant listeners. *Journal of the Acoustical Society of America, 103,* 2515–2519.

Cherry, E. C. (1953). Some experiments upon the recognition of speech, with one and with two ears. *Journal of the Acoustical Society of America, 25,* 975–979.

Cohen, W., Hodson, A., O'Hare, A., Boyle, J., Durrani, T., McCartney, E., . . . Watson, J. (2005). Effects of computer-based intervention through acoustically modified speech (Fast ForWord) in severe mixed receptive-expressive language impairment: Outcomes from a randomized controlled trial. *Journal of Speech, Language, and Hearing Research, 48,* 715–729.

Creese, I. (1999). Rate processing constraints may underlie developmental language impairments and also hemispheric specialization for speech. *Brain Research Bulletin, 50,* 431–432.

Creutzfeldt, O., Hellweg, F.-C., & Schreiner, C. (1980). Thalamocortical transformation of responses to complex auditory stimuli. *Experimental Brain Research, 39,* 87–104.

Dennett, D. C. (1991). *Consciousness explained.* Boston, MA: Little, Brown.

Diamond, D. M., & Weinberger, N. M. (1986). Classical conditioning rapidly induces specific changes in frequency receptive fields of single neurons in secondary and ventral ectosylvian auditory cortical fields. *Brain Research, 372,* 357–360.

Divenyi P. L. (2004). The times of Ira Hirsh: Multiple ranges of auditory temporal perception. *Seminars in Hearing, 25,* 229–239.

Divenyi, P. L., & Danner, W. F. (1977). Discrimination of time intervals marked by brief acoustic pulses of various intensities and spectra. *Perception and Psychophysics, 21,* 125–142.

Eddins, D. A., Hall, J. W., & Grose, J. H. (1992). The detection of temporal gaps as a function of frequency region and absolute noise bandwidth. *Journal of the Acoustical Society of America, 91,* 1069–1077.

Eggermont, J. J. (1990). *The correlative brain. Theory and experiment in neural interaction.* Berlin, Germany: Springer-Verlag.

Eggermont, J. J. (1991). Rate and synchronization measures of periodicity coding in cat primary auditory cortex. *Hearing Research, 56,* 153–167.

Eggermont, J. J. (1994). Temporal modulation transfer functions for AM and FM stimuli in cat auditory cortex. Effects of carrier type, modulating waveform and intensity. *Hearing Research, 74,* 51–66.

Eggermont, J. J. (1996). How homogeneous is cat primary auditory cortex? Evidence from simultaneous single-unit recordings. *Auditory Neuroscience, 3,* 79–96.

Eggermont, J. J. (1997). Firing rate and firing synchrony distinguish dynamic from steady state sound. *NeuroReport, 8,* 2709–2713.

Eggermont, J. J. (1999). Neural correlates of gap detection in three auditory cortical fields in the cat. *Journal of Neurophysiology, 81,* 2570–2581.

Eggermont, J. J. (2000). Neural responses in primary auditory cortex mimic psychophysical, across-frequency channel, gap-detection thresholds. *Journal of Neurophysiology, 84,* 1453–1463.

Eggermont, J. J. (2002). Temporal modulation transfer functions in cat primary auditory cortex: Separating stimulus effects from neural mechanisms. *Journal of Neurophysiology, 87,* 305–321.

Eimas, P. D., & Corbit, J. D. (1973). Selective adaptation of linguistic feature detectors. *Cognitive Psychology, 4,* 99–109.

Elangovan, S., & Stuart, A. (2008). Natural boundaries in gap detection are related to categorical perception of stop consonants. *Ear and Hearing, 29,* 761–774.

Eramudugolla, R., Irvine, D. R. F., McAnally, K. I., Martin, R. L., & Mattingley, J.B. (2005). Directed attention eliminates "change deafness" in complex auditory scenes. *Current Biology, 15,* 1108–1113.

Farmer, M. E., & Klein, R. M. (1995). The evidence for a temporal processing deficit linked to dyslexia: A review. *Psychological Bulletin and Review, 2,* 460–493.

Fitzgibbons, P. J., Pollatsek, A., & Thomas, I. B. (1974). Detection of temporal gaps within and between perceptual tonal groups. *Perception and Psychophysics, 16,* 522–528.

Florentine, M., Buus, S., & Geng, W. (1999). Psychometric functions for gap detection in a yes-no procedure. *Journal of the Acoustical Society of America, 106,* 3512–3520.

Formby, C., & Forrest, T. G. (1991). Detection of silent temporal gaps in sinusoidal markers. *Journal of the Acoustical Society of America, 89,* 830–837.

Formby, C., Gerber, M. J., Sherlock, L. P., & Magder, L. S. (1998). Evidence for an across-frequency, between-channel process in asymptotic monaural temporal gap detection. *Journal of the Acoustical Society of America, 103,* 3554–3560.

Formby, C., Sherlock, L. P., & Forrest, T. G. (1996). An asymmetric Roex filter model for describing detection of silent temporal gaps in sinusoidal markers. *Auditory Neuroscience, 3,* 1–20.

Formby, C., Sherlock, L. P., & Li, S. (1998). Temporal gap detection measured with multiple sinusoidal markers: Effects of marker number, frequency, and temporal position. *Journal of the Acoustical Society of America, 104,* 984–998.

Forrest, T. G., & Formby, C. (1996). Detection of silent temporal gaps in sinusoidal markers simulated with a single-channel envelope detector model. *Auditory Neuroscience, 3,* 21–33.

Forrest, T. G., & Green, D. M. (1987). Detection of partially filled gaps in noise and the temporal modulation transfer function. *Journal of the Acoustical Society of America, 82,* 1933–1943.

Freyman, R. L., Zurek, P. M., Balakrishnan, U., & Chiang, Y-C. (1997). Onset dominance in lateralization. *Journal of the Acoustical Society of America, 101,* 1649–1659.

Geldard, F.A. (1976). The saltatory effect in vision. *Sensory Processes, 1,* 77–86.

Geldard, F. A., & Sherrick, C. E. (1972). The cutaneous "rabbit": A perceptual illusion. *Science, 178,* 178–179.

Gordon, J. W. (1987). The perceptual attack time of musical tones. *Journal of the Acoustical Society of America, 82,* 88–105.

Grantham, D. W., & Wightman, F. L. (1979). Detectability of a pulsed tone in the presence of a masker with time-varying interaural correlation. *Journal of the Acoustical Society of America, 65,* 1509–1517.

Greenberg, S. (1999). Speaking in shorthand—a syllable-centric perspective for understanding pronunciation variation. *Speech Communication, 29,* 159–176.

Griffiths, T. D., Rees, A., Witton, C., Shakir, R.A., Henning, G. B., & Green, G. G. R. (1996). Evidence for a sound movement area in the human cerebral cortex. *Nature, 383,* 425–427.

Grose, J. H. (1991). Gap detection in multiple narrow bands of noise as a function of spectral configuration. *Journal of the Acoustical Society of America, 90,* 3061–3068.

Grose, J. H., Hall, J. W. III, & Buss, E. (1999). Modulation gap detection: Effects of modulation rate, carrier separation, and mode of presentation. *Journal of the Acoustical Society of America, 106,* 946–953.

Grose, J. H., Hall, J. W. III, Buss, E., & Hatch, D. (2001). Gap detection for similar and dissimilar gap markers. *Journal of the Acoustical Society of America, 109,* 1587–1595.

Hafter, E. R., & Buell, T. N. (1990). Restarting the adapted binaural system. *Journal of the Acoustical Society of America, 88,* 806–812.

Hall, J. W., Grose, J. H., & Saju, J. (1996). Gap detection for pairs of noise bands: Effects of stimulus level and frequency separation. *Journal of the Acoustical Society of America, 99,* 1091–1095.

Hari, R. (1995). Illusory directional hearing in humans. *Neuroscience Letters, 189,* 29–30.

Hari, R., & Kiesilä, P. (1996). Deficit of temporal auditory processing in dyslexic adults. *Neuroscience Letters, 205,* 138–140.

Hari, R., & Renvall, H. (2001). Impaired processing of rapid stimulus sequences in dyslexia. *Trends in Cognitive Neuroscience, 5,* 525–532.

Hawkins, J. E., & Stevens, S.S. (1950). The masking of pure tones and of speech by white noise. *Journal of the Acoustical Society of America, 22,* 6–13.

Heil, P. (1997a). Auditory onset responses revisted. I. First-spike timing. *Journal of Neurophysiology, 77,* 2616–2641.

Heil, P. (1997b). Auditory onset responses revisted. II. Response strength. *Journal of Neurophysiology, 77,* 2642–2660.

Heinz, M. G., Goldstein, M. H. Jr., & Formby, C. (1996). Temporal gap detection thresholds in sinusoidal markers simulated with a multi-channel, multi-resolution model of the auditory periphery. *Auditory Neuroscience, 3,* 35–56.

Helenius, P., Uutela, K., & Hari, R. (1999). Auditory stream segregation in dyslexic adults. *Brain, 122,* 907–913.

Hirsh, I. J. (1959). Auditory perception of temporal order. *Journal of the Acoustical Society of America, 31,* 759–767.

Houtgast, T., & Aoki, S. (1994). Stimulus-onset dominance in the perception of binaural information. *Hearing Research, 72,* 29–36.

Howell, P., & Rosen, S. (1983). Production and perception of rise time in the voiceless affricate/fricative distinction. *Journal of the Acoustical Society of America, 73,* 976–984.

Irino, T., & Patterson, R. D. (1996). Temporal asymmetry in the auditory system. *Journal of the Acoustical Society of America, 99,* 2316–2331.

Ishigami, Y., & Phillips, D. P. (2008). Effect of stimulus hemifield on free-field auditory saltation. *Hearing Research, 241,* 97–102.

Ison, J. R., Castro, J., Allen, P., Virag, T. M., & Walton, J. P. (2002). The relative detectability for mice of gaps having different ramp durations at their onset and offset boundaries. *Journal of the Acoustical Society of America, 112,* 740–747.

Jenkins, W. M., & Masterton, R. B. (1982) Sound localization: Effects of unilateral lesions in central auditory pathways. *Journal of Neurophysiology, 47,* 987–1016.

Jenkins, W. M., & Merzenich, M. M. (1984). Role of cat primary auditory cortex for sound localization behavior. *Journal of Neurophysiology, 52,* 819–847.

Joris, P.X., & Yin, T. C. T. (1992). Responses to amplitude-modulated tones in the auditory nerve of the cat. *Journal of the Acoustical Society of America, 91,* 215–232.

Kavanagh, G. L., & Kelly, J. B. (1987). Contribution of auditory cortex to sound localization by the ferret (*Mustela putorius*). *Journal of Neurophysiology, 57,* 1746–1766.

Kidd, G., Mason, C. R., Rothla, T. L., & Deliwala, P. S. (1998). Release from masking due to spatial separation of sources in the identification of nonspeech auditory patterns. *Journal of the Acoustical Society of America, 104,* 422–431.

Kidd, J. C., & Hogben, J. H. (2007). Does the auditory saltation stimulus distinguish dyslexic from competently reading adults? *Journal of Speech, Language and Hearing Research, 50,* 982–998.

Kitzes, L. M. (2008). Binaural interactions shape binaural response structures and frequency response functions in primary auditory cortex. *Hearing Research, 238,* 68–76.

Klein, R. M. (2002). Observations on the temporal correlates of reading failure. *Reading and Writing, 15,* 207–232.

Kuhl P. K., & Miller J. D. (1978). Speech perception by the chinchilla: Identification functions for synthetic VOT stimuli. *Journal of the Acoustical Society of America, 63,* 905–917.

Kunov, H., & Abel, S. M. (1981). Effects of rise/decay time on the lateralization of interaurally delayed 1-kHz tones. *Journal of the Acoustical Society of America, 69,* 769–776.

Levitt, H. (1971). Transformed up-down methods in psychoacoustics. *Journal of the Acoustical Society of America, 49,* 467–477.

Liang, L., Lu, T., & Wang, X. (2002). Neural representations of sinusoidal amplitude and frequency modulations in the primary auditory cortex of awake primates. *Journal of Neurophysiology, 87,* 2237–2261.

Lister, J. J., Koehnke, J. D., & Besing, J. M. (2000). Binaural gap duration discrimination in listeners with impaired hearing and normal hearing. *Ear and Hearing, 21,* 141–150.

Lu, T., Liang, L., & Wang, X. (2001). Neural representations of temporally asymmetric stimuli in the auditory cortex of awake primates. *Journal of Neurophysiology, 85,* 2364–2380.

Massaro, D. W. (1972). Preperceptual images, processing time, and perceptual units in auditory perception. *Psychological Review, 79,* 124–145.

McAnally, K., & Stein, J. (1996). Auditory temporal coding in dyslexia. *Proceedings of the Royal Society of London, Series B, 263,* 961–965.

McArthur, G. M., & Bishop, D. V. M. (2001). Auditory perceptual processing in people with reading and oral language impairments: Current issues and recommendations. *Dyslexia, 7,* 150–170.

Merzenich, M. M., Jenkins, W. M., Johnston, P., Schreiner, C., Miller, S. L., & Tallal, P. (1996). Temporal processing deficits of language-learning impaired children ameliorated by training. *Science, 271,* 77–81.

Miyasaka, E., & Sakai, H. (1982). Detectability of switching transients. *NHK Laboratories Note No. 275.* Tokyo, Japan: NHK Science & Technical Research Labs, pp. 2–11 (English translation).

Moore, B. C. J. (1993). Temporal analysis in normal and impaired hearing. *Annals of the New York Academy of Sciences, 682,* 119–136.

Moore, B. C. J. (2003). *An introduction to the psychology of hearing* (5th ed.). London, UK: Academic Press.

Moore, B.C.J., & Glasberg, B. R. (1988). Gap detection with sinusoids and noise in normal, impaired, and electrically stimulated ears. *Journal of the Acoustical Society of America, 83,* 1093–1101.

Moore, B. C. J., Glasberg, B. R., Plack, C. J., & Biswas, A. K. (1988). The shape of the ear's temporal window. *Journal of the Acoustical Society of America, 83,* 1102–1116.

Moray, N. (1969). *Attention: Selective processes in vision and hearing.* London, UK: Hutchinson Educational Ltd.

Nagarajan, S., Mahncke, H., Salz, T., Tallal, P., Roberts, T., & Merzenich, M. M. (1999). Cortical auditory signal processing in poor readers. *Proceedings of the National Academy of Sciences of the United States of America, 96,* 6483–6488.

Nicholls, M. E. R., Schier, M., Stough, C. K. K., & Box, A. (1999). Psychophysical and electrophysiological support for a left hemisphere temporal processing advantage. *Neuropsychiatry, Neuropsychology and Behavioral Neurology, 12,* 11–16.

Nilsson, M., Soli, S., & Sullivan, J. A. (1994). Development of the Hearing In Noise Test for the measurement of speech reception thresholds in quiet and in noise. *Journal of the Acoustical Society of America, 95,* 1085–1099.

Nørretranders, T. (1991). *The user illusion. Cutting consciousness down to size.* New York, NY: Penguin Books.

Oxenham, A. J. (1997). Increment and decrement detection in sinusoids as a measure of temporal resolution. *Journal of the Acoustical Society of America, 102*, 1779–1790.

Oxenham, A. J. (2000). Influence of spatial and temporal coding on auditory gap detection. *Journal of the Acoustical Society of America, 107*, 2215–2223.

Patterson, R. D. (1994a). The sound of a sinusoid: Spectral models. *Journal of the Acoustical Society of America, 96*, 1409–1418.

Patterson, R. D. (1994b). The sound of a sinusoid: Time-interval models. *Journal of the Acoustical Society of America, 96*, 1419–1428.

Pavani, F., & Turatto, M. (2008). Change perception in complex auditory scenes. *Perception and Psychophysics, 70*, 619–629.

Penner, M. J. (1977). Detection of temporal gaps in noise as a measure of decay in auditory sensation. *Journal of the Acoustical Society of America, 61*, 552–557.

Peretz, I., Kolinsky, R., Tramo, M., Labrecque, R., Hublet, C., Demeurisse, G., & Belleville, S. (1994). Functional dissociations following bilateral lesions of auditory cortex. *Brain, 117*, 1283–1301.

Phillips, D. P. (1985). Temporal response features of cat auditory cortex neurons contributing to sensitivity to tones delivered in the presence of continuous noise. *Hearing Research, 19*, 253–268.

Phillips, D. P. (1987). Stimulus intensity and loudness recruitment: neural correlates. *Journal of the Acoustical Society of America, 82*, 1–12.

Phillips, D. P. (1990). Neural representation of sound amplitude in the auditory cortex: Effects of noise masking. *Behavioral Brain Research, 37*, 197–214.

Phillips, D. P. (1995). Central auditory processing: A view from auditory neuroscience. *American Journal of Otology, 16*, 338–352.

Phillips, D. P. (1998). Sensory representations, the auditory cortex, and speech perception. *Seminars in Hearing, 19*, 319–332.

Phillips, D. P. (2001). Introduction to the central auditory nervous system. In A. F. Jahn, & J. Santos-Sacchi (Eds.), *Physiology of the ear* (2nd ed., pp. 613–638). San Diego, CA: Singular.

Phillips, D. P. (2002). Central auditory system and central auditory processing disorders: Some conceptual issues. *Seminars in Hearing, 23*, 251–262.

Phillips, D. P. (2008). A perceptual architecture for sound lateralization in man. *Hearing Research, 238*, 124–132.

Phillips, D. P., & Brugge, J. F. (1985). Progress in neurophysiology of sound localization. *Annual Review of Psychology, 36*, 245–274.

Phillips, D. P., & Cynader, M. S. (1985). Some neural mechanisms in the cat's auditory cortex underlying sensitivity to combined tone and wide-spectrum noise stimuli. *Hearing Research, 18*, 87–102.

Phillips, D. P., & Hall, S. E. (1987). Responses of single neurons in cat auditory cortex to time-varying stimuli: Linear amplitude modulations. *Experimental Brain Research, 67*, 479–492.

Phillips, D. P., & Hall, S. E. (1990). Response timing constraints on the cortical representation of sound time structure. *Journal of the Acoustical Society of America, 88*, 1403–1411.

Phillips, D. P., & Hall, S. E. (1992). Multiplicity of inputs in the afferent path to cat auditory cortex neurons revealed by tone-on-tone masking. *Cerebral Cortex, 2*, 425–433.

Phillips, D. P., & Hall, S. E. (2000). Independence of frequency channels in auditory temporal gap detection. *Journal of the Acoustical Society of America, 108*, 2957–2963.

Phillips, D. P., & Hall, S. E. (2001). Spatial and temporal factors in auditory saltation. *Journal of the Acoustical Society of America, 110*, 1539–1547.

Phillips, D. P., & Hall, S. E. (2002). Auditory temporal gap detection for noise markers with partially-overlapping and non-overlapping spectra. *Hearing Research, 174*, 133–141.

Phillips, D. P., Hall, S. E., & Boehnke, S. E. (2002). Central auditory onset responses, and temporal asymmetries in auditory perception. *Hearing Research, 167*, 192–205.

Phillips, D. P., Hall, S. E., Boehnke, S. E., & Rutherford, L. E. D. (2002). Spatial stimulus cue information supplying auditory saltation. *Perception, 31*, 875–885.

Phillips, D. P., Hall, S. E., Harrington, I. A., & Taylor, T. L. (1998). "Central" auditory gap detection: A spatial case. *Journal of the Acoustical Society of America, 103*, 2064–2068.

Phillips, D. P., & Irvine, D. R. F. (1981). Responses of neurons in physiologically defined area AI of cat cerebral cortex: Sensitivity to interaural intensity differences. *Hearing Research, 4*, 299–307.

Phillips, D. P., Mendelson, J. R., Cynader, M. S., & Douglas, R. M. (1985). Responses of single neurons in cat auditory cortex to time-varying stimuli: Frequency-modulated tones of narrow excursion. *Experimental Brain Research, 58*, 443–454.

Phillips, D. P., Reale, R. A., & Brugge, J. F. (1991). Stimulus processing in the auditory cortex. In R. A. Altschuler, R. P. Bobbin, B. M. Clopton, & D. W. Hoffman (Eds.), *Neurobiology of hearing. The central auditory system* (pp. 335–365). New York, NY: Raven Press.

Phillips, D. P., & Sark, S. A. (1991). Separate mechanisms control spike numbers and inter-spike intervals in transient responses of cat auditory cortex neurons. *Hearing Research, 53*, 17–27.

Phillips, D. P., Semple, M. N., Calford, M. B., & Kitzes, L. M. (1994). Level-dependent representation of stimulus frequency in cat primary auditory cortex. *Experimental Brain Research, 102*, 210–226.

Phillips, D. P., & Smith, J. C. (2004). Correlations among within- and between-channel auditory gap detection thresholds in normal listeners. *Perception, 33*, 371–378.

Phillips, D. P., Taylor, T. L., Hall, S. E., Carr, M. M., & Mossop, J. E. (1997). Detection of silent intervals between noises activating different perceptual channels: Some properties of "central" auditory gap detection. *Journal of the Acoustical Society of America, 101*, 3694–3705.

Phillips, D. P., Vigneault-MacLean, B., Hall, S. E., & Boehnke, S. E. (2003). Acoustic hemifields in the spatial release from masking of speech by noise. *Journal of the American Academy of Audiology, 14*, 518–524.

Plack, C. J. (2005). *The sense of hearing*. Mahwah, NJ: Lawrence Erlbaum.

Plack, C. J., Gallun, F. J., Hafter, E. R., & Raimond, A. (2006). The detection of increments and decrements is not facilitated by abrupt onsets or offsets. *Journal of the Acoustical Society of America, 119*, 3950–3959.

Plack, C. J., & Moore, B. C. J. (1990). Temporal window shape as a function of frequency and level. *Journal of the Acoustical Society of America, 87*, 2178–2187.

Plomp, R. (1964). Rate of decay of auditory sensation. *Journal of the Acoustical Society of America, 36*, 277–282.

Rhode, W. S., & Smith, P. H. (1986). Encoding timing and intensity in the ventral cochlear nucleus of the cat. *Journal of Neurophysiology, 56*, 261–286.

Rosen, S. (1992). Temporal information in speech: Acoustic, auditory and linguistic aspects. *Philosophical Transactions of the Royal Society of London, Series B, 336*, 367–373.

Rosen, S. (1999). Language disorders: A probem with auditory processing? *Current Biology, 9*, 698–700.

Rosen, S. M., & Howell, P. (1981). Plucks and bows are not categorically perceived. *Perception and Psychophysics, 30*, 156–168.

Ruggero, M. A. (1992). Physiology and coding of sound in the auditory nerve. In A. N. Popper & R. R. Fay (Eds.), *The mammalian auditory pathway: Neurophysiology* (pp. 34–93). New York, NY: Springer-Verlag.

Saberi, K., Dostal, L., Sadralodabai, T., Bull, V., & Perrott, D. R. (1991). Free-field release from masking. *Journal of the Acoustical Society of America, 90*, 1355–1370.

Saldanha, E. L., & Corso, J. F. (1964). Timbre cues and the identification of musical instruments. *Journal of the Acoustical Society of America, 36*, 2021–2026.

Sanchez-Longo, L. P., & Forster, F. M. (1958). Clinical significance of impairment of sound localization. *Neurology, 8*, 119–125.

Scharf, B., Quigley, S., Aoki, C., Peachey, N., & Reeves, A. (1987). Focused auditory attention and frequency selectivity. *Perception and Psychophysics, 42*, 215–223.

Schneider, B. A., & Hamstra, S. J. (1999). Gap detection thresholds as a function of tonal duration for younger and older listeners. *Journal of the Acoustical Society of America, 106*, 371–380.

Schulte-Körne, G., Deimel, W., Bartling, J., & Remschmidt, H. (1998). Role of auditory temporal processing for reading and spelling disability. *Perceptual and Motor Skills, 86*, 1043–1047.

Semple, M. N., & Kitzes, L. M. (1993). Binaural processing of sound pressure level in cat primary auditory cortex: Evidence for a representation based on absolute levels rather than level differences. *Journal of Neurophysiology, 69*, 449–461.

Shailer, M. J., & Moore, B. C. J. (1983). Gap detection as a function of frequency, bandwidth and level. *Journal of the Acoustical Society of America, 74*, 467–473.

Shore, D. I., Hall, S. E., & Klein, R. M. (1998). Auditory saltation: A new measure for an old illusion. *Journal of the Acoustical Society of America, 103*, 3730–3733.

Sidiropoulos, K., Ackermann, H., Wannke, M., & Hertrich, I. (2010). Temporal processing capabilities in repetition conduction aphasia. *Brain and Cognition, 73*, 194–202.

Sininger, Y. S., & de Bode, S. (2008). Asymmetry of temporal processing in listeners with normal hearing and unilaterally deaf subjects. *Ear and Hearing, 29*, 228–238.

Smith, R. L. (1977). Short-term adaptation in single auditory nerve fibers: Some poststimulatory effects. *Journal of Neurophysiology, 40*, 1098–1112.

Snell, K. B., & Hu, H-L. (1999). The effect of temporal placement on gap detectability. *Journal of the Acoustical Society of America, 106*, 3571–3577.

Soli, S. D. (1983). The role of spectral cues in the discrimination of voice onset time differences. *Journal of the Acoustical Society of America, 73*, 2150–2165.

Soli, S., & Nilsson, M. (1994). Assessment of communication handicap with the HINT. *Hearing Instruments, 45*, 12–16.

Stecker, G. C., & Hafter, E. R. (2000) An effect of temporal asymmetry on loudness. *Journal of the Acoustical Society of America, 107*, 3358–3368.

Stecker, G. C., Harrington, I. A., & Middlebrooks, J. C. (2005). Location coding by opponent neural populations in the auditory cortex. *Public Library of Science, 3*, 520–528, e78.

Stark, R.E., & Tallal, P. (1979). Analysis of stop consonant production errors in developmentally dysphasic children. *Journal of the Acoustical Society of America, 66*, 1703–1712.

Stefanatos, G. A., Braitman, L. E., & Madigan. S. (2007). Fine-grain temporal analysis in aphasia: Evidence from auditory gap detection. *Neuropsychologia, 45*, 1127–1133.

Stefanatos, G. A., Gershkoff, A., & Madigan, S. (2005). On pure word deafness, temporal processing and the left hemisphere. *Journal of the International Neuropsychological Society, 11*, 456–470.

Stefanatos, G. A., Green, G. G. R., & Ratcliff, G. G. (1989). Neurophysiological evidence of auditory channel anomalies in developmental dysphasia. *Archives of Neurology, 46*, 871–875.

Steinschneider, M., Arezzo, J., & Vaughan, H. G. (1982). Speech evoked activity in the auditory radiations and cortex of the awake monkey. *Brain Research, 252*, 353–365.

Suga, N., Yan, J., & Zhang, Y. (1997). Cortical maps for hearing and egocentric selection for self-organization. *Trends in Cognitive Sciences, 1*, 13–20.

Sulakhe, N., Elias, L. J., & Lejbak, L. (2003). Hemispheric asymmetries for gap detection depend on noise type. *Brain and Cognition, 53*, 372–375.

Tallal, P. (1980). Auditory temporal perception, phonics, and reading disabilities in children. *Brain and Language, 9*, 182–198.

Tallal, P., Miller, S., & Fitch, R. H. (1993). Neurobiological basis of speech: A case for the preeminence of temporal processing. *Annals of the New York Academy of Sciences, 682,* 27–47.

Tallal, P., & Piercy, M. (1974). Developmental aphasia: Rate of auditory processing and selective impairment of consonant perception. *Neuropsychologia, 12,* 83–93.

Tallal, P., & Stark, R. E. (1980). Speech acoustic-cue discrimination abilities of normally developing and language-impaired children. *Journal of the Acoustical Society of America, 69,* 568–574.

Tallal, P., Stark, R., Kallman, C., & Mellits, D. (1981). A reexamination of some nonverbal perceptual abilities of language-impaired and normal children as a function of age and sensory modality. *Journal of Speech and Hearing Research, 24,* 351–357.

Tallal, P., Stark, R. E., & Mellits, D. (1985). The relationship between auditory temporal analysis and receptive language development: Evidence from studies of developmental language disorder. *Neuropsychologia, 23,* 527–534.

Taylor, T. L., Hall, S. E., Boehnke, S. E., & Phillips, D. P. (1999). Additivity of perceptual channel-crossing effects in auditory gap detection. *Journal of the Acoustical Society of America, 105,* 563–566.

Turgeon, M., Bregman, A. S., & Ahad, P. A. (2002). Rhythmic masking release: Contribution of cues for perceptual organization to the cross-spectral fusion of concurrent narrowband noises. *Journal of the Acoustical Society of America, 111,* 1819–1831.

Van Wieringen, A., & Wouters, J. (1999). Gap detection in single- and multiple-channel stimuli by LAURA cochlear implantees. *Journal of the Acoustical Society of America, 106,* 125–1939.

Viemeister, N. F. (1979). Temporal modulation transfer functions based upon modulation thresholds. *Journal of the Acoustical Society of America, 66,* 1364–1380.

Walker, K. M. M., Hall, S. E., Klein, R. M., & Phillips, D. P. (2006). Development of perceptual correlates of reading performance. *Brain Research, 1124,* 126–141.

Walton, J. P., Frisina, R.D., Ison, J. R., & O'Neill, W. E. (1997). Neural correlates of behavioral gap detection in the inferior colliculus of the young CBA mouse. *Journal of Comparative Physiology [A], 181,* 161–176.

Warren, R. M. (1970). Perceptual restoration of missing speech sounds. *Science, 167,* 392–393.

Watson, C. S., & Kidd, G. R. (2002). On the lack of association between basic auditory abilities, speech processing, and other cognitive skills. *Seminars in Hearing, 23,* 83–93.

Weinberger, N.M. (1997). Learning-induced receptive field plasticity in the primary auditory cortex. *Seminars in Hearing, 9,* 59–67.

Williams, K. N., & Perrott, D. R. (1972). Temporal resolution of tonal pulses. *Journal of the Acoustical Society of America, 51,* 644–647.

Winkler, I., Czigler, I., Jaramillo, M., Paavilainen, P., & Näätänen, R. (1998). Temporal constraints of auditory event synthesis: Evidence from ERPs. *NeuroReport, 9,* 495–499.

Witton, C., Talcott, J. B., Hansen, P. C., Richardson, A. J., Griffiths, T. D., Rees, A., . . . Green, G. G. R. (1998). Sensitivity to dynamic auditory and visual stimuli predicts nonwod reading ability in both dyslexic and normal readers. *Current Biology, 8,* 791–797.

Wright, B. A., Lombardino, L. J., King, W. M., Puranik, C. S., Leonard, C. M., & Merzenich, M. M. (1997). Deficits in auditory temporal and spectral resolution in language-impaired children. *Nature, 387,* 176–178.

Yabe, H., Tervaniemi, M., Sinkkonen, J., Huotilainen, M., Ilmoniemi, R. J., & Näätänen, R. (1998). Temporal window of integration of auditory information in the human brain. *Psychophysiology, 35,* 615–619.

Yost, W. A., Dye, R. H., & Sheft, S. (1996). A simulated "cocktail party" with up to three sound sources. *Perception and Psychophysics, 58,* 1026–1036.

Zhang, W., Salvi, R. J., & Saunders S. S. (1990). Neural correlates of gap detection in auditory nerve fibers of the chinchilla. *Hearing Research, 46,* 181–200.

4

Translational Perspectives: Current Issues in Inner Ear Regeneration

Jennifer S. Stone and Clifford R. Hume

LEARNING OBJECTIVES

■ To understand the cellular basis of hearing loss and to gain insight into the current state of hair cell regeneration research.

■ To explore the different types of animal models used to study hair cell regeneration in the laboratory.

■ To learn about supporting cells and their important role in hair cell regeneration.

■ To understand potential strategies for repairing hair cells and their connections with spiral ganglion neurons after injury.

Key Words. Hair cell, supporting cell, regeneration, gene therapy, stem cell, cell division, direct conversion

INTRODUCTION

Hearing loss is the most common disability affecting over 28 million Americans and 312 million people worldwide (http://www.who.int/mediacentre/factsheets/fs300/en/index.html). Because hearing loss directly affects communication, this impact can be far-reaching and affect social interactions, access to education, and employment opportunities. While hearing aids and cochlear implants can provide remarkable benefits, they do not restore the full spectrum of hearing and remain underutilized and inaccessible to some. With advances in auditory science and genetics over the past several decades, hope has emerged that regenerative medicine may eventually supplant these technologies and restore the functions of the inner ear that are responsible for the exquisite specificity and sensitivity that we associate with normal hearing and balance.

In this chapter, we review some of the advances in regenerative biology relevant to inner ear disorders and outline some of the challenges affecting the speed at which these advances will be able to be translated into new treatments for patients. We also introduce some of the research in animal model systems that form the foundation for the optimism that regenerative medicine has a future in the treatment of inner ear disorders.

WHAT NEEDS TO BE REPAIRED?

Acquired hearing loss can occur from damage-induced changes at multiple points along the auditory pathway and dysfunction or loss of multiple cell types (see Chapter 1 on noise-induced hearing loss). Similarly, in genetic forms of hearing loss, mutations may in some cases affect hair cells, supporting cells, or nonsensory cells. Although injury of hair cells and neurons underlies most forms of hearing loss, several other cell types that serve important functions in hearing also sustain injury and lose proper function.

These include fibrocytes and cells of the stria vascularis (which regulate endolymph composition), cells of Reissner's membrane, cells of the spiral limbus forming the tectorial membrane, and other unknown cellular targets. Therefore, effective repair of an injured inner ear will most likely require repair of several cell types. The complex pathology of hearing loss suggests that selecting the appropriate type of treatment may also require advances in diagnostic testing to allow identification of specific defects in individual patients. It is unlikely that a single therapy will be applicable to all forms of hearing loss. Once targets for repair are well understood, an additional hurdle will be the reassembly of these cells into tissues that can integrate in the auditory end organ and restore function. However, for the sake of simplicity, our chapter focuses on the restoration of sensory hair cells and their neural connections, whose loss is the major direct cause of hearing loss.

Question 1

Does the damaged inner ear normally repair itself?

Answer 1

Some forms of damage are readily repaired. This includes injury to the stereociliary bundles on hair cells following intense noise exposure. However, extreme injury can lead to degeneration and loss of hair cells, and this type of damage cannot be repaired in mammals, such as humans. By contrast, nonmammalian vertebrates are capable of restoring auditory and vestibular hair cells throughout their lives.

HOW MUCH REPAIR IS NEEDED?

The normal human ear contains approximately 3,500 inner hair cells, 12,000 outer hair cells, and over 30,000 auditory (spiral ganglion) neurons (Spoendlin & Schrott, 1990). Despite this apparent overwhelming complexity, several studies with cochlear implants have demonstrated that users may perform very well in speech testing with limited numbers of electrodes under optimal (quiet) listening environments. In contrast to normal-hearing listeners, cochlear implant user performance degrades dramatically with the addition of noise. Current cochlear implant devices have from 12 to 22 intracochlear electrodes, capable of stimulation at over 1000 pulses per electrode per second. Each electrode stimulates multiple spiral ganglion neurons simultaneously at suprathreshold levels. Patient performance seems to show a ceiling where no significant benefits of more channels are measured beyond 8 electrodes (Friesen et al., 2001; Friesen et al., 2005). Several models have been proposed to explain these limitations, including the number of surviving neurons, the distance of the stimulating electrodes from the target neurons, and the spread of electrical stimulation across the turns of the cochlea.

Together, these findings suggest that a limited number of repaired, regenerated, or transplanted hair cells with appropriate innervation may be sufficient to enable perception that would approach the level of cochlear implant users in a quiet environment. Since hair cells are a principal source of electrical and chemical trophic support to neurons, retention or restoration of hair cells would also likely have potent and lasting supportive effects on the cochlear ganglion population. Further regeneration of injured inner ear structures, perhaps combined with optimization of cochlear implant electrodes, may lead to improvements in performance in more complex, noisy environments and enhance music perception.

NONMAMMALS READILY REGENERATE HAIR CELLS AFTER DAMAGE

Restoration of auditory function could occur by stimulating the repair of existing damaged inner ear cells, by forming replacement cells from stem cells residing within the inner ear, or by transplanting stem cells derived from outside the ear that then differentiate into appropriate cell types.

The degree to which the inner ear cells of mammals, including humans, are capable of self-repair is not well understood. In some cases, threshold shifts in response to loud noise exposure are temporary, and repair of hair cell stereocilia, synaptic dysfunction, tectorial membrane, or endocochlear potential may account for the return of function (Gao et al., 1992; Hirose & Liberman, 2003; Saunders et al., 1985). In some cases of sudden hearing loss, high doses of anti-inflammatory steroids, administered either systemically or transtympanically, may promote recovery of hearing (http://www.clinicaltrials.gov/ct/show/NCT00097448?order=16). The mechanism through which steroids act is unknown, but this observation suggests that inflammation at some level impacts the repair process. It is clear that in many cases the innate repair mechanisms are inadequate, and formation of new cell types is critical for complete recovery of hearing.

The replacement of lost cells in a damaged tissue is called regeneration. Stem cells are cells with the capacity to divide and give rise to more than one cell type in addition to their ability to self-renew. The ability of stem cells to self-renew is critical, since it prevents stem cell depletion and allows regeneration, sometimes throughout the life of the animal. Stem cells are retained in tissues that turn over continuously, such as the columnar epithelium of the gut, keratinocytes in the epidermis (skin), and the hematopoietic system. In general, stem cells are present at low numbers, even in continuously regenerating tissues. Tissues that have limited ability to regenerate, such as the mammalian central nervous system, either lack stem cells or lack the ability to mobilize them adequately. Later in this chapter we discuss the potential use of stem cells for therapy of the inner ear.

It has been known for many years that cold-blooded vertebrates readily regenerate complex tissues, including bone, muscle, and neurons. In fact, the process of hair cell regeneration was first documented in lateral line neuromasts. These collections of hair cells and supporting cells are distributed in regularly spaced patches along the body wall of aquatic species and act as sensor organs to detect fluid movement in the surrounding environment. Following tail amputation, salamanders regenerate a well-formed tail, including neuromasts with the correct number and morphology of hair cells (Stone, 1933, 1937). Salamanders accomplish this by first generating a collection of undifferentiated cells called the blastema along the cut edge of the tail stump. Stem cell intermediaries in the blastema then differentiate into all of the original tissue types found in the tail, including hair cells. Although humans are not capable of this type of repair, these studies demonstrated that cells capable of giving rise to hair cells exist in some mature vertebrates.

Three groups discovered that birds form new auditory hair cells after damage and, perhaps more strikingly, that birds also generate new vestibular hair cells on an ongoing basis, much like humans form new skin cells. The observation that birds can regenerate auditory hair cells was discovered by two groups of scientists who were studying mechanisms of hair cell damage after acoustic overstimulation or treatment with ototoxic aminoglycoside antibiotics. In the first study, investigators exposed posthatch chickens to different pure-tone stimuli at high levels to determine where each tone generated the largest basilar membrane movements and, therefore, the highest degree of hair cell damage (Cotanche et al., 1987). When chickens were allowed to survive several days after the stimulus, it became increasingly difficult to identify where the hair cell lesion had occurred, because it had come to be occupied by immature-looking hair cells (Cotanche, 1987). In the second study, the ototoxic antibiotic gentamicin was administered to posthatch chickens, and auditory epithelia were examined at different times afterward (Cruz et al., 1987). Numbers of hair cells were highly reduced at early time points after drug treatment, but they increased to near-normal levels a couple weeks later. These studies suggested chickens could regenerate new hair cells after damage. These findings were confirmed in two studies showing that replacement hair cells were in fact formed by renewed cell division (discussed below). The importance of this discovery is underscored by the fact that the birds forming new hair cells had mature hearing. Furthermore, regenerated hair cells restored auditory sensitivity in the frequency range where hair cell loss occurred within several weeks of damage (Bermingham-McDonogh & Rubel, 2003).

In the third study alluded to above, Jørgensen and Mathiesen demonstrated for the budgerigar bird utricle in 1988 (Jorgensen & Mathiesen, 1988) that hair cells are renewed on an ongoing basis in vestibular epithelia of the inner ear. As vestibular hair cells die, they are replaced by division of supporting cells surrounding them. In the normal avian ear, precise temporal and spatial regulation of hair cell death and regeneration results in a stable functioning vestibular organ. Hair cells can also be replaced when large numbers are damaged by aminoglycosides (Weisleder & Rubel, 1992), and regenerated hair cells restore vestibular function (Carey et al., 1996b, 1996a).

Findings such as these in non-mammalian vertebrates, perhaps most importantly in warm-blooded birds, underlie the optimism for functional regeneration of the inner ear in humans. Unfortunately, as we discuss below, the capacity for hair cell replacement is significantly more limited in the mammalian vestibular epithelia and appears to be absent in the organ of Corti of mature mammals.

Question 2

What strategies could be used to regenerate the damaged inner ear?

Answer 2

Current research is aimed at two approaches for promoting hair cell regeneration in laboratory mammals, such as mice. First, investigators are attempting to promote supporting cells, the cells that form new hair cells in nonmammals, to either divide and form new hair cells or to directly convert into hair cells without dividing. Second, investigators are examining the capacity of various types of stem cells to form new hair cells when they are transplanted into the inner ear. Both approaches are in early stages of development, and it will likely be several years before they could be developed into therapies.

SUPPORTING CELLS SERVE AS HAIR CELL PROGENITORS

Studies in birds and cold-blooded animals have been instrumental in defining mechanisms that may

someday allow for hair cell regeneration in humans. Perhaps most relevant have been investigations into the identity of the cells that give rise to new hair cells, the hair cell progenitors. New auditory hair cells are formed from cells that divide shortly after damage (Corwin & Cotanche, 1988; Ryals & Rubel, 1988). The newly formed cells differentiate into new hair cells and supporting cells (Figure 4–1). Since new supporting cells were generated after damage, investigators hypothesized that supporting cells

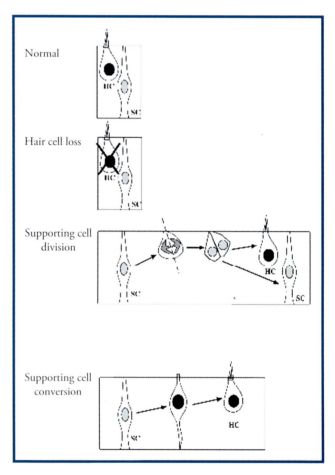

Figure 4–1. Pathways for hair cell regeneration. In the normal inner ear, hair cells (HC) and supporting cells (SC) reside in different layers of the sensory epithelium. After hair cell loss from aging, noise, or ototoxic drugs, hair cells in the nonmammalian vertebrate inner ear are regenerated by two primary mechanisms: supporting cell division and supporting cell conversion. The relative importance of these mechanisms may differ according to the type of damage and species, but both have potential for mammalian hair cell regeneration.

function as limited stem cells, or progenitor cells. This model was confirmed a few years later for the avian auditory epithelium (Hashino & Salvi, 1993; Raphael, 1992; Stone & Cotanche, 1994), vestibular epithelium (Tsue et al., 1994), the amphibian lateral line (Jones & Corwin, 1993, 1996), and saccule (Baird et al., 1993). Supporting cells are nonsensory cells that are organized in a network surrounding individual hair cells. They have many important normal functions, including structural support of the epithelium, sequestration and recycling of ions within the cochlea, and formation and secretion of the tectorial and basement membranes. Supporting cells also secrete important neurotrophic factors, such as neuregulin and brain-derived neurotrophic factor (BDNF), which nourish and maintain cochlear ganglion neurons (Farinas et al., 2001; Rubel & Fritzsch, 2002; Sugawara et al., 2007). This is critical since the continued secretion of these factors by supporting cells may help keep neurons alive after hair cells have degenerated (discussed below).

Identification of supporting cells as hair cell progenitors raised questions: Is there a subpopulation of supporting cells specialized to serve as progenitor cells? Is there a similar cell type in the mammalian inner ear that is capable of dividing after hair cell damage, or is this cell absent? In fact, very little is known about supporting cell specialization vis-à-vis their ability to form new hair cells in any animals, including birds. Although there is variation in cell size and nuclear position among non-mammalian supporting cells, very few other overt distinctions are evident. In contrast, supporting cells in the mammalian organ of Corti are highly specialized, and clear morphologic subpopulations exist. However, the capacity of each cell type for regeneration is not understood.

Although nonmammalian supporting cells readily divide under moderate damage, they fail to do so when damage is severe. For example, prolonged exposure to intense noise in chickens causes massive extrusion of auditory hair cells and de-differentiation of supporting cells to a cuboidal or squamous appearance (Cotanche et al., 1995; Girod et al., 1989). It is suspected that once supporting cells transition to this state, they cannot respond to signals promoting cell division. If this is true in mammals, it could pose a significant problem for late-stage repair of injured

tissues. Even in long-term deafened mammals, some cells with supporting cell features persist, but it remains possible that their capacity to respond to innate pro-regenerative signals has become highly limited (Oesterle & Campbell, 2009).

NONMAMMALIAN REGENERATION DOES NOT REQUIRE CELL DIVISION

Remarkably, it has been demonstrated that cell division is not actually required for the generation of new hair cells in the avian auditory epithelium (Roberson et al., 2004; Rubel et al., 1995; Shang et al., 2010) and the amphibian vestibular epithelia (Baird et al., 2000; Baird et al., 1996; Taylor & Forge, 2005). Regeneration without cell division occurs because supporting cells are able to directly convert into hair cells, a process called *direct transdifferentiation*. During this process, supporting cells undergo stepwise changes in their morphological and molecular features to acquire the form and function of hair cells (see Figure 4–1). It is estimated that between 35 and 50% of new hair cells are formed by direct transdifferentiation (Roberson et al., 2004; Rubel et al., 1995). Thus, new hair cells can be made by two possible mechanisms that could potentially be harnessed to restore hearing function in mammals (see Figure 4–1). Importantly, production of a new hair cell via direct transdifferentiation involves the loss of a supporting cell. Therefore, extensive regeneration using only direct transdifferentiation could eventually deplete the supporting cell progenitor population, if these cells are not replaced. In the chicken auditory epithelium, conversion of supporting cells into hair cells occurs quite early and is followed by a wave of cell division (Cafaro et al., 2007; Roberson & Rubel, 1994). This delayed period of new cell production replenishes the supporting cells lost during direct transdifferentiation. A similar phenomenon, if triggered in mammals, could successfully lead to the regeneration of the correct number and type of cells in the damaged inner ear. Alternatively, we may be able to trigger only moderate levels of hair cell regeneration via direct transdifferentiation, avoiding depletion of supporting cells to a degree that would affect function.

STEM CELLS IN NONMAMMALIAN HAIR CELL EPITHELIA

Multiple studies indicate that supporting cells serve as hair cell progenitors. However, there is much speculation as to whether multipotential stem cells exist in inner ear epithelia or lateral line neuromasts. The continued production of new hair cells and supporting cells in avian vestibular epithelia supports the existence of stem cells in the mature avian inner ear. In addition, birds regenerate auditory hair cells after repeated injuries (Marean et al., 1993; Niemiec et al., 1994), suggesting that progenitor cell renewal occurs. Perhaps most significantly, studies have shown that after a single injury, some supporting cells in the epithelium undergo at least two rounds of cell division (Stone et al., 1999; Wilkins et al., 1999). However, a definitive stem cell has not yet been identified in any hair cell epithelium, and specific cell lineages in mature epithelia have not been described. This is in contrast to other tissues that regenerate, such as the olfactory epithelium (Chen et al., 2004). Therefore, future studies should use markers for stem cells or measures of stem cell behaviors (such as clonal analysis in culture) to search for evidence of this important cell type in nonmammalian inner ear epithelia. Characterization of stem cell properties would stimulate important studies toward hair cell regeneration in mammals.

FACTORS CONTROLLING HAIR CELL REGENERATION IN NONMAMMALIAN VERTEBRATES

In the posthatch avian auditory epithelium, supporting cells and hair cells are normally a stable population; they are fully differentiated, and little new cell production occurs (Corwin & Cotanche, 1988; Oesterle & Rubel, 1993; Ryals & Rubel, 1988). Shortly after hair cell damage is initiated, however, some supporting cells convert into hair cells, whereas others remain quiescent. A few days later, more supporting cells leave their state of growth arrest, enter the cell cycle, and divide. Thus, hair cell damage triggers a series of changes in supporting cells resulting in the re-establishment of the original cellular types, numbers, and patterning in the epithelium.

The signals that direct supporting cells to stay in growth arrest or to transition to either directly transdifferentiate into hair cells or to divide are of critical importance, since it is the apparent inertia of supporting cells after damage that prevents hair cell regeneration in mammals. Considerable progress has been made in identifying markers for dividing cells and regenerated cells, and in developing methods for culturing hair cell epithelia that permit hair cell regeneration. A few studies have utilized these tools to identify factors controlling supporting cell behavior. For example, growth factors, such as insulin-like growth factor-1, fibroblast growth factor-2, activin, and cytokines such as TNF-alpha appear to regulate supporting cell division in damaged chicken auditory and vestibular epithelia (McCullar et al., 2010; Oesterle et al., 1997; Oesterle et al., 2000; Warchol, 1999). Intracellular signaling molecules that may mediate this signaling have been identified, including cAMP, PI-3 Kinase, and TOR (Navaratnam et al., 1996; Witte et al., 2001). In addition, after damage, signaling through the Notch receptor antagonizes proliferation-dependent hair cell regeneration in the zebrafish lateral line (Ma et al., 2008), and it blocks both proliferation-dependent regeneration and direct transdifferentiation in the chicken basilar papilla (Daudet et al., 2009).

A lot of work remains to be done in this area. Identification of stem cells and tools for purifying them will lead to progress in understanding how hair cell regeneration is controlled in non-mammals. Also, large scale bioinformatics studies of genes that are turned on or off after hair cell damage will help to identify signaling pathways that promote or block new hair cell production in non-mammals. These efforts will provide new leads toward biological cures for hearing loss in humans.

HAIR CELL REGENERATION IS BLOCKED IN MATURE MAMMALS

Limited Capacity for Hair Cell Regeneration in Mature Mammalian Organ of Corti

Shortly after the discovery that new hair cells can be formed in birds after damage, several laboratories began to examine the degree to which the mature mammalian auditory epithelium also regenerates hair cells. Most of these studies were conducted in rodents with large and easily dissected ears, such a guinea pigs. Investigators have used acoustic overstimulation and ototoxic drugs to trigger hair cell damage in these studies. Unfortunately, investigators have consistently found that new auditory hair cells are not formed after damage in mammals. In fact, only rare, if any, supporting cells in the mature organ of Corti re-enter the cell cycle after hair cell loss (Roberson & Rubel, 1994), and little or no spontaneous direct transdifferentiation occurs in the mature organ of Corti after hair cell loss (Forge et al., 1998).

In contrast to the auditory epithelium, low levels of supporting cell division are triggered after hair cell damage in the mammalian vestibular epithelia (Rubel et al., 1995; Warchol et al., 1993). This is interesting in light of the fact that vestibular epithelia are morphologically and functionally less divergent across species than the auditory epithelia. A few of the limited new cells that are generated appear to initiate differentiation of hair cell features (Oesterle et al., 2003; Warchol et al., 1993), but these rarely acquire mature hair cell characteristics, as do avian vestibular epithelia. Direct transdifferentiation may be a much larger player in vestibular hair cell regeneration in mammals (Forge et al., 1993; Forge et al., 1998; Kawamoto et al., 2009; Li & Forge, 1997). For instance, careful morphological analyses of the utricular epithelium of adult guinea pigs at several time-points after gentamicin treatment revealed that original hair cells quickly disappear from the striolar region, the zone of polarity reversal for hair cell stereociliary bundles (Forge et al., 1998). Two weeks later, immature-appearing hair cells are evident in this region, suggesting newly differentiating hair cells have emerged there. At later times, this population of hair cells seems to have matured.

In the immature mammalian auditory and the vestibular systems, there is an innate capacity for hair cell regeneration in immature organs. For example, in vitro ablation of hair cells in the embryonic mouse cochlea triggers adjacent cells to differentiate into replacement hair cells (Kelley et al., 1995). Under appropriate conditions, supporting cells isolated from neonatal mice divide and form new hair cells in culture as late as the onset of hearing (White et al., 2006). Furthermore, a small number of cells isolated from the organ of Corti of neonatal mice is able to form cellular clusters containing hair cells when treated with a mixture of growth factors, suggesting that they arise from a stem cell (Malgrange et al., 2002; Oshima et al., 2007). However, in these cultures, the capacity for cell proliferation and hair cell production falls off steeply during the early postnatal period. These observations suggest that stem or progenitor cells are lost from the supporting cell population over time, or that regenerative capacity in supporting cells declines during maturation. Future studies should be aimed at determining how properties of the organ of Corti progressively become more restrictive to new hair cell production as the mammalian ear matures. In contrast to humans who are born with hearing function, mice develop hearing during the early postnatal period. There may be some link between loss of regenerative capacity and the acquisition of hearing.

MODELS FOR BIOLOGICAL INTERVENTION TO PROMOTE HAIR CELL REGENERATION IN MAMMALS

Given the limited degree of spontaneous hair cell regeneration that occurs after damage in the mature mammalian inner ear, several investigators have turned toward identifying new ways to induce the replacement of sensory hair cells. Two general approaches are being taken: (1) to promote higher numbers of cells *within the inner ear* to form new hair cells, by cell division or direct transdifferentiation; and (2) to introduce cells from outside the ear that have the capacity to proliferate and differentiate into new hair cells (Figure 4–2). In both approaches, emphasis is placed on determining if newly formed cells restore auditory (or vestibular) function. Investigators must consider both the initial cause of hair cell damage and the time that has elapsed since that damage has occurred when selecting which types of treatments to investigate and develop. Each of these factors weighs heavily on the status of the inner ear and is likely to have a large impact on the effectiveness of a given treatment. Specific experiments using the two approaches are discussed below.

Regeneration from the Inside: Teaching Old Supporting Cells New Tricks

As hair cell regeneration is robust and spontaneous in birds and other nonmammals, there is considerable excitement about the feasibility of stimulating resident supporting cells, or other cells, to form new hair cells in mammals. However, because mammalian supporting cells fail to form any new auditory hair cell after damage, investigators are faced with identifying manipulations that promote supporting cells to respond in more favorable ways. Research toward this goal has focused on two general strategies: (1) promoting proliferation of supporting cells by exposing them to substances that trigger cell division (growth factors, cytokines, or activators of second messenger signalers); and (2) triggering supporting cells to convert directly into new hair cells (via direct transdifferentiation) by introducing genes, or inducing genes, that promote this process.

The first demonstration that specific growth factors can stimulate cell division in the damaged inner ear epithelia was first performed in cultured utricles from mature rats and mice (Lambert, 1994; Yamashita & Oesterle, 1995). Several growth factors, including insulin and transforming growth factor alpha, were shown to have limited although significant effects on supporting cell division in these cultures. Utricles were studied because of their ease of culture relative to the mature organ of Corti. In fact, the extreme challenge of removing intact organ of Corti tissue in animals after the first postnatal week is a huge impediment for research on auditory hair cell regeneration in mammals and has biased investigators toward studying immature animals in which dissections are easier and have a higher success rate. Unfortunately, molecules that show dramatic effects in promoting supporting cell division in young rodents have little or no effect on mature rodents (Gu et al., 2007; Hume et al., 2003; Kuntz & Oesterle, 1998; Saffer et al., 1996;). This finding suggests that control of cell division becomes more stringent with time and that manipulation of more than one pathway may be required to promote new hair cell production. There is also concern that unregulated stimulation of cell division may have detrimental effects on function or may pose a risk for malignant transformation.

To identify signals that promote supporting cells to convert into hair cells, or to trigger cells regenerated via new cell division to differentiate into hair cells, investigators have studied the molecules that regulate hair cell differentiation during embryogenesis. Of the numerous genes identified, *atoh1* (also called *math1*), appears to have the most potential.

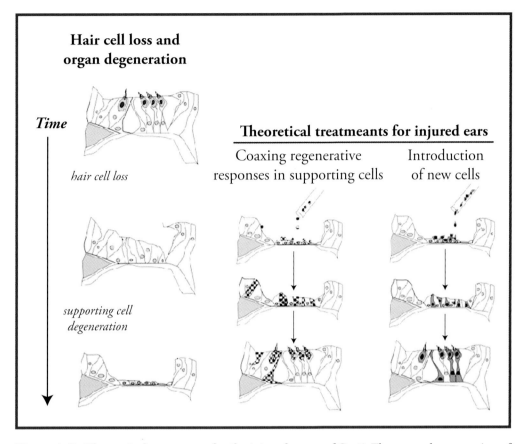

Figure 4–2. Theoretical treatments for the injured organ of Corti. The general progression of organ of Corti degeneration is depicted in the left panel. Two theoretical strategies for treating the degenerated organ of Corti are presented in the two panels on the right. The first treatment ("Coaxing regenerative responses in supporting cells") involves the delivery of genes or other molecules to supporting cells that, as a result, drive supporting cells toward regenerating new hair cells, either by cell division or conversion. The second treatment ("Introduction of new cells") entails transplantation of stemlike or differentiated cells into the organ of Corti that subsequently differentiate into hair cells and/or supporting cells.

Atoh1 is a transcription factor that is required for hair cell formation during development in mice (Bermingham et al., 1999) and fish (Millimaki et al., 2007). Transcription factors are proteins that control and coordinate the expression of specific sets of genes and thereby create the unique molecular identity of each cell type. In cultures of the developing rodent organ of Corti, forced expression of *atoh1* can trigger targeted cells to differentiate into hair cells, demonstrating the power of this transcription factor in directing hair cell–specific gene programs (Zheng & Gao, 2000). A similar effect is seen in cultures of

the adult rat utricle (Shou et al., 2003). These exciting findings in vitro prompted investigators to see if similar effects of *atoh1* misexpression could induce hair cell differentiation in mature damaged cochleae.

Kawamoto et al. injected adenovirus encoding *atoh1* into the scala media of deafened adult guinea pigs (Kawamoto et al., 2003). When performed soon after deafening, this treatment appears to either protect hair cells from damage or trigger limited hair cell regeneration in some regions of the cochlea. Furthermore, newly formed hair cell–like cells appeared to attract auditory neural processes, and *atoh1*-treated animals exhibited improved hearing thresholds (Izumikawa et al., 2005). In a similar study, adenoviral *atoh1* was shown to promote vestibular hair cell regeneration and recovery of vestibular function in aminoglycoside-treated rodents (Baker et al., 2009; Staecker et al., 2007).

One very important finding is that there is only a narrow time window after hair cell damage during which misexpression of *atoh1* gene alone is sufficient to trigger the regenerative process. At later time points after damage, no new hair cell differentiation occurs (Izumikawa et al., 2008). This finding suggests the milieu of the organ of Corti or the supporting cells themselves undergoes progressive changes after damage that render supporting cells less receptive to the pro-regenerative influence afforded by *atoh1* misexpression. It remains to be determined if *atoh1*-induced hair cells will continue to survive and function in the organ of Corti, or if they eventually undergo cell death or immune attack.

The identification of *atoh1* is only a starting point to explore the potential of genetic cellular reprogramming to regenerate hair cells. The promotion of regeneration in a long-damaged inner ear may require more complex manipulations, such as the delivery of a cocktail of transcription factors to coordinate the differentiation and assembly of multiple cell types critical for inner ear function.

Regeneration from the Outside-In: Cell Transplantation

There is much optimism that researchers will find ways to trigger mature supporting cells residing in the ear to form new hair cells, even a long time postinjury. Nonetheless, some investigators are looking into how cells derived from outside the inner ear can be used to promote hair cell replacement. This approach may be more efficient at producing large numbers of differentiated hair cells than intrinsic regeneration. The clear drawback to this approach is that transplanted cells must integrate appropriately into the damaged inner ear.

The main types of cells considered for transplantation into the injured inner ear are stem cells. As discussed above, stem cells are multipotent (they

form many cell types) and under appropriate conditions can divide for long periods of time. Several types of stem cells exist. Embryonic stem (ES) cells and induced pluripotent stem (iPS) cells appear to be capable of forming all cell types in the body. Other stem cells, such as mesenchymal or neural stem cells, are more restricted with respect to their potential. ES cells are derived from the inner cell mass of very early embryos from humans or mice. All other stem cells are derived from progenitor-like or terminally differentiated somatic cells that have been coaxed to have stemlike properties by forced misexpression of transcription factors that induce de-differentiation and restore cells to more primitive identities. Stem cells are easily amplified in culture, and treatment with growth factors and other compounds stimulates their differentiation along specific developmental pathways so that specific cell types can be generated.

Several types of stem cells have been transplanted into the injured inner ear to study their regenerative properties. In the earliest studies, investigators used neural stem cells (Ito et al., 2001; Parker et al., 2007; Tateya et al., 2003), which are more differentiated and restricted than ES and iPS cells. Neural stem cells were injected into the perilymph of the rodent cochlea, and their incorporation into inner ear epithelia and other regions was monitored. Although some cells were able to incorporate into the spiral ganglion and the vestibular epithelia, few transplanted cells found their way to the organ of Corti. Additional avenues for cell delivery, such as via the endolymph, may be required to achieve high-efficiency transplantation to the organ of Corti. Alternatively, transplantation of less restricted cell types may be the key. ES cells can be coaxed stepwise to differentiate into hair cell–like cells in vitro (Li et al., 2003). ES cells and iPS cells, when stimulated with a specific cocktails and grown on mesenchyme derived from the inner ear, form hair cell–like cells with the ability to mechanotransduce (Li et al., 2003; Oshima et al., 2010. Although these in vitro studies are promising, it remains unclear whether transplanted ES or iPS cells will be able to integrate into damaged sensory epithelia, differentiate hair cell features, and re-establish appropriate neural connections, or whether they will be capable of restoring function to the damaged injured inner ear.

Question 4

What risks might there be to using viruses or other gene therapy vectors to treat hearing loss?

Answer 4

Viruses are powerful delivery systems for gene therapy. Several steps can be taken to minimize risks to patients, such as improving viral targeting (i.e., limiting the types of cells that are infected) and reducing viral spread (e.g., by using viruses that cannot replicate). Nonetheless, viruses do pose risks for patients. Some risks can be anticipated. For example, viruses stimulate immune reactions that could theoretically rid the ear of treated cells, thereby abolishing positive effects of gene therapy, or worse, that could trigger immunological responses that are injurious to the patient. Additional risks are impossible to predict, since viral gene therapy has not been applied to inner ear tissues.

Any gene therapy poses risks by its very nature: it represents an intrusion on the normal genetic programs of cells and tissues. Accordingly, it will be important to determine ways to turn target genes on and off, in specific cell types and at specific times, to obtain the best results for improving function in the injured ear.

REGENERATION OF AUDITORY NEURONS

The auditory nerve is the final common pathway for transmission of signals from hair cells and cochlear implant electrodes to the brainstem. An important side effect of hair cell loss is the subsequent degeneration of auditory nerve fibers and cell bodies that occurs because hair cells and supporting cells are a major source of neurotrophic factors nourishing cochlear ganglion neurons (Fayad & Linthicum, 2006; Linthicum & Fayad, 2009; Nadol, 1997; Nadol &

Eddington, 2006; White et al., 2000). Once significant neuronal loss has occurred, the potential for improvements in hearing that are mediated by hearing aids or cochlear implants may decrease. However, human temporal bone studies show there is little correlation between the number of surviving auditory neurons and cochlear implant performance. This emphasizes that the critical variables that determine how well cochlear implant electrodes interface with surviving neurons are still poorly understood (Fayad & Linthicum, 2006, reviewed in Nadol & Eddington, 2006; Kawano et al., 1998). Research on auditory neuron regeneration can be divided into two general areas of interest (discussed below): (1) promoting neurite outgrowth in surviving neurons, and (2) increasing the number of auditory neurons either through regeneration or transplantation.

Neurite Regeneration

Several strategies have been used to deliver neurotrophic agents to the inner ear and to promote auditory neuron survival and neurite outgrowth. These include direct infusion of agents via osmotic pumps, delivery of viral vectors encoding agents, and implantation of exogenous cells producing agents. The major site of neural stimulation by conventional cochlear implants is the neuronal cell body, with a small contribution by the peripheral neurites (Briaire & Frijns, 2006; Clopton et al., 1980). It has been shown that moving the array closer to the spiral ganglion in the modiolus results in both a decrease in the threshold of the electrically evoked auditory brainstem response and an increase in the dynamic range (Shepherd et al., 1993). Closing the distance between the stimulating electrodes and their targets is expected to have the benefit of more localized stimulation of auditory neurons and reduced power consumption (Frijns et al., 2001; Snyder et al., 2008). One strategy to accomplish this goal is to specifically attract neurites to electrodes by engineering them to release neural guidance molecules (neurotropic factors). Alternatively, surviving supporting cells in the deafened organ of Corti may be stimulated by gene therapy to release neurotropic factors and to act as surrogate targets to coax neurites closer to cochlear implant electrodes or regenerated hair cells (Figure 4–3).

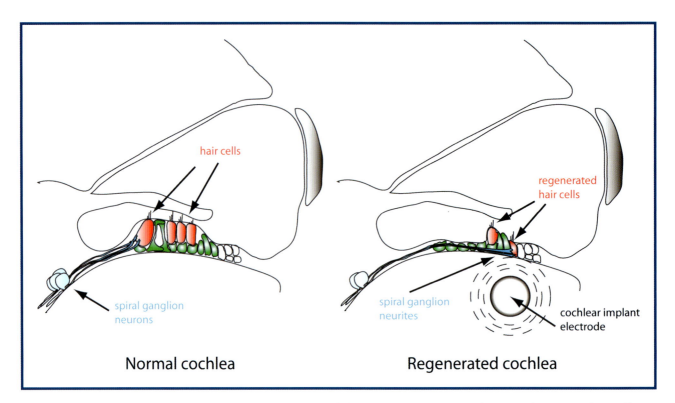

Figure 4–3. Additional strategies to improve hearing through hair cell regeneration. In the normal inner ear, hair cells are innervated by afferent type I spiral ganglion neurons. In one regeneration scenario, spiral ganglion neurons could be coaxed to reinnervate regenerated or transplanted hair cells. Alternatively, these new hair cells or cells engineered to express neurotropic factors could attract neurites to locations where they can be more specifically stimulated by cochlear implant electrodes.

NT3 and BDNF act as neural guidance factors for sensory neurons (Genc et al., 2004; O'Connor & Tessier-Lavigne, 1999). Intracochlear infusion of BDNF and NT3 or neurotrophin-producing viruses into deafened guinea pigs promotes survival of spiral ganglion neurons and resprouting of peripheral fibers (Chikar et al., 2008; Ernfors et al., 1996; Miller et al., 1997; Ruan et al., 1999; Shibata et al., 2010; Shinohara et al., 2002; Wise et al., 2005; Wise et al., 2010). In some cases, electrically evoked thresholds from cochlear implants improve after neurotrophin treatment (Chikar et al., 2008). However, it remains unknown whether the peripheral fibers regenerate in a sufficiently organized manner to improve functional performance (Shibata et al., 2010; Wise et al., 2005; Wise et al., 2010). In addition to NT3 and BDNF, a number of other growth factors also hold promise to promote regeneration of auditory neurons (Roehm & Hansen, 2005). Because the tonotopic specificity of the normal inner ear and the pitch cod-

ing of cochlear implants are both dependent on this organization, the disorganized growth may compromise function. This loss of specificity may not be revealed in electrically evoked auditory brainstem response thresholds, but it may be evident in physiologic studies of upper auditory pathways by looking at the spread of activation (Middlebrooks and Snyder, 2008). Localized sources of a neurotrophic molecule in the cochlea may provide adequate signals for appropriate regeneration of the normally precisely oriented afferent fibers, enabling improvements in cochlear implant function.

Neuronal Replacement Via Transplantation

In addition to their ability to form hair cells in vitro, ES cells and cells derived from the fetal cochlea can also be coaxed in vitro to acquire neuronlike properties (Chen et al., 2009; Corrales et al., 2006). Injection of ES-derived or iPS-derived neuronal cells into the injured spiral ganglion in vivo leads to incorporation and growth of neurites from the transplanted cells toward the organ of Corti of gerbils (Corrales et al., 2006; Nishimura et al., 2009). This suggests that some of the necessary signals to guide auditory neuron axons remain intact, even in the deafened inner ear. Again, it remains unknown if the specificity of the regenerated neurons is sufficient to improve auditory function. Delivery of drugs directly into the inner ear may improve the outcomes of cell transplantaion by promoting cellular integration and maturation of transplanted cells (McCall et al., 2010).

Question 5

What might the drawbacks be to transplantation of cells to the inner ear?

Answer 5

Some theoretical downsides of cell transplantation include potential worsening of inner ear function due to proliferation of transplanted cells within the target tissue and/or migration of cells out of the target tissue and into areas where they negatively impact function. In addition, transplanted cells may not differentiate all features required to restore function, or they may not be stable once they have differentiated. It will be critical to characterize the behavior of all types of transplanted cells once they have been introduced into the inner ear compartments, in the short and long term.

FUTURE AREAS FOR RESEARCH

New Animal Models for Studying Hair Cell Regeneration

For many years, most studies on hair cell regeneration were conducted in birds and mammals. Recently, zebrafish have developed into an exciting model to study hair cell regeneration (Harris et al., 2003). As described above, in addition to inner ear hair cells, fish have clusters of neuromasts arrayed along the outside of their bodies. Compared to traditional vertebrate models of inner ear hair cell regeneration, neuromast regeneration is amenable to rapid in vivo imaging in real time and space using fluorescent tracers. Combined with well-characterized genetics and short generation times, zebrafish have proven a powerful model for high throughput screens for new drugs. Using molecular techniques (morpholinos), it is also possible to manipulate the expression of individual genes to test hypotheses about candidate regulatory molecules. These strengths of zebrafish as an animal model should hasten discovery into hair cell progenitors and the molecules that promote their regenerative behaviors after hair cell loss.

Gene Therapy and Inner Ear Disorders

Gene therapy to increase or decrease expression of specific genes or sets of genes may provide a way to eventually restore function to hard of hearing and dizzy patients. The potential for this strategy has already been hinted at above, where overexpression of *atoh1* under specific conditions can stimulate some degree of regeneration in the adult mammalian inner ear (Izumikawa et al., 2005; Kawamoto et al., 2001; Kawamoto et al., 2003). The inner ear has several advantages compared to other organ systems. For example, the relative isolation of the inner ear in the temporal bone provides a natural barrier to the spread of gene therapy reagents to other parts of the body where they could have unintended side effects. The fluid-filled scalae allow some degree of diffusion throughout the labyrinth from a single site of injection (Praetorius et al., 2007; Salt & DeMott, 1997, 1998). Several disadvantages also exist. The minute size of the inner ear, its encapsulation in dense bone, and its delicate structure result in inevitable surgical trauma when one gains access to its fluid spaces. Therefore, surgical manipulation of the ear can have the unfortunate side effect of causing additional loss of hearing and balance function.

Delivery of a therapeutic agent to a specific inner ear compartment will likely be preferred with most regenerative approaches. Delivery of genes to the inner ear was first reported in 1996 (Raphael et al., 1996). Since then, the field has progressed on multiple fronts and a variety of viral and non-viral gene transfer vectors such as cationic liposomes, adeno-associated virus (AAV), adenovirus, lentivirus, herpes simplex virus and vaccinia virus have been studied (Derby et al., 1999; Han et al., 1999; Komeda et al., 1999; Lalwani et al., 1997; Lalwani et al., 1996; Luebke et al., 2001a, 2001b; Raphael et al., 1996; Staecker et al., 2001). Multiple surgical approaches to deliver chemicals, viruses, or cells to the inner ear have also been described. These include delivery via a semicir-

cular canalostomy, injection into the ampulla, injection through the round window, and a basal-turn cochleostomy (Chen et al., 2006; Iguchi et al., 2004; Lalwani et al., 1996; Liu et al., 2005; Praetorius et al., 2003; Raphael et al., 1996; Wenzel et al., 2007). One example is shown in Figure 4–4. There is considerable variability in the specificity, efficiency, and toxicity of gene therapies delivered by each approach to the different scalae and the vestibular labyrinth. Therefore, in future studies it will be critical to evaluate the best approach for a given patient based on the target for gene therapy, the condition of the patient's inner ear, and the specific symptoms targeted for treatment.

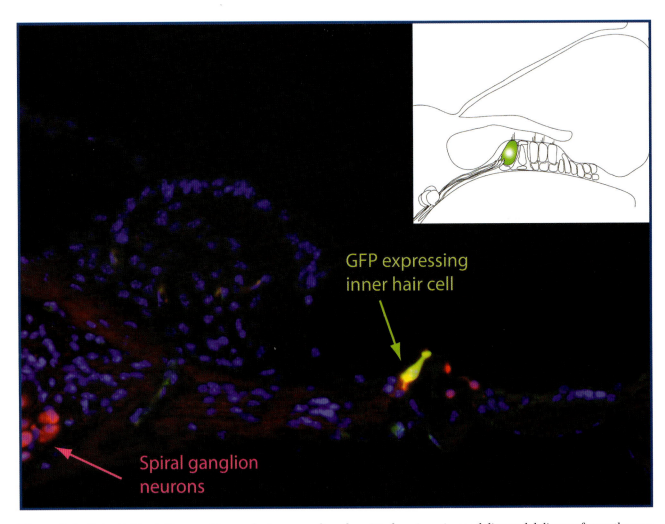

Figure 4–4. Potential tools for gene therapy for inner ear disorders. Viral engineering and directed delivery of gene therapy reagents to the inner ear enables targeting of specific inner ear cell types. In this example, Adeno-Associated Virus-6 expressing a green fluorescent protein reporter gene (GFP) was delivered to the scala tympani. Only inner hair cells were found to express GFP, demonstrating they can be targeted for gene therapy.

CONCLUSION

Over the past several decades, there have been dramatic advances in our understanding of the pathways and molecules that regulate the regeneration of the mammalian inner ear. At the same time, a number of powerful new techniques for delivery of drugs, gene therapy vectors, and cells to the inner ear have been developed using animal models for human hearing and balance disorders. The combination of these approaches have led to promising studies demonstrating that inner ear cells can be regenerated by direct transdifferentiation using gene therapy or by cell transplantation under appropriate conditions. The next challenge will be how to improve the efficiency of this process and to coordinate the integration of regenerated cells into the functional architecture of the ear without causing further damage.

Although these techniques are still far from direct application to human patients, even a modest degree of regeneration may provide significant improvement in function. Because the underlying inner ear pathology is diverse, there is a critical need to improve physiologic/anatomic diagnostic audiology, so that we can know which specific abnormalities need to be treated in individual patients with hearing loss and dizziness, to allow for the best possible targeting of therapy.

Question 6

How does the current state of diagnostic audiology limit approaches to treatment of human hearing loss?

Answer 6

Current diagnostics are unable to pinpoint which cell types are impacted in patients with hearing loss (or loss of balance function). Therefore, delivery of therapy at this time would involve educated guesses and may prove to be insufficient or off-target. For this reason, it is essential to define better tests for determining the site(s) of injury in the inner ear that are noninvasive.

FURTHER READINGS

Brignull, H. R., Raible, D. W., & Stone, J. S. (2009). Feathers and fins: Non-mammalian models for hair cell regeneration. *Brain Research, 1277*, 12–23.

Groves A. K. (2010). The challenge of hair cell regeneration. *Experimental Biology and Medicine, 235*, 434–446.

Stone, J. S., & Oesterle, E. O. (2008). Cell determinants of proliferation and differentiation during hair cell regeneration. In R. Salvi, R. Fay, & A. Popper (Eds.), *Auditory hair cell protection and regeneration*. New York, NY: Springer-Verlag.

Kwan, T., White, P. M., & Segil, N. (2009). Development and regeneration of the inner ear. *Annals of the New York Academy of Sciences, 1170*, 28–33.

REFERENCES

Baird, R. A., Burton, M. D., Fashena, D. S., & Naeger, R. A. (2000). Hair cell recovery in mitotically blocked cultures of the bullfrog saccule. *Proceedings of the National Academy of Sciences of the United States of America, 97*, 11722–11729.

Baird, R. A., Steyger, P. S., & Schuff, N. R. (1996). Mitotic and nonmitotic hair cell regeneration in the bullfrog vestibular otolith organs. *Annals of the New York Academy of Sciences, 781*, 59–70.

Baird, R. A., Torres, M. A., & Schuff, N. R. (1993). Hair cell regeneration in the bullfrog vestibular otolith organs following aminoglycoside toxicity. *Hearing Research, 65*, 164–174.

Baker, K., Brough, D. E., & Staecker, H. (2009). Repair of the vestibular system via adenovector delivery of Atoh1: A potential treatment for balance disorders. *Advances in Otorhinolaryngology, 66*, 52–63.

Bermingham-McDonogh, O., & Rubel, E. W. (2003). Hair cell regeneration: Winging our way towards a sound future. *Current Opinion in Neurobiology, 13*, 119–126.

Bermingham, N. A., Hassan, B. A., Price, S. D., Vollrath, M. A., Ben-Arie, N., Eatock, R. A., . . . Zoghbi, H. Y. (1999). Math1: An essential gene for the generation of inner ear hair cells. *Science, 284*, 1837–1841.

Briaire, J. J., & Frijns, J. H. (2006). The consequences of neural degeneration regarding optimal cochlear implant position in scala tympani: A model approach. *Hearing Research, 214*, 17–27.

Cafaro, J., Lee, G. S., & Stone, J. S. (2007). Atoh1 expression defines activated progenitors and differentiating hair cells during avian hair cell regeneration. *Developmental Dynamics, 236*, 156–170.

Carey, J. P., Fuchs, A. F., & Rubel, E. W. (1996a). Hair cell regeneration and recovery of the vestibuloocular reflex in the avian vestibular system. *Journal of Neurophysiology, 76*, 3301–3312.

Carey, J. P., Fuchs, A. F., & Rubel, E. W. (1996b). Hair cell regeneration and vestibulo-ocular reflex recovery. *Annals of the New York Academy of Sciences, 781*, 47–58.

Chen, W., Johnson, S. L., Marcotti, W., Andrews, P. W., Moore, H. D., & Rivolta, M. N. (2009). Human fetal auditory stem cells can be expanded in vitro and differentiate into functional auditory neurons and hair cell-like cells. *Stem Cells, 27*, 1196–1204.

Chen, X., Fang, H., & Schwob, J. E. (2004). Multipotency of purified, transplanted globose basal cells in olfactory epithelium. *Journal of Comparative Neurology, 469*, 457–474.

Chen, Z., Mikulec, A. A., McKenna, M. J., Sewell, W. F., & Kujawa, S. G. (2006). A method for intracochlear drug delivery in the mouse. *Journal of Neuroscience Methods, 150*, 67–73.

Chikar, J. A., Colesa, D. J., Swiderski, D. L., Di Polo, A., Raphael, Y., & Pfingst, B. E. (2008). Over-expression of BDNF by adenovirus with concurrent electrical stimulation improves cochlear implant thresholds and survival of auditory neurons. *Hearing Research, 245*, 24–34.

Clopton, B. M., Spelman, F. A., & Miller, J. M. (1980). Estimates of essential neural elements for stimulation through a cochlear prosthesis. *Annals of Otology, Rhinology, and Laryngology (Suppl.), 89*, 5–7.

Corrales, C. E., Pan, L., Li, H., Liberman, M. C., Heller, S., & Edge, A. S. (2006). Engraftment and differentiation of embryonic stem cell-derived neural progenitor cells in the cochlear nerve trunk: Growth of processes into the organ of Corti. *Journal of Neurobiology, 66*, 1489–1500.

Corwin, J. T., & Cotanche, D. A. (1988). Regeneration of sensory hair cells after acoustic trauma. *Science, 240*, 1772–1774.

Cotanche, D. A. (1987). Regeneration of hair cell stereociliary bundles in the chick cochlea following severe acoustic trauma. *Hearing Research, 30*, 181–195.

Cotanche, D. A., Messana, E. P., & Ofsie, M. S. (1995). Migration of hyaline cells into the chick basilar papilla during severe noise damage. *Hearing Research, 91*, 148–159.

Cotanche, D. A., Saunders, J. C., & Tilney, L. G. (1987). Hair cell damage produced by acoustic trauma in the chick cochlea. *Hearing Research, 25*, 267–286.

Cruz, R. M., Lambert, P. R., & Rubel, E. W. (1987). Light microscopic evidence of hair cell regeneration after gentamicin toxicity in chick cochlea. *Archives of Otolaryngology-Head and Neck Surgery, 113*, 1058–1062.

Derby, M. L., Sena-Esteves, M., Breakefield, X. O., & Corey, D. P. (1999). Gene transfer into the mammalian inner ear using HSV-1 and vaccinia virus vectors. *Hearing Research, 134*, 1–8.

Ernfors, P., Duan, M. L., ElShamy, W. M., & Canlon, B. (1996). Protection of auditory neurons from aminoglycoside toxicity by neurotrophin-3. *Nature Medicine, 2*, 463–467.

Farinas, I., Jones, K. R., Tessarollo, L., Vigers, A. J., Huang, E., Kirstein, M., . . . Fritzsch, B. (2001). Spatial shaping of cochlear innervation by temporally regulated neurotrophin expression. *Journal of Neuroscience, 21*, 6170–6180.

Fayad, J. N., & Linthicum, F. H. J. (2006). Multichannel cochlear implants: Relation of histopathology to performance. *Laryngoscope, 116*, 1310–1320.

Forge, A., Li, L., Corwin, J. T., & Nevill, G. (1993). Ultrastructural evidence for hair cell regeneration in the mammalian inner ear. *Science, 259*, 1616–1619.

Forge, A., Li, L., & Nevill, G. (1998). Hair cell recovery in the vestibular sensory epithelia of mature guinea pigs. *Journal of Comparative Neurology, 397*, 69–88.

Friesen, L. M., Shannon, R. V., Baskent, D., & Wang, X. (2001). Speech recognition in noise as a function of the number of spectral channels: Comparison of acoustic hearing and cochlear implants. *Journal of the Acoustical Society of America, 110*, 1150–1163.

Friesen, L. M., Shannon, R. V., & Cruz, R. J. (2005). Effects of stimulation rate on speech recognition with cochlear implants. *Audiology and Neurootology, 10*, 169–184.

Frijns, J. H., Briaire, J. J., & Grote, J. J. (2001). The importance of human cochlear anatomy for the results of modiolus-hugging multichannel cochlear implants. *Otology and Neurotology, 22*, 340–349.

Gao, W. Y., Ding, D. L., Zheng, X. Y., Ruan, F. M., & Liu, Y. J. (1992). A comparison of changes in the stereocilia between temporary and permanent hearing losses in acoustic trauma. *Hearing Research, 62*, 27–41.

Genc, B., Ozdinler, P. H., Mendoza, A. E., & Erzurumlu, R. S. (2004). A chemoattractant role for NT-3 in proprioceptive axon guidance. *PLoS Biology, 2*, e403.

Girod, D. A., Duckert, L. G., & Rubel, E. W. (1989). Possible precursors of regenerated hair cells in the avian cochlea following acoustic trauma. *Hearing Research, 42*, 175–194.

Gu, R., Montcouquiol, M., Marchionni, M., & Corwin, J. T. (2007). Proliferative responses to growth factors decline rapidly during postnatal maturation of mammalian hair cell epithelia. *European Journal of Neuroscience, 25*, 1363–1372.

Han, J. J., Mhatre, A. N., Wareing, M., Pettis, R., Gao, W. Q., Zufferey, R. N., . . . Lalwani, A. K. (1999). Transgene expression in the guinea pig cochlea mediated by a lentivirus-derived gene transfer vector. *Human Gene Therapy, 10*, 1867–1873.

Harris, J. A., Cheng, A. G., Cunningham, L. L., MacDonald, G., Raible, D. W., & Rubel, E. W. (2003). Neomycin-induced hair cell death and rapid regeneration in the lateral line of zebrafish (Danio rerio). *Journal of the Association for Research in Otolaryngology, 4*, 219–234.

Hashino, E., & Salvi, R. J. (1993). Changing spatial patterns of DNA replication in the noise-damaged chick cochlea. *Journal of Cell Science, 105*, 23–31.

Hirose, K., & Liberman, M. C. (2003). Lateral wall histopathology and endocochlear potential in the noise-damaged mouse cochlea. *Journal of the Association for Research in Otolaryngology, 4*, 339–352.

Hume, C. R., Kirkegaard, M., & Oesterle, E. C. (2003). ErbB expression: The mouse inner ear and maturation of the mitogenic response to heregulin. *Journal of the Association for Research in Otolaryngology, 4*, 422–443.

Iguchi, F., Nakagawa, T., Tateya, I., Endo, T., Kim, T. S., Dong, Y., . . . Ito, J. (2004). Surgical techniques for cell transplantation into the mouse cochlea. *Acta Otolaryngologica (Suppl.),* pp. 43–47.

Ito, J., Kojima, K., & Kawaguchi, S. (2001). Survival of neural stem cells in the cochlea. *Acta Otolaryngology, 121,* 140–142.

Izumikawa, M., Batts, S. A., Miyazawa, T., Swiderski, D. L., & Raphael, Y. (2008). Response of the flat cochlear epithelium to forced expression of Atoh1. *Hearing Research, 240,* 52–56.

Izumikawa, M., Minoda, R., Kawamoto, K., Abrashkin, K. A., Swiderski, D. L., Dolan, D. F., . . . Raphael, Y. (2005). Auditory hair cell replacement and hearing improvement by Atoh1 gene therapy in deaf mammals. *Nature Medicine, 11,* 271–276.

Jones, J. E., & Corwin, J. T. (1993). Replacement of lateral line sensory organs during tail regeneration in salamanders: Identification of progenitor cells and analysis of leukocyte activity. *Journal of Neuroscience, 13,* 1022–1034.

Jones, J. E., & Corwin, J. T. (1996). Regeneration of sensory cells after laser ablation in the lateral line system: Hair cell lineage and macrophage behavior revealed by time-lapse video microscopy. *Journal of Neuroscience, 16,* 649–662.

Jorgensen, J. M., & Mathiesen, C. (1988). The avian inner ear. Continuous production of hair cells in vestibular sensory organs, but not in the auditory papilla. *Naturwissenschaften, 75,* 319–320.

Kawamoto, K., Izumikawa, M., Beyer, L. A., Atkin, G. M., & Raphael, Y. (2009). Spontaneous hair cell regeneration in the mouse utricle following gentamicin ototoxicity. *Hearing Research, 247,* 17–26.

Kawamoto, K., Ishimoto, S., Minoda, R., Brough, D. E., & Raphael, Y. (2003). Math1 gene transfer generates new cochlear hair cells in mature guinea pigs in vivo. *Journal of Neuroscience, 23,* 4395–4400.

Kawamoto, K., Kanzaki, S., Yagi, M., Stover, T., Prieskorn, D. M., Dolan, D. F., . . . Raphael, Y. (2001). Gene-based therapy for inner ear disease. *Noise Health, 3,* 37–47.

Kelley, M. W., Talreja, D. R., & Corwin, J. T. (1995). Replacement of hair cells after laser microbeam irradiation in cultured organs of corti from embryonic and neonatal mice. *Journal of Neuroscience, 15,* 3013–3026.

Komeda, M., Roessler, B. J., & Raphael, Y. (1999). The influence of interleukin-1 receptor antagonist transgene on spiral ganglion neurons. *Hearing Research, 131,* 1–10.

Kuntz, A. L., & Oesterle, E. C. (1998). Transforming growth factor-alpha with insulin induces proliferation in rat utricular extrasensory epithelia. *Otolaryngology-Head and Neck Surgery, 118,* 816–824.

Lalwani, A. K., Han, J. J., Walsh, B. J., Zolotukhin, S., Muzyczka, N., & Mhatre, A. N. (1997). Green fluorescent protein as a reporter for gene transfer studies in the cochlea. *Hearing Research, 114,* 139–147.

Lalwani, A. K., Walsh, B. J., Reilly, P. G., Muzyczka, N., & Mhatre, A. N. (1996). Development of in vivo gene therapy for hearing disorders: Introduction of adeno-associated virus into the cochlea of the guinea pig. *Gene Therapy, 3,* 588–592.

Lambert, P. R. (1994). Inner ear hair cell regeneration in a mammal: Identification of a triggering factor. *Laryngoscope, 104,* 701–718.

Li, H., Liu, H., & Heller, S. (2003). Pluripotent stem cells from the adult mouse inner ear. *Nature Medicine, 9,* 1293–1299.

Li, L., & Forge, A. (1997). Morphological evidence for supporting cell to hair cell conversion in the mammalian utricular macula. *International Journal of Developmental Neuroscience, 15,* 433–446.

Linthicum, F. H. J., & Fayad, J. N. (2009). Spiral ganglion cell loss is unrelated to segmental cochlear sensory system degeneration in humans. *Otology and Neurotology, 30,* 418–422.

Liu, Y., Okada, T., Sheykholeslami, K., Shimazaki, K., Nomoto, T., Muramatsu, S., . . . Ozawa, K. (2005). Specific and efficient transduction of cochlear inner hair cells with recombinant adeno-associated virus type 3 vector. *Molecular Therapy, 12,* 725–733.

Luebke, A. E., Foster, P. K., Muller, C. D., & Peel, A. L. (2001a). Cochlear function and transgene expression in the guinea pig cochlea, using adenovirus- and adeno-associated virus-directed gene transfer. *Human Gene Therapy, 12,* 773–781.

Luebke, A. E., Steiger, J. D., Hodges, B. L., & Amalfitano, A. (2001b). A modified adenovirus can transfect cochlear hair cells in vivo without compromising cochlear function. *Gene Therapy, 8,* 789–794.

Ma, E. Y., Rubel, E. W., & Raible, D. W. (2008). Notch signaling regulates the extent of hair cell regeneration in the zebrafish lateral line. *Journal of Neuroscience, 28,* 2261–2273.

Malgrange, B., Rigo, J. M., Coucke, P., Thiry, M., Hans, G., Nguyen, L., . . . Lefebvre, P. P. (2002). Identification of factors that maintain mammalian outer hair cells in adult organ of Corti explants. *Hearing Research, 170,* 48–58.

Marean, G. C., Burt, J. M., Beecher, M. D., & Rubel, E. W. (1993). Hair cell regeneration in the European starling (Sturnus vulgaris): Recovery of pure-tone detection thresholds. *Hearing Research, 71,* 125–136.

McCall, A. A., Swan, E. E., Borenstein, J. T., Sewell, W. F., Kujawa, S. G., & McKenna, M. J. (2010). Drug delivery for treatment of inner ear disease: Current state of knowledge. *Ear and Hearing, 31,* 156–165.

McCullar, J. S., Ty, S., Campbell, S., & Oesterle, E. C. (2010). Activin potentiates proliferation in mature avian auditory sensory epithelium. *Journal of Neuroscience, 30,* 478–490.

Middlebrooks, J. C., & Snyder, R. L. (2008). Intraneural stimulation for auditory prosthesis: Modiolar trunk and intracranial stimulation sites. *Hearing Research, 242,* 52–63.

Miller, J. M., Chi, D. H., O'Keeffe, L. J., Kruszka, P., Raphael, Y., & Altschuler, R. A. (1997). Neurotrophins can enhance spiral ganglion cell survival after inner hair cell loss. *International Journal of Developmental Neuroscience, 15,* 631–643.

Millimaki, B. B., Sweet, E. M., Dhason, M. S., & Riley, B. B. (2007). Zebrafish atoh1 genes: Classic proneural activity in the inner ear and regulation by Fgf and Notch. *Development, 134,* 295–305.

Nadol, J. B. J. (1997). Patterns of neural degeneration in the human cochlea and auditory nerve: Implications for cochlear implantation. *Otolaryngology-Head and Neck Surgery, 117,* 220–228.

Nadol, J. B. J., & Eddington, D. K. (2006). Histopathology of the inner ear relevant to cochlear implantation. *Advances in Otorhinolaryngology, 64,* 31–49.

Navaratnam, D. S., Su, H. S., Scott, S. P., & Oberholtzer, J. C. (1996). Proliferation in the auditory receptor epithelium mediated by a cyclic AMP-dependent signaling pathway [See comments]. *Nature Medicine, 2,* 1136–1139.

Niemiec, A. J., Raphael, Y., & Moody, D. B. (1994). Return of auditory function following structural regeneration after acoustic trauma: Behavioral measures from quail. *Hearing Research, 79,* 1–16.

Nishimura, K., Nakagawa, T., Ono, K., Ogita, H., Sakamoto, T., Yamamoto, N., . . . Ito, J. (2009). Transplantation of mouse induced pluripotent stem cells into the cochlea. *NeuroReport, 20,* 1250–1254.

O'Connor, R., & Tessier-Lavigne, M. (1999). Identification of maxillary factor, a maxillary process-derived chemoattractant for developing trigeminal sensory axons. *Neuron, 24,* 165–178.

Oesterle, E. C., Bhave, S. A., & Coltrera, M. D. (2000). Basic fibroblast growth factor inhibits cell proliferation in cultured avian inner ear sensory epithelia. *Journal of Comparative Neurology, 424,* 307–326.

Oesterle, E. C., & Campbell, S. (2009). Supporting cell characteristics in long-deafened aged mouse ears. *Journal of the Association for Research in Otolaryngology, 10,* 525–544.

Oesterle, E. C., Cunningham, D. E., Westrum, L. E., & Rubel, E. W. (2003). Ultrastructural analysis of [3H]thymidine-labeled cells in the rat utricular macula. *Journal of Comparative Neurology, 463,* 177–195.

Oesterle, E. C., & Rubel, E. W. (1993). Postnatal production of supporting cells in the chick cochlea. *Hearing Research, 66,* 213–224.

Oesterle, E. C., Tsue, T. T., & Rubel, E. W. (1997). Induction of cell proliferation in avian inner ear sensory epithelia by insulin-like growth factor-I and insulin. *Journal of Comparative Neurology, 380,* 262–274.

Oshima, K., Grimm, C. M., Corrales, C. E., Senn, P., Martinez Monedero, R., Geleoc, G. S., . . . Heller, S. (2007). Differential distribution of stem cells in the auditory and vestibular organs of the inner ear. *Journal of the Association for Research in Otolaryngology, 8*(1), 18–31.

Oshima, K., Suchert, S., Blevins, N. H., & Heller, S. (2010). Curing hearing loss: Patient expectations, health care practitioners, and basic science. *Journal of Communication Disorders, 43,* 311–318. Epub 2010 Apr 7.

Parker, M. A., Corliss, D. A., Gray, B., Anderson, J. K., Bobbin, R. P., Snyder, E. Y., & Cotanche, D. A. (2007). Neural stem cells injected into the sound-damaged cochlea migrate throughout the cochlea and express markers of hair cells, supporting cells, and spiral ganglion cells. *Hearing Research, 232,* 29–43.

Praetorius, M., Baker, K., Brough, D. E., Plinkert, P., & Staecker, H. (2007). Pharmacodynamics of adenovector distribution within the inner ear tissues of the mouse. *Hearing Research, 227,* 53–58.

Praetorius, M., Baker, K., Weich, C. M., Plinkert, P. K., & Staecker, H. (2003). Hearing preservation after inner ear gene therapy: The effect of vector and surgical approach. *ORL: Journal for Otorhinolaryngology and Its Related Specialties, 65,* 211–214.

Raphael, Y. (1992). Evidence for supporting cell mitosis in response to acoustic trauma in the avian inner ear. *Journal of Neurocytology, 21,* 663–671.

Raphael, Y., Frisancho, J. C., & Roessler, B. J. (1996). Adenoviral-mediated gene transfer into guinea pig cochlear cells in vivo. *Neuroscience Letters, 207,* 137–141.

Roberson, D. W., Alosi, J. A., & Cotanche, D. A. (2004). Direct transdifferentiation gives rise to the earliest new hair cells in regenerating avian auditory epithelium. *Journal of Neuroscience Research, 78,* 461–471.

Roberson, D. W., & Rubel, E. W. (1994). Cell division in the gerbil cochlea after acoustic trauma. *American Journal of Otology, 15,* 28–34.

Roehm, P. C., & Hansen, M. R. (2005). Strategies to preserve or regenerate spiral ganglion neurons. *Current Opinion in Otolaryngology-Head and Neck Surgery, 13,* 294–300.

Ruan, R. S., Leong, S. K., Mark, I., & Yeoh, K. H. (1999). Effects of BDNF and NT-3 on hair cell survival in guinea pig cochlea damaged by kanamycin treatment. *NeuroReport, 10,* 2067–2071.

Rubel, E. W., Dew, L. A., & Roberson, D. W. (1995). Mammalian vestibular hair cell regeneration. *Science, 267,* 701–707.

Rubel, E. W., & Fritzsch, B. (2002). Auditory system development: Primary auditory neurons and their targets. *Annual Review of Neuroscience, 25,* 51–101.

Ryals, B. M., & Rubel, E. W. (1988). Hair cell regeneration after acoustic trauma in adult Coturnix quail. *Science, 240,* 1774–1776.

Saffer, L. D., Gu, R., & Corwin, J. T. (1996). An RT-PCR analysis of mRNA for growth factor receptors in damaged and control sensory epithelia of rat utricles. *Hearing Research, 94,* 14–23.

Salt, A. N., & DeMott, J. (1997). Longitudinal endolymph flow associated with acute volume increase in the guinea pig cochlea. *Hearing Research, 107,* 29–40.

Salt, A. N., & DeMott, J. E. (1998). Longitudinal endolymph movements induced by perilymphatic injections. *Hearing Research, 123,* 137–147.

Saunders, J. C., Dear, S. P., & Schneider, M. E. (1985). The anatomical consequences of acoustic injury: A review and tutorial. *Journal of the Acoustical Society of America, 78,* 833–860.

Shang, J., Cafaro, J., Nehmer, R., & Stone, J. (2010). Supporting cell division is not required for regeneration of auditory hair cells after ototoxic injury in vitro. *Journal of the Association for Research in Otolaryngology, 11,* 203–222.

Shepherd, R. K., Hatsushika, S., & Clark, G. M. (1993). Electrical stimulation of the auditory nerve: The effect of electrode position on neural excitation. *Hearing Research, 66,* 108–120.

Shibata, S. B., Cortez, S. R., Beyer, L. A., Wiler, J. A., Di Polo, A., Pfingst, B. E., & Raphael, Y. (2010). Transgenic BDNF induces nerve fiber regrowth into the auditory epithelium in deaf cochleae. *Experimental Neurology, 223*(2), 464–472.

Shinohara, T., Bredberg, G., Ulfendahl, M., Pyykko, I., Olivius, N. P., Kaksonen, R., . . . Miller, J. M. (2002). Neurotrophic factor intervention restores auditory function in deafened animals. *Proceedings of the National Academy of Sciences of the United States of America, 99,* 1657–1660.

Shou, J., Zheng, J. L., & Gao, W. Q. (2003). Robust generation of new hair cells in the mature mammalian inner ear by adenoviral expression of Hath1. *Molecular and Cellular Neuroscience, 23,* 169–179.

Snyder, R. L., Middlebrooks, J. C., & Bonham, B. H. (2008). Cochlear implant electrode configuration effects on activation threshold and tonotopic selectivity. *Hearing Research, 235,* 23–38.

Spoendlin, H., & Schrott, A. (1990). Quantitative evaluation of the human cochlear nerve. *Acta Otolaryngologica (Suppl.), 470,* 61–69; discussion 69–70.

Staecker, H., Li, D., O'Malley, B. W., Jr., & Van De Water, T. R. (2001). Gene expression in the mammalian cochlea: A study of multiple vector systems. *Acta Otolaryngologica, 121,* 157–163.

Staecker, H., Praetorius, M., Baker, K., & Brough, D. E. (2007). Vestibular hair cell regeneration and restoration of balance function induced by math1 gene transfer. *Otology and Neurotology, 28,* 223–231.

Stone, J. S., Choi, Y. S., Woolley, S. M., Yamashita, H., & Rubel, E. W. (1999). Progenitor cell cycling during hair cell regeneration in the vestibular and auditory epithelia of the chick. *Journal of Neurocytology, 28,* 863–876.

Stone, J. S., & Cotanche, D. A. (1994). Identification of the timing of S phase and the patterns of cell proliferation during hair cell regeneration in the chick cochlea. *Journal of Comparative Neurology, 341,* 50–67.

Stone, L. S. (1933). The development of the lateral-line sense organs in amphibians observed in living and vital stained preparations. *Journal of Comparative Neurology, 57,* 507–540.

Stone, L. S. (1937). Further experimental studies of the development of the lateral-line sense organs in amphibians observed in living and vital stained preparations. *Journal of Comparative Neurology, 68,* 83–115.

Sugawara, M., Murtie, J. C., Stankovic, K. M., Liberman, M. C., & Corfas, G. (2007). Dynamic patterns of neurotrophin 3 expression in the postnatal mouse inner ear. *Journal of Comparative Neurology, 501,* 30–37.

Tateya, I., Nakagawa, T., Iguchi, F., Kim, T. S., Endo, T., Yamada, S., . . . Ito, J. (2003). Fate of neural stem cells grafted into injured inner ears of mice. *NeuroReport, 14,* 1677–1681.

Taylor, R. R., & Forge, A. (2005). Hair cell regeneration in sensory epithelia from the inner ear of a urodele amphibian. *Journal of Comparative Neurology, 484,* 105–120.

Tsue, T. T., Watling, D. L., Weisleder, P., Coltrera, M. D., & Rubel, E. W. (1994). Identification of hair cell progenitors and intermitotic migration of their nuclei in the normal and regenerating avian inner ear. *Journal of Neuroscience, 14,* 140–152.

Warchol, M. E. (1999). Immune cytokines and dexamethasone influence sensory regeneration in the avian vestibular periphery. *Journal of Neurocytology, 28,* 889–900.

Warchol, M. E., Lambert, P. R., Goldstein, B. J., Forge, A., & Corwin, J. T. (1993). Regenerative proliferation in inner ear sensory epithelia from adult guinea pigs and humans. *Science, 259,* 1619–1622.

Weisleder, P., & Rubel, E. W. (1992). Hair cell regeneration in the avian vestibular epithelium. *Experimental Neurology, 115,* 2–6.

Wenzel, G. I., Xia, A., Funk, E., Evans, M. B., Palmer, D. J., Ng, P., . . . Oghalai, J. S. (2007). Helper-dependent adenovirus-mediated gene transfer into the adult mouse cochlea. *Otology and Neurotology, 28,* 1100–1108.

White, J. A., Burgess, B. J., Hall, R. D., & Nadol, J. B. (2000). Pattern of degeneration of the spiral ganglion cell and its processes in the C57BL/6J mouse. *Hearing Research, 141,* 12–18.

White, P. M., Doetzlhofer, A., Lee, Y. S., Groves, A. K., & Segil, N. (2006). Mammalian cochlear supporting cells can divide and trans-differentiate into hair cells. *Nature, 441,* 984–987.

Wilkins, H. R., Presson, J. C., & Popper, A. N. (1999). Proliferation of vertebrate inner ear supporting cells. *Journal of Neurobiology, 39,* 527–535.

Wise, A. K., Hume, C. R., Flynn, B. O., Jeelall, Y. S., Suhr, C. L., Sgro, B. E., . . . Richardson, R. T. (2010). Effects of localized neurotrophin gene expression on spiral ganglion neuron resprouting in the deafened cochlea. *Molecular Therapy, 18,* 1111–1122.

Wise, A. K., Richardson, R., Hardman, J., Clark, G., & O'Leary, S. (2005). Resprouting and survival of guinea pig cochlear neurons in response to the administration of the neurotrophins brain-derived neurotrophic factor and neurotrophin-3. *Journal of Comparative Neurology, 487,* 147–165.

Witte, M. C., Montcouquiol, M., & Corwin, J. T. (2001). Regeneration in avian hair cell epithelia: Identification of intracellular signals required for S-phase entry. *European Journal of Neuroscience, 14,* 829–838.

Yamashita, H., & Oesterle, E. C. (1995). Induction of cell proliferation in mammalian inner ear sensory epithelia by transforming growth factor alpha and epidermal growth factor. *Proceedings of the National Academy of Sciences of the United States of America, 92,* 3152–3155.

Zheng, J. L., & Gao, W. Q. (2000). Overexpression of Math1 induces robust production of extra hair cells in postnatal rat inner ears. *Nature Neuroscience, 3,* 580–586.

5

Current Issues in Tinnitus

Jos J. Eggermont

LEARNING OBJECTIVES

- Understanding the origin of the phantom sound that is called subjective tinnitus, and separating this from objective tinnitus resulting from physical, body-generated, sounds.
- Knowing the relationship between physiological and behavioral correlates of tinnitus, and how this forms the basis for sound treatment.
- Appreciating the molecular and pharmacological substrates of tinnitus and their potential for drug treatment of tinnitus.
- Thoroughly understanding the psychoacoustic characterization of tinnitus and how this differs from the distress aspects of tinnitus as quantified by tinnitus questionnaires.
- Understanding the basis for behavioral treatment of tinnitus distress.

Key Words. Alcohol, amygdala, animal models, annoyance, auditory evoked potentials, cochlear implants, caffeine, cognitive behavioral therapy, cortical plasticity, etiology, functional magnetic resonance imaging (fMRI), head and neck injuries, hearing aids, hyperacusis, ion channels, immediate early genes, limbic system, loudness, magnetoencephalography (MEG), masking, neural synchrony, neuromodulators, neurotransmitters, noise-induced hearing loss (NIHL), objective tinnitus, oto-acoustic emissions, phantom sound, pitch, positron emission tomography (PET), questionnaires, quality of life, quinine, residual inhibition, tonotopic maps, salicylate, smoking, sound therapy, spontaneous firing rates, subjective tinnitus, tinnitus retraining therapy (TRT), transcranial magnetic stimulation (TMS)

INTRODUCTION

In common English, tinnitus stands for "ringing in the ears," but hissing and roaring sounds also fall under the rubric of tinnitus. A commonly adapted scientific definition reads, "tinnitus is the conscious expression of a sound that originates in an involuntary manner in the head of its owner, or may appear to him to do so."

A PERSONAL HISTORY OF TINNITUS RESEARCH

I approach the history of research on the topic of tinnitus through a narrative centered on the topics presented at six International Tinnitus Seminars (ITS) that I attended over a 25-year span.

In 1983, the second ITS was held in New York City. I presented a talk on the presumed physiological background of tinnitus (Eggermont, 1984). The dominant topics at the seminar were the etiology of tinnitus, which makes sense if one wants to establish the topic of study, and psychoacoustical studies on the percept of tinnitus. Tinnitus masking, drug treatments, electrical stimulation and surgical approaches were part of the series of talks, but any presentations on cognitive-based treatment were lacking.

The fourth ITS was held in Bordeaux in 1991. Psychological aspects including cognitive therapy started to be featured in a prominent way at this seminar, whereas etiological studies were on the decline. At that time I was still leaning more toward a peripheral than central origin of tinnitus (Eggermont, 1990), but was convinced that correlated neural activity was at the source of tinnitus. We subsequently found a clear dose-related effect of quinine on neural correlation strength in auditory cortex (AC). Ochi and Eggermont (1995) presented this at the 5th ITS held in 1995 in Portland, Oregon, the birthplace of behavioral tinnitus research and treatment. This Portland seminar and the next were the most prominent for the emergence of animal models of tinnitus. We subsequently found that salicylate and quinine did produce increased spontaneous activity in the secondary auditory cortex (SAC), but not in primary auditory cortex (PAC) (Eggermont & Kenmochi, 1998).

Permanent hearing loss resulting from noise trauma caused, besides increased spontaneous firing rates (SFR) and increased neural synchrony, a reorganization of the cortical tonotopic map in PAC (Eggermont & Komiya, 2000). We presented the initial results at the 6th ITS in Cambridge, UK in 1999, where Tinnitus Retraining Therapy (TRT) was the most discussed topic, with epidemiology and demographic studies a close second.

We (Noreña & Eggermont, 2005, 2006) then started using an enhanced acoustic environment, that is, presenting sounds in the frequency range of the hearing loss, to balance the uneven output of the auditory nerve (AN) after noise-induced hearing loss (the same effect would be obtained with a well-fitted hearing aid with very good high-frequency output, but that is not practical in animals). This acoustic environment prevented the triad of tonotopic map changes, increased SFR and increased neural synchrony from occurring. Around this time (2005), the 8th ITS was held in Pau, France, and featured the emergence of imaging (fMRI and PET) techniques to study tinnitus in human subjects as well as neu-

rosurgical approaches to tinnitus treatment based on direct stimulation of AC. The first results of transcranial magnetic stimulation (TMS) to treat tinnitus were also presented.

Important future avenues to investigate tinnitus will combine genetic and molecular studies, animal behavioral models and electrophysiologic recordings, on one hand, and improved structural and functional imaging methods in humans with tinnitus on the other hand. Some results of this approach were presented at the ninth ITS held in Göteborg, Sweden in 2008. However, the most-presented topic was on cognitive therapy, whereas the number of presentations featuring TRT continued their decline, suggesting either the maturity of this approach or a paucity of controlled clinical trials to report. The number of imaging studies was only slightly increased over that at the previous seminar.

This chapter focuses on what is known about tinnitus, based on human research and how to interpret this in the light of animal research. A large, but not exhaustive, number of treatments will be reviewed and this is meant to indicate that although there is currently no cure, there are some surprisingly promising methods to alleviate tinnitus.

Question 1

When I fit a tinnitus masker on a patient, how does that affect the physiology?

Answer 1

Masking does several things in the auditory nervous system. First of all, the masking sound activates neurons and prevents them from firing to a probe sound (e.g., tinnitus). Secondly, masking provides a suppression effect where the masker interferes with the cochlear mechanical activity pattern of the probe sound. This suppression causes the basilar membrane to vibrate less than normal to the probe tone in the masker-frequency region and thus produces less firing to the probe tone in the ANFs innervating the IHCs in that region. These are all fast-occurring (within milliseconds) phenomena. If the tinnitus does not originate in the cochlea, then the suppression effect is absent. In addition there is a potential plastic effect of the masking sound on the central auditory system when the masker is continuously on for a week or more. In that case the masking noise decreases the gain of the synapses in the brain for those neurons that are tuned to frequencies contained in the masker (Formby et al., 2003). If the masker is on for, for example, for 12 hours and off for 12 hours, there still may be a noticeable plastic effect, especially if used for months (Pienkowski & Eggermont, 2010). I only can see an effect on tinnitus if the masking sound matches the frequency region of the hearing loss and has a level that balances the output of the ANFs across frequency. The level that is appropriate for getting the auditory system potentially back to normal may not necessarily mask the tinnitus, at least not in the first few months. If the masker level is too high, another asymmetry occurs and a "new" tinnitus may result at off-masker frequencies.

SUBJECTIVE VERSUS OBJECTIVE TINNITUS

Objective tinnitus can be heard both by the patient and the examiner. Subjective tinnitus can only be perceived by the patient, and represents a percept experienced in the absence of any external or internal physical sound source.

Clicking tinnitus may indicate a mechanical cause for the tinnitus, often resulting from repetitive contractions of muscles in the middle ear or nasopharynx. An open eustachian tube can result in pulsatile tinnitus, as a consequence of inward and outward movement of the tympanic membrane in association with respiration (Liyanage, Singh, Savundra, & Kalan, 2006). Objective pulsatile tinnitus has numerous causes, including benign intracranial hypertension, glomus tumors, and atherosclerotic carotid arteries. Pulsatile tinnitus can thus be the result of the sound of turbulent blood flow that is

transmitted to the inner ear (Waldvogel, Mattle, Sturzenegger, & Schroth, 1998). Hearing one's own heart murmur has been reported in adults, and Anderson, Teitel, and Wu (2008) reported the case of a young child who clearly heard her own venous hum, causing her to complain of pulsatile tinnitus.

The remainder of this chapter is restricted to subjective tinnitus, which, from now on, I call tinnitus. Some further distinctions in tinnitus type are sometimes made. Transient or reversible tinnitus is often distinguished from chronic tinnitus because it typically does not need treatment and may have a source that is different from that of chronic tinnitus. Very short transient tonal tinnitus, accompanied by fullness in the ear and transient hearing loss, is experienced by nearly everyone. It is not clear what the underlying mechanism is, but it combines three of the symptoms that define Ménière's disease. Acute application of salicylates typically produces a reversible form of tinnitus. Only after prolonged salicylate use will the tinnitus become chronic, but that may likely be attributed to the development of a hearing loss as a result of the drug use. Tinnitus accompanied by sensorineural hearing loss (Chapter 6) is typically chronic and generally irreversible. The distinction of peripheral versus central tinnitus is, in my opinion, similar to that for transient versus chronic tinnitus (Eggermont, 2003). I hold that all chronic tinnitus is central in origin, but of course is often triggered by hearing loss or, in substantial numbers, also by somatic injuries (Levine, 1999).

SYMPTOMS

Descriptive Quality of Tinnitus

Two representative and well-documented early studies give two very different illustrations of tinnitus quality. 1800 tinnitus cases were studied by Meikle and Taylor-Walsh (1984) and more than 500 persons with tinnitus were investigated by Stouffer and Tyler (1990). The various characterizations of their tinnitus, as reported by the patients, are shown in Table 5–1. Although the distributions for unilateral and bilateral tinnitus are very similar in the two studies, it is

Table 5–1. The Sound of Tinnitus

	Meikle and Taylor-Walsh (1984) $N = 1800$	Stouffer and Tyler (1990) $N = 500$
Bilateral, ear-localized	52%	44%
Unilateral	37%	34%
In the head	11%	22%
Ringing	25%	37.5%
Clear tone (humming)	4.4%	5.3%
Chirping (cricket like)	1.2%	8.5%
Whistling	1%	6.6%
Hissing	4.3%	7.8%
Ocean waves	1.7%	
Buzzing	1.4%	11.2%

clear that ocean waves are characterizations used by persons living close to the Pacific, but not by landlocked people in Iowa. It is also obvious that cricket sounds are more familiar in Iowa compared to Oregon. Although both studies find a ringing sound the most common, reminiscent of the English description of tinnitus as ringing in the ears, otherwise there is not much common in the characterization of the tinnitus sound in these two large surveys.

To investigate this proliferation of descriptions, Wahlström and Axelsson (1996) presented pure tones to tinnitus patients and asked them to describe what they heard. It appeared that the description of these external sounds was not an easy task, and sometimes tinnitus patients even labeled pure tones as noise. Pure tones were labeled differently according to their frequency. For instance, a 4 kHz tone was listed in 34% of cases as a tone, in 26% as a hissing sound, in 18% as a roaring sound, and in the remaining 22% as whistling, squeaking, and so forth. An 8 kHz tone did not result in any tonal quality: 48% described it as rushing, 16% as beeping, 12% as ringing, the remainder as whistling, a cricket sound, a dentist drill, and so forth. Buzzing sounds were identified for a 250 Hz tone (10%), and 4 kHz narrowband noise (12%). Roaring sounds were heard to 250 Hz tones (18%) and 250 Hz narrowband noise

(8%). There was no correlation between the person's own tinnitus sound and the above descriptions of the external sound. This suggests that the characterization of external sounds, and likely also internal sounds such as tinnitus, is not an easy task for people with tinnitus. Hence the proliferation of labels (see Table 5–1) to describe what tinnitus sounds like.

Del Bo et al. (2008) showed that it is also not easy for normal-hearing subjects to characterize low-level tinnituslike sounds. Normal-hearing persons were confined to an anechoic chamber for 4 minutes, and when they came out reported hearing buzzing and humming sounds mostly, followed by squeaking, whirling, sound of ocean waves, clicking, heartbeat, crickets, flowing water, and so forth.

Tinnitus and Hyperacusis

Often tinnitus is accompanied by hyperacusis, an intolerance of ordinary environmental sounds even of low intensity. Loudness recruitment can be distinguished from hyperacusis. If the individual perceives only sound of moderate intensity as rapidly increasing in loudness, then they are experiencing recruitment; if sound of low-to-high intensities are uncomfortably loud, they are experiencing hyperacusis. However, recruitment and hyperacusis can occur together. Among patients attending tinnitus clinics with a primary complaint of tinnitus, the prevalence of hyperacusis is about 40%; and in patients with a primary complaint of hyperacusis the prevalence of tinnitus has been reported as 86% (Baguley, 2003).

Psychological Aspects of Tinnitus

There is wide agreement that tinnitus severity (quality) is not closely related to its perceived loudness (quantity). Perceived severity does depend on loudness but also includes the degree of annoyance and associated disability resulting from tinnitus. Although some patients do not spontaneously report any unpleasant emotional or behavioral consequences of their tinnitus, others experience considerable distress. Hiller and Goebel (2006) found a moderate correlation between tinnitus loudness and annoyance. Both factors were generally more prevalent in men, and in people older than 50 years. In addition, those with binaural tinnitus or tinnitus in the head, those who had continuous tinnitus, and those with hyperacusis, complained the most. The coexistence of tinnitus with hearing loss and hyperacusis seems to be of clinical relevance for the prediction of high annoyance levels (Folmer, Griest, Meikle, & Martin, 1999). The severity of tinnitus was generally related to hearing thresholds, and tinnitus loudness in sensation level (SL) provides little clinically useful information (Andersson, 2003). Thus, factors other than loudness often contribute to tinnitus severity and annoyance.

Stress and Tinnitus

Emotional or physical stress initiates the release of corticotrophin-releasing factor, which in turn leads to the release of cortisol and adrenalin from the adrenal gland and the activation of the sympathetic nervous system. Hébert, Paiement, and Lupien (2004) measured cortisol levels in saliva in tinnitus patients and controls. The high tinnitus-related distress group had chronic cortisol levels that were greater than both the low tinnitus-related distress and control groups, and also displayed greater intolerance to external sounds (hyperacusis?). This suggests a link between intolerance to both internal (tinnitus) and external sounds in persons with tinnitus, which is compatible with the clinical observation that severe tinnitus is associated with high stress levels. Predictive factors for tinnitus severity include anxiety disorders and a poor sense of well-being at tinnitus onset (Holgers, Erlandsson, & Barrenäs, 2000; Holgers, Zöger, & Svedlund, 2005). Psychosocial stress and social problems are also more common in patients with severe tinnitus than in patients with less severe tinnitus (Holgers et al., 2005).

ETIOLOGY

Hearing Loss

Tinnitus most often accompanies noise-induced hearing loss (NIHL: Chapter 1), but also co-occurs in patients with hearing loss due to presbycusis, otosclerosis, otitis media, impacted cerumen, sudden deafness, Meniere's disease, and other forms of hearing loss. Conductive losses likely result in tinnitus by reducing environmental sounds, which normally act as tinnitus maskers. It has been suggested that the conductive hearing loss could unmask the tinnitus that is potentially present in every normal hearing subject, where it only becomes audible in very quiet environments (Mills, Albert, & Brain, 1986). Infections such as otitis media, and other infectious or inflammatory processes that affect hearing, comprise about 8% of tinnitus cases.

About 20% of tinnitus is due to NIHL. Regulations of the Occupational Safety and Health Administration, or equivalent, limit the level of noise exposure in the workplace. However, regulations about admissible sound levels do not generally apply to recreational areas such as bars and concert venues, and if they do apply, only to what is audible outside the venue. Ear protection inside these establishments is advisable but not considered a social grace, and generally not complied with. Personal listening devices are new and potentially harmful sources of recreational noise that could cause or exacerbate hearing loss, especially when used for an extended time period on a daily basis. Yet, in a study that surveyed hearing loss in a group ($N = 2526$) of young workers entering the workforce in a large company, with workplaces widely distributed across the United States, over a 20-year period ending in 2004, Rabinowitz, Slade, Galusha, Dixon-Ernst, and Cullen (2006) found no difference in the prevalence of hearing loss over this 20-year period. One might argue that the personal listening device fashion was not adequately sampled, as this had barely started around 2000, but these data suggest that the presumption of increased hearing loss in young adults does not apply to all groups. A survey of a group of 2015 Australians aged 55+ years found that a significant increase in the risk of tinnitus was caused not only by poorer hearing and cochlear function, and self-reported work-related noise exposure, but also by a history of middle ear or sinus infections, severe neck injury, or migraine (Sindhusake et al., 2003).

Vestibular schwannoma and cerebellopontine angle tumors can also cause tinnitus by putting pressure on the high-frequency auditory nerve fibers

(ANFs) that lie on the outside of the nerve, thereby causing a partial conduction block that limits output to the brain. In addition, a vestibular schwannoma may disrupt cochlear blood flow, thereby creating a sensory hearing loss.

In about 40% of tinnitus cases, the etiology is unknown. Henry, Dennis, and Schechter (2005, p. 1205) wrote: "in many patients, the emergence of tinnitus as a problem occurs long after the underlying medical condition (most commonly hearing loss). The trigger for the adverse or intrusive effects of tinnitus is sometimes unrelated to the associated condition."

A considerable number of patients (about 8% in a study by Barnea, Attias, Gold, & Shahar, 1990; 18% in Stouffer & Tyler, 1990) complain about tinnitus in the absence of hearing loss or obvious somatic problems. Tinnitus without hearing loss and no obvious signs of somatic tinnitus remains something of a mystery. One possibility already mentioned could be undetectable venous hum. Another one could be that there are narrow dead regions in the cochlea that cannot be detected by standard audiometry. A test has been developed (Moore, Huss, Vickers, Glasberg, & Alcántara, 2000) to detect these dead regions, and Weisz, Hartmann, Dohrmann, Schlee, and Noreña (2006) used this technique to demonstrate that most high-pitched tinnitus in the absence of hearing loss could be the result of the presence of such dead regions. These dead regions may cause mini-reorganizations and disinhibition in the central auditory system (see later). One also wonders whether some of the persons with tinnitus in the absence of hearing loss could have suffered from prolonged conductive hearing loss in childhood. This causes tinnitus whose pitch is related to the shape of the audiogram (Savastano, 2007), and after recovering from this childhood hearing disorder the tinnitus might have retreated temporarily, only to show up again in adulthood. This would be due to the same mechanisms that induce tinnitus following mild NIHL (described above). However, mild NIHL is here to stay and the conductive loss usually disappears, and one would expect brain plasticity to return aberrant neural activity back to normal as soon as the hearing loss disappears, so this remains speculative. Plasticity aspects of tinnitus are discussed later on in this chapter.

Head and Neck Injuries

Head and neck injuries, including whiplash, cause about 10% of tinnitus cases (Folmer & Griest, 2003). Head and neck injuries may in various ways affect the auditory system as injured cranial and spinal nerves affect both the vascular supply to the cochlea and also innervate the granule cells in the dorsal cochlear nucleus (DCN) (Shore & Zhou, 2006). Temporo-mandibular-joint dysfunction and other dental disorders also frequently co-occur with tinnitus, suggesting a role of the trigeminal nerve in tinnitus.

Hearing dysfunction can occur as a consequence of head injuries because of damage to the AN, the cochlea, or middle ear. Whiplash injuries can cause abnormal firing activity in the medullary somatosensory nuclei (MSN) that is located in the lower medulla and upper cervical spinal cord. The MSN normally provides inhibitory innervation to the DCN. During some whiplash accidents, MSN to DCN pathways are damaged. Subsequent disinhibition of the DCN and associated auditory structures causes higher spontaneous and induced neural activity in these structures, and could result in the generation and perception of tinnitus (Levine, 1999).

Cutaneous- and Gaze-Evoked Tinnitus

Complete and acute unilateral deafferentation of the auditory periphery (auditory and vestibular afferents) can induce changes in the central nervous system that may result in unique forms of tinnitus. These tinnitus perceptions can be controlled (turned on and off) or modulated (changed in pitch or loudness) by certain overt behaviors in other sensory/motor systems.

Baguley et al. (2006) studied a cohort of 359 patients who had undergone translabyrinthine removal of a vestibular schwannoma. Gaze modulation of tinnitus after vestibular schwannoma removal was identified in 19% of patients in this series. Explanations for this form of tinnitus include crossmodal plasticity, which has been hypothesized to involve neural sprouting between the para-abducens nucleus, or medial longitudinal fasciculus, and the auditory pathway, perhaps at the level of the cochlear nucleus. Alternatively, the development of gaze-evoked tinnitus may involve the unmasking of a previously inhibited pathway linking auditory gain and eye movement. The deafferentation associated with vestibular schwannoma removal would potentially disinhibit such a pathway (Cacace et al., 1999). The timing of the onset of tinnitus might help distinguish between these suggested mechanisms. An immediate onset of gaze-evoked tinnitus might be attributed to unmasking, whereas a later onset, even after the first year, might indicate aberrant reinnervation or plastic change in the auditory and/or oculo-motor systems. The onset data in the above study did not favor a specific mechanism.

Drugs

Tinnitus is a common side effect of many commonly used or prescribed drugs, including salicylates (aspirin), nonsteroidal anti-inflammatory drugs, quinine, aminoglycoside antibiotics, loop diuretics such as furosemide, chemotherapeutic agents such as cisplatin and carboplatin, and commonly accepted recreational drugs such as nicotine, caffeine, and alcohol. However, as most of this tinnitus is reversible when the drug use is stopped (except tinnitus accompanying the permanent hearing loss caused by aminoglycoside antibiotics, cisplatin, and carboplatin), it contributes only 2% to chronic tinnitus cases. Some of the most common tinnitus-causing drugs are now briefly reviewed.

Salicylates

Ototoxicity is a common side effect of high-dose aspirin treatment in patients with rheumatoid arthritis. Low-dose daily aspirin administration in animal models presumably causes tinnitus without hearing loss (Bauer et al., 2000), so it is possible that it could occur in humans who use a maintenance dose for cardiovascular reasons and show oversensitivity. Hearing loss and tinnitus intensity generally increase progressively with the aspirin dosage and increasing plasma salicylate concentrations (Day et al., 1989; Halla, Atchison, & Hardin, 1991).

Quinine

Quinine, used in the past to prevent night cramps (e.g., in marathon runners or prospective ones) and as an antimalaria drug, is a potent potassium-channel blocker. Quinine works on the cochlea by partially blocking the sensory gates at the tips of the hair cell sterocilia, thereby producing a hearing loss. By its interference with K^+ channels in the axons it also prolongs the duration of action potentials (Lin, Chen, & Tee, 1998), which could result in a stronger depolarizing effect on postsynaptic neurons, and hence increased firing rates.

Cisplatin and Carboplatin

Cisplatin, a drug with antitumor activity used in the treatment of recurrent pediatric brain tumors, produces a high-frequency hearing loss not unlike that caused by aminoglycosides (Coupland, Ponton, Eggermont, Bowen, & Grant, 1991) by initially affecting predominantly the OHCs. In contrast, carboplatin at moderate dose dominantly affects the inner hair cells (IHCs) (so far only shown in chinchillas), thereby reducing the output of ANFs in specific frequency regions accompanied by a mild audiometric hearing loss (Takeno, Harrison, Mount, Wake, & Harada, 1994).

Caffeine, Alcohol, and Smoking

Sininger, Eggermont, and King (1992) reported tinnitus in an individual that could be induced by drinking a cup of good strong coffee, and presented some objective indicators for its presence. However, no general correlation appears to exist between enjoying or abstaining from coffee and changes in the nature of existing tinnitus (Juliano & Griffiths, 2004; Kemp & George, 1992).

The data on a relationship between alcohol and tinnitus are also insufficient to draw any firm conclusions. Goodey (1981) found a positive correlation between alcohol consumption and tinnitus. On the other hand Kemp and George (1992) found no statistically significant effects of alcohol consumption on tinnitus.

Nicotine affects the cochlea (Maffei and Miani, 1962) and smoking is accompanied by a higher incidence of high-frequency hearing loss (Zelman, 1973). However, direct correlations between smoking and tinnitus have not been established. Hoffman and Reed (2004) classified both alcohol use and smoking under possible risk factors for tinnitus.

Question 2

Why do hearing aids sometimes decrease a patient's complaint of tinnitus? What is happening with the physiology?

Answer 2

Hearing aid fitting depends on the intended effect. Hearing aids are usually fitted with the goal of improving speech perception. The hearing aid fitting would likely be different for appreciating music. Hearing aid fitting for alleviation of tinnitus may be very different from that for improving speech perception. In addition, most hearing aids do not provide enough output in the high-frequency region, which is important for affecting tinnitus. The frequency region to amplify for speech is generally below the frequency range where the tinnitus occurs. So there will only be an effect on tinnitus when there is an overlap of the amplified frequency region and the tinnitus frequency range. The latter typically starts one-third of an octave above the high-frequency edge of the audiogram. Hearing aids do, in principle, the same thing as masking sounds, that is, balancing the output of the cochlea. Again, the difference is the frequency range that is activated and the amount of activity produced in the ANFs.

SUBJECTIVE QUANTIFICATION

Questionnaires

The objective for any tinnitus questionnaire is to accurately identify and quantify the patient's tinnitus-associated problems. Assessing the effects of tinnitus on an individual's quality of life is a complex issue that is due to a variety of factors. First of all, tinnitus is an entirely subjective percept of the patient. Psychological factors may play a critical role in determining an individual's reactions to tinnitus (e.g., some people are accustomed to solving their own problems whereas others are largely dependent on support; Erlandsson, 2000). There are gender differences: women appear more likely to report emotional reactions to their tinnitus than men (Dineen, Doyle, & Bench, 1997; Hallberg & Erlandsson, 1993; Meikle & Griest, 1989), and the incidence of personality disturbances is greater for male than for female tinnitus patients (Erlandsson, 2000). Individual differences in daily lifestyle, as well as individual acoustic environments, may make some patients more likely to experience problematic tinnitus. Quality of life is likely reduced for anyone with chronic tinnitus. Sleep disturbance is reported by about one-half of those individuals who complain of tinnitus.

The use of written, self-administered questionnaires is important for any tinnitus assessment, but should be used with care. There are at least a dozen published outcome instruments that are used to obtain tinnitus severity ratings, and there is no consensus regarding their use across tinnitus treatment centers (Newman & Sandridge, 2004). The questionnaires most often used in North America are the Tinnitus Severity Index (TSI) (Meikle, 1992), the Tinnitus Handicap Inventory (THI) (Newman, Sandridge, & Jacobson, 1998), and the Tinnitus Handicap Questionnaire (THQ) (Kuk, Tyler, Russell, & Jordan, 1990; Tyler, 1993). The baseline index scores for THI, THQ, and TSI show comparable intersubject variability. However, an examiner cannot rely solely on one index score to make a clinical severity judgment (Newman & Sandridge, 2004).

Tinnitus, just like pain, may cause emotional and psychological distress that is often out of proportion with the magnitude of the injury. In this regard, tinnitus is similar to other phantom sensations such as phantom pain and phantom limb (Jastreboff, 1990). The strong emotional implications of sound in general may be the basis for psychological distress in some tinnitus patients (Hallam, Rachman, & Hinchcliffe, 1984; Jastreboff, Gray, & Gold, 1996).

Psychoacoustics: Listening to Tinnitus

We have seen above that there are no unique subjective descriptors of the tinnitus sound. It may be that tinnitus patients do hear sounds differently then other people. This can be evaluated by psychoacoustic methods.

Pitch

The spectral characteristics of tinnitus have been recognized as fundamentally important for many years. Fowler (1944) argued that it was important to match the loudness and pitch of tinnitus using tones presented to the contralateral ear. For pitch matching, the importance of presenting matching tones at levels equal to the perceived tinnitus loudness was stressed. Pitch matching to a pure tone indicates the most prominent pitch, and pitch matching could be obtained in 92% of 1,033 patients (Meikle, 1995). Pitch matching reliability varies widely across patients. Pitch can vary from day-to-day or within a day (Stouffer & Tyler, 1990a). Tinnitus pitch increased over time in 20% of patients. Pitch matches occur often in the frequency region of maximum hearing loss or at the edge frequency (Penner, 1980), and the most common tinnitus pitch with noise-induced hearing loss appears to match that of a 3 kHz tone (Penner, 2000).

Tinnitus sounds can be synthesized by combining pure tones (Penner, 1993) in the following way (Figure 5–1; based on Noreña, Micheyl, Chéry-Croze, & Collet, 2002). After threshold determination, subjects adjusted the intensity of tones within the hearing loss range (one randomly selected tone at a time) to match the loudness of their tinnitus. The persons then stated whether the frequency corresponded to one of the components of their tinnitus spectrum and, if it did, gave a rating on a 10-point scale (10 = tinnitus) of the extent to which the frequency was part of their tinnitus sensation. Frequencies were selected randomly from the tested range and repeated until a total of three measurements had been obtained for each frequency. Tones were presented monaurally either to the tinnitus ear or to the ear where tinnitus was most pronounced. In each of the ten cases tested, the rated tinnitus spectrum spanned the region of hearing loss with no dominance of edge-frequency ratings. The tones are then combined according to their rated importance into a spectrum, and the sound corresponding to that spectrum can be presented to the person for feedback

about the degree of similarity to his/her tinnitus. Two idealized and hypothetical examples are shown. In the top panel we show a high-frequency hearing loss (black dots) and the tinnitus spectrum (open circles) that is approximately the inverse of the hearing loss. Here we expect a hissing tinnitus with a pitch between 4 and 12 kHz. In the bottom panel there is a notched hearing loss centered around 4 to 6 kHz. The tinnitus spectrum suggests a tonal tinnitus pitch in that same range. The predicates "hissing" and "tonal" that I use here are purely inferential as this likely cannot be predicted from the audiogram and is a truly subjective predicate (see under Symptoms).

Loudness

Loudness relates to the number of neurons activated, their rate of firing, and likely also the degree of synchrony of their firings. Tinnitus loudness is usually measured by rating on a scale from 1 to 10, or by matching to external sounds. Loudness matching is typically done by adjusting the level of a pure tone. Fowler (1944) commented that patients described their tinnitus as very loud, yet the tinnitus could usually be matched at levels of only 5 to 10 dB SL. One has to realize that sensation levels (SL) represent a sound level in dB above the person's threshold at a particular frequency and are not a measure of loudness. It is clear that the experienced loudness will include the recruitment phenomenon, that is, the abnormal increase in the loudness for a given increase in sound level. Tyler and Conrad-Armes (1983) converted sensation level into conventional HL (taking into account the hearing loss) and then into loudness (sones), based on a standard theoretical recruitment function. This of course resulted in much higher loudness values than the SL indicated.

Just as tinnitus pitch fluctuates, so does its loudness (Stouffer & Tyler, 1990b). This fluctuation likely represents the cumulative effects of test-retest variability, actual fluctuation of the tinnitus loudness, and changes in tinnitus pitch or loudness produced by the measurement stimulus if presented to the tinnitus ear. Presenting a matching stimulus to the contralateral ear might also influence certain aspects of the tinnitus because of central interactions. One way to avoid this sound-tinnitus interaction is to use cross-modal loudness matching. Cross-modal

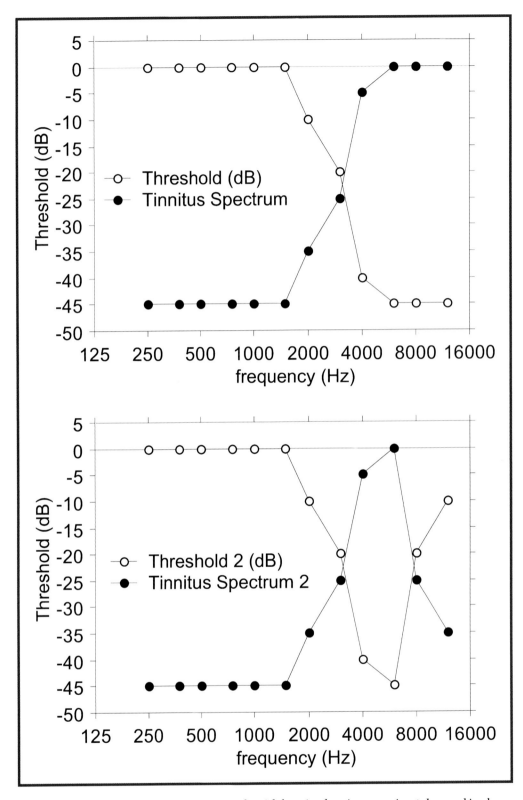

Figure 5–1. The tinnitus spectrum in people with hearing loss is approximately equal in shape to the inverted audiogram. Two idealized and hypothetical examples are shown. In the top panel there is a high-frequency hearing loss (*black dots*) and the tinnitus spectrum shown (*open circles*) is approximately the inverse of the hearing loss. Here we expect a hissing tinnitus with a pitch between 4 and 12 kHz. In the bottom panel there is a notched hearing loss centered around 4 to 6 kHz. The tinnitus spectrum suggests a tinnitus pitch in that same range.

matching compares tinnitus loudness to either the brightness of a visual stimulus, the length of a bar, etc. Somatosensory stimuli as comparators however, should be avoided because of their potential modulation of tinnitus properties.

Masking

Masking is based on two mechanisms: a "line-busy" effect where the masking sound activates the neurons and prevents them from firing to a probe sound (e.g., tinnitus), and a suppression effect where the masker interferes with the cochlear mechanical activity pattern of the probe sound (Delgutte, 1990). This suppression causes the basilar membrane to vibrate less than normal to the probe tone in the masker-frequency region and thus produces less firing to the probe tone in the ANFs innervating the IHCs in that region.

Although pure tones were reported to mask tinnitus completely in 91% of patients, masking of tinnitus does not produce the standard effects that a masker has on a probe sound. Tyler and Conrad-Armes (1984) found that the psychophysical masking curve for a real tone (matched in pitch and loudness to the tinnitus) was different from the tinnitus-masking pattern (see also Burns, 1984). Penner (1980) found that lateral-suppression mechanisms were impaired in tinnitus patients (based on psychoacoustic tuning curve measurements). If the changes, and the generation of tinnitus, were at the cochlear level, the masking of an external pure tone would be similar to the masking of tinnitus. Thus the difference of the tuning curve approach and the tinnitus masking profile points to central tinnitus. For tinnitus, even of peripheral origin, the suppressive effects of the masker at the level of the basilar membrane are absent and the overall masking effect is very different than that seen with external tones as stimuli.

From these studies it became clear that tinnitus is best masked with frequencies in the region of the hearing loss. Noreña et al. (2002) elucidated this by showing that the tinnitus spectrum resembles the hearing loss frequencies (see Figure 5–1).

Residual Inhibition

Residual inhibition is a postmasking effect (Feldman, 1971; Tyler & Conrad-Armes, 1984). As residual inhibition often lasts for a long time (usually seconds, but can last for minutes to hours), it likely is of central origin. If the origin were cochlear, then the standard time scale of forward masking would determine the duration of the inhibition, and this is rarely longer than 200 ms. Roberts, Moffat, Baumann, Ward, and Bosnyak (2008) found that psychoacoustic functions relating the depth and duration of tinnitus suppression ("residual inhibition") to the center frequency of band-passed noise masking sounds appear to span the region of hearing loss, as do psychoacoustic measurements of the tinnitus spectrum. The residual inhibition was generally largest for sounds in the hearing loss range and for sounds that resembled the tinnitus spectrum. The results suggested that cortical map reorganization induced by hearing loss, which results in an overrepresentation of the edge frequency(ies) in the audiogram, is not the principal source of the tinnitus sensation. Were that the case, one would expect the tinnitus pitch to match the edge frequency and that these edge frequencies would result in the largest residual inhibition.

OBJECTIVE QUANTIFICATION

Objective measurements of human auditory system activity can be done at nearly all levels from cochlea to cortex, that is, with techniques as diverse as otoacoustic emission recording and brain imaging.

Otoacoustic Emissions

Spontaneous otoacoustic emissions (SOAEs) are low-level sounds emitted by the healthy normal ear that are recordable with sensitive microphones inserted in the ear canal. In at least 4% (Penner & Jastreboff, 1996) of normal hearing persons, SOAEs are considered partially responsible for the tinnitus (Norton, Schmidt & Stover, 1990). In most cases, however, SOAEs and tinnitus are independent phenomena (Penner, 1992; Penner & Burns, 1987). Although spontaneous emissions could theoretically produce increased "spontaneous firing" in neurons innervating the basilar membrane at the emission site, central nervous system adaptation may preclude their audibility. Occasionally, some subjects hear intermittent SOAEs as intermittent tinnitus (Burns & Keefe, 1992). Aspirin administration was reported to abolish OAE-related tinnitus, likely by interfering with the outer hair cell amplifier (Coles & Penner, 1992). This could potentially be used as a test to eliminate SOAEs as the source of tinnitus.

Stimulated OAEs are sensitive indicators of outer hair cell loss and the influence of the efferent system on the cochlea. Patients with normal hearing acuity who have acute tinnitus seem to have a less effective functioning of the cochlear efferent system, because the application of contralateral noise either enhanced the distortion product OAEs (DPOAEs) or suppressed them less intensely than it did in a control group (Riga, Papadas, Werner, & Dalchow, 2007). Nottet, Moulin, Brossard, Suc, and Job (2006) found, 24 hours after an acute acoustic trauma, that OAEs appeared to be a better predictor of the persistence of tinnitus than hearing thresholds alone. After head injury, significantly higher spontaneous and stimulated OAE amplitudes, and reduced medial olivocochlear suppression, were reported in patients with tinnitus, as compared to subjects without tinnitus (Ceranic, Prasher, Raglan, & Luxon, 1998). Thus, stimulated OAEs are sensitive indicators of subthreshold hearing loss and changes in efferent activity at the cochlear level, but only rarely are the cause of tinnitus.

Findings in Tinnitus with Brain Imaging

Brain imaging in humans would ideally provide an accurate representation of increased neural brain activity during silence, which is generally considered the crucial neural substrate linked to tinnitus. This problem cannot readily be solved at the group comparison level between tinnitus patients and normal controls because of high variability in resting metabolic activity levels among people.

It has been addressed indirectly by focusing on people who can modulate the strength of their tinnitus by either changing eye gaze direction (Giraud et al., 1999; Lockwood et al., 2001) or by making orofacial movements (Cacace, 2003). For these groups, it has been demonstrated by using positron emission tomography (PET) that increased tinnitus loudness corresponds to increased neural activity in several auditory areas. Group analysis of PET data (Plewnia et al., 2007) also showed tinnitus-related increases of regional cerebral blood flow in the left middle- and inferior-temporal cortex as well as right temporo-parietal cortex and posterior cingulum, when compared to activity following intravenous lidocaine that induced a suppression of tinnitus (Figure 5–2). Like prior imaging studies, the group data showed no significant tinnitus-related hyperactivity of the PAC. These findings support the notion that tinnitus-related neuroplastic changes, as documented in the PAC by electrophysiologic methods that are more sensitive to neural synchrony, are not necessarily associated with enhanced cortical oxygen demands.

How does one measure spontaneous activity level in the human brain? Typically, sound-induced blood-oxygen-level dependent (BOLD) responses reflect the difference with the nonstimulus baseline activity. In the case of tinnitus, this baseline activity could be higher than normal, leaving fewer neurons that can be activated with the sound ("line-busy" effect). In the inferior colliculus (IC) Melcher et al. (2000) found that external sound produced abnormally low further activation in the IC contralateral to the tinnitus ear. Smits et al. (2007) found the same in IC, auditory thalamus and AC. So indirectly this points to increased spontaneous activity levels in these brain structures. The problem with this method is that the sound likely interacts with the spontaneous activity related to tinnitus, such that the estimated spontaneous levels may be biased. Contradicting these findings, Lanting, De Kleine, Bartels, and Van Dijk (2008) observed increased responses to sound in the IC of tinnitus patients. However, methodological differences, such as continuous sampling versus sparse sampling, may explain this.

A potentially promising method of measuring resting levels of activity that does not use sound stimulation and that would be applicable to investigate substrates of tinnitus has been proposed by Haller, Wetzel, Radue, and Bilecen (2006). They used inhaled CO_2 as a vasodilator to induce a "global" blood oxygenation level-dependent (BOLD) response. They implied, although indirectly, that spontaneously active brain areas in subjects with tinnitus will exhibit a reduced CO_2-induced change in the BOLD response due to pre-existing tinnitus-induced BOLD response. This putative reduction in the change of

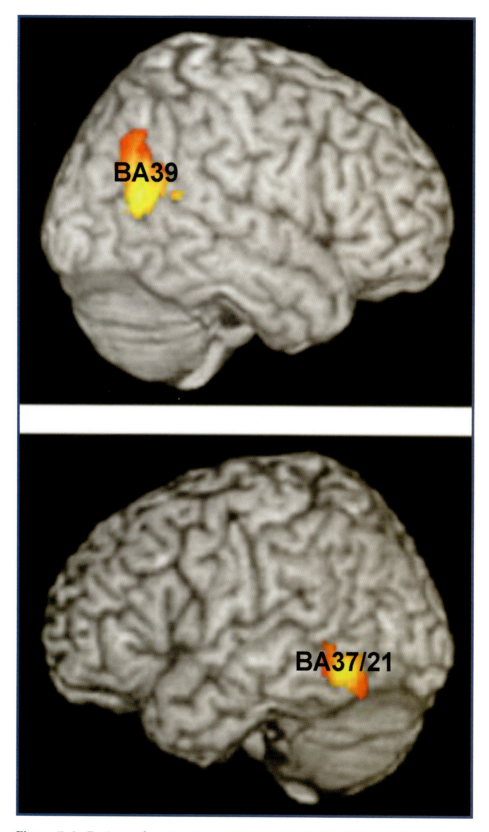

Figure 5–2. Regions where tinnitus activity is abolished by lidocaine. Note that the involved regions are not primary auditory areas. BA39 is angular gyrus; Ba37/21 represents middle and lower temporal cortex. Modified from Plewnia et al. (2007) with permission from the Publisher.

the BOLD response compared to nonauditory areas might then be exploited for mapping of a continuous neuronal activation that putatively exists in tinnitus. The comparison with the effect in nonauditory areas could provide a within-subject control, which obviously is not possible when using a sound to obtain a BOLD response. This, however, assumes that central manifestations of tinnitus are limited to the auditory nervous system, which as we will see later is not always the case.

EEG and MEG Findings in Tinnitus

If large numbers of neurons are activated simultaneously, the changes in the membrane potential occur synchronously across neurons. The corresponding currents then add up in phase and become so large that they can be detected at the scalp (Eggermont, 2006). The compound membrane potential from a large number of cortical neurons recorded from the scalp is called the electroencephalogram (EEG). Its magnetic equivalent is called the magnetoencephalogram (MEG). Traditionally, the EEG is quantified by the power in discrete frequency bands, labeled in the order that they were discovered; the first one was the alpha rhythm.

The spontaneous MEG in a group of individuals with tinnitus was characterized by a marked reduction in alpha (8 to 12 Hz) power together with an enhancement in delta (1.5 to 4 Hz) power as compared to normal-hearing controls. This pattern was especially pronounced over the temporal cortex. Moreover, correlations with tinnitus-related distress revealed strong associations with this abnormal spontaneous activity pattern, particularly in right temporal and left frontal areas (Weisz, Moratti, Meinzer, Dohrmann, & Elbert, 2005a).

High-frequency (gamma band, 30 to 60 Hz) oscillations have been linked to conscious sensory perception and positive symptoms in a variety of neurologic disorders (Llinás, Urbano, Leznik, Ramírez, & van Marle, 2005). With that in mind, Weisz et al. (2007) examined gamma-band activity during brief periods of marked enhancement of slow-wave (delta) activity (see Weisz et al., 2005a). Results revealed that both control and tinnitus groups showed significant increases in gamma-band activity after the onset of slow waves. However, gamma-band activity was more prominent in tinnitus subjects than in controls. The hemispheric lateralization of the gamma-band activity did correlate with the lateralization of the perceived tinnitus.

AEP and AEF Findings in Tinnitus

In tinnitus patients, magnetically recording the stimulus-evoked P_2, which originates largely from secondary and association cortex, was found to be delayed and low in amplitude (or even completely missing), whereas the amplitude of the N_1 was significantly augmented (Hoke, Feldmann, Pantev, Lütkenhöner, & Lehnertz, 1989). However, Jacobson et al. (1991) and Colding-Jørgensen, Lauritzen, Johnsen, Mikkelsen, and Saermark (1992) could not confirm these findings. Attias, Urbach, Gold, and Shemesh (1993) found that, in tinnitus subjects, the N_1 and P_2 were both reduced in amplitude compared to a group of controls matched for hearing loss and age. Weisz, Wienbruch, Dohrmann, and Elbert (2005b) compared tinnitus subjects with normal controls and used tonal stimuli at the edge of their hearing loss as well as tonal stimuli with a frequency one-octave below the edge frequency. They found that the N_1 dipole strength for tinnitus subjects and controls was not different for the audiogram edge-frequency tones, but that the N_1 responses were significantly larger for tonal stimuli that were one-octave below the edge-frequency of the audiogram in the right hemisphere of the tinnitus subjects. This points to a reduced inhibition originating from the neurons whose best frequencies are in the hearing-loss range. The data from Weisz et al. (2005b) also suggest increased neural synchrony (larger N_1) but in the normal-hearing range, partially in contrast to the interpretation of the Attias et al. (1993) data.

Weisz, Voss, Berg, and Elbert (2004) found an increased mismatch-negativity (MMN) in tinnitus sufferers with high-frequency hearing loss that was associated with subjective distress level. The enlarged MMN may be related to the enhanced frequency discrimination that sometimes accompanies the broadened central representation of edge frequencies in steep-sloping hearing loss. But how that would be related to distress level is unclear. Subjects with hearing loss exhibit slightly reduced detection thresholds (Irvine, Rajan, & McDermott, 2000) and slightly enhanced frequency discrimination (Thai-Van, Micheyl, Moore, & Collet, 2003) for sound frequencies at the edge of the affected frequency region.

Question 3

Is tinnitus related to central and/or peripheral damage?

Answer 3

Tinnitus is typically the result of damage to the cochlea, or (possibly) to peripheral nerves of the somatosensory system (trigeminal nerve and ganglion) that innervate the dorsal cochlear nucleus and give rise to somatic tinnitus. Although the damage is peripheral, this gives rise to changes in the central auditory nervous system, causing increased spontaneous firing rates, increased neural synchrony and reorganization of the cortical frequency-place (tonotopic) map. In addition, there will be changes in the interaction between the auditory system and the limbic system, especially with the amygdala that provides for the strong emotional or annoyance component related to tinnitus. It is possible that more central damage underlies tinnitus; for instance that following vestibular schwannoma or cerebellopontine angle surgery that can give rise to gaze-induced tinnitus. Thus, most of the causes of tinnitus appear to be peripheral or in the lower brainstem, and likely all the transient forms of tinnitus are. Chronic tinnitus most likely involves altered thalamocortical activity. What makes things so difficult is that the AC exerts frequency-specific influences down to the cochlear nucleus (see Figure 5–4; Luo et al., 2008), and a cortex with a changed tonotopic map will send different signals to the brainstem compared to a normal one.

ANIMAL MODELS

Behavioral Models

The neural substrate of tinnitus can only be studied in depth in animal models that show behavioral evidence of tinnitus under conditions similar to those that cause tinnitus in humans. The question is: do animals have tinnitus and, furthermore, can it be demonstrated? A myriad of behavioral test models have been devised for rats (Bauer & Brozoski, 2001; Guitton et al., 2003; Jastreboff, Brennan, Coleman, & Sasaki, 1988; Lobarinas, Sun, Cushing, & Salvi, 2004; Rüttiger, Ciuffani, Zenner, & Knipper, 2003; Turner et al., 2006), hamsters (Heffner & Harrington, 2002), mice (Prosen & May, 2005), and chinchillas (Bauer et al., 2008). For a critical comparison of some of the earlier models see Moody (2004).

The first behavioral test of tinnitus in animals was developed by Jastreboff et al. (1988). The basic procedure involved training rats to stop licking a waterspout whenever a broadband noise was turned off for 1 minute by presenting a brief foot shock at the end of the "noise off" or silent interval. Animals with tinnitus were expected to hear a sound (i.e., tinnitus) and be more likely to continue licking during silent intervals.

Bauer and Brozoski (2001) trained rats to press a lever in the presence of broadband noise (105-dB SPL noise band centered at 16 kHz in one ear for 1 or 2 hours) to obtain food, but to stop pressing the lever during silent intervals to avoid foot shock. The animal was subsequently tested by presenting four intervals containing a tone, but no shock is given, and four silent intervals followed by shock if the animal does not stop lever pressing. The tone is varied in frequency and intensity with the expectation that animals with tinnitus will respond to the tones matching the tinnitus pitch differently than will control animals.

A modification of the Jastreboff et al. (1988) procedure was designed by Heffner and Harrington (2002) for use in hamsters. The animals received extensive training using sounds that, while clearly audible, were as low as 33 dB above threshold, and varied the location of the loudspeakers so that the animals learned to respond to sound regardless of its location. The hamsters were trained to stop drinking during silence but were more likely to continue drinking following exposure to a loud 10-kHz tone for 2 or 4 h. In other words, they behaved as though they hear a sound when no external sound is presented.

Another behavioral technique utilized "false positive" responses that occurred during a quiet interval to infer the presence or absence of tinnitus. The approach utilized a shock avoidance conditioning procedure in which rats learned to climb a pole during the presentation of a sound to avoid foot shock. Animals could remain on the cage floor during quiet intervals since the shock was turned off (Guitton et al., 2003). During salicylate treatment, rats climbed the pole (false positive) during quiet, which was interpreted as evidence of tinnitus.

Rüttiger et al. (2003) introduced a positive reinforcement technique in which responses made in the presence of sound were reinforced with a fluid reward, but not during quiet. Salicylates induced a high false response rate in quiet; the false alarm rate was equivalent to the access rate evoked by a 30 dB SPL white noise.

The schedule-induced polydipsia avoidance conditioning procedure (Lobarinas et al., 2004) combines shock avoidance associated with an audible stimulus. Therefore, animals continued to suppress licking during sound trials. High doses of salicylate suppressed licks-in-quiet; this was interpreted as evidence of tinnitus.

Turner et al. (2006) described another method for tinnitus screening in rats by a modified prepulse inhibition of the startle reflex. Detection of a gap in an acoustic background functioned as the prepulse and induced an inhibition of a loud noise-burst induced startle reflex. The authors hypothesized that if the background acoustic signal was qualitatively similar to the rat's tinnitus, poorer detection of a silent gap in this background would be expected and the startle reflex would not be inhibited.

Are these behavioral tests measuring the presence of tinnitus? Tinnitus-inducing agents will likely induce a certain amount of hyperacusis. For instance, salicylate increases serotonergic activity in the brain (see later section in this chapter on brain chemistry) that has been linked to central hyperacusis, and noise trauma produces release from inhibition in the neighboring unaffected frequency regions that also greatly increases activity therein, and causes hyperacusis in those regions (Noreña, Gourévitch, Aizawa, & Eggermont, 2006). Thus, animals will as likely respond to weak previously ignored sounds in the environment as to the also weak internally generated tinnitus. Hearing loss and hyperacusis both will affect the audibility and loudness of low-level stimuli and behavioral tests might not be able to successfully discriminate between the two. The potential confound caused by hyperacusis in all test outcomes makes animal behavioral tests less than ideal, unless one can be sure that hyperacusis implies tinnitus and vice versa. This reinforces the notion that the best experimental animal in which to study tinnitus is the human, where one might be more able to successfully differentiate hyperacusis from tinnitus.

Neural Substrates

Electrophysiologic studies in awake versus anesthetized animals showed potentially larger effects of tinnitus-inducing agents in awake animals (Yang et al., 2007). One reason may be that in anesthetized animals the spontaneous activity is often (surprisingly) much higher than in awake animals (Shoham, O'Connor, & Segev, 2006). This could make the detection of changes in SFR (especially increases in SFR) more difficult in anesthetized animals. Different levels of corticofugal activity to subcortical structures cannot be excluded either, although the anesthesia effect on corticofugal activity appears small (Yan & Ehret, 2002).

Spontaneous Firing Rates

There is limited support for the assumption that tinnitus is the result of increased spontaneous firing rates (SFR) in ANFs: evidence is only found after acute high-dose application of salicylate in cats (Evans, Wilson, & Borerwe, 1981), but moderate doses in the same species do not increase the SFR

(Stypulkowski, 1990). However, chronic salicylate application may result in increased SFR in ANFs (Cazals, 2000), consistent with the behavioral indication of tinnitus even for low doses of salicylate in rats (Bauer, Brozoski, Holder, & Caspary, 2000). Other drugs that cause tinnitus, such as quinine (Mulheran, 1999) and aminoglycosides (Kiang, Moxon, & Levine, 1970), produced a consistent decrease in the SFR of ANFs. A similar decrease was found in NIHL (Liberman & Kiang, 1978; Salvi, Hamernik, Henderson, & Ahroon, 1983). Thus, there is an "edge" in the distribution of spontaneous activity that corresponds to the boundary of the hearing loss.

These results, showing reduced SFR in ANFs following noise exposure or ototoxicity (Table 5–2), point to a central cause of tinnitus, possibly related to changes in the balance of excitatory and inhibitory inputs conveyed to central auditory structures. Two important qualifications are that tinnitus can be prevented if *N*-methyl-D-aspartate (NMDA) receptor blockers are infused into the cochlea before salicylate application (Guitton et al., 2003), and that prior administration of NMDA receptor blockers can limit hearing loss resulting from noise trauma (Duan, Agerman, Ernfors, & Canlon, 2000). It seems that by reducing the extent of the hearing loss, probably by preventing neurotoxic effects at cochlear α-amino-3-hydroxy-5-methyl-4-isoxalone propinoic acid (AMPA) or NMDA receptors, the tinnitus is also prevented. These findings are consistent with the view that the origin of tinnitus may be an imbalance of firing patterns across the tonotopic array of ANFs

(Kiang et al., 1970), but not with the alternative view that tinnitus is always the result of increased spontaneous activity generated in ANFs. The data, however, do suggest two different models for the generation of tinnitus; a peripheral-salicylate model and a central-noise trauma model.

The Salicylate Model for Peripheral Tinnitus. Acute salicylate application has two effects in the cochlea; one is that it blocks the outer hair cell motor by affecting the prestin expression in the hair cell wall and thereby abolishes the positive feedback to the basilar membrane motion and thus produces a hearing loss. The other effect is that salicylate inhibits cochlear cyclooxygenase, which increases levels of arachidonate and so activates NMDA receptors and thereby potentially increases spontaneous and driven firing rates (Guitton et al., 2003; Ruel et al., 2008). Acute salicylate application at a dose of 200 mg/kg failed to increase SFR in cat (Stypulkowski, 1990) and gerbil ANFs (Müller, Klinke, Arnold and Oestreicher, 2003). In contrast, chronic salicylate administration even in high doses increases spontaneous firing rates (Cazals, 2000), consistent with an observed increase in DPOAEs (Huang et al., 2005). Obviously acute and chronic salicylate applications activate different mechanisms to generate tinnitus.

Central Effects of Salicylate. Salicylate attenuates inhibitory postsynaptic currents in the AC, suggesting that this may be one way to increase SFR in the central auditory regions and so produce tinnitus

Table 5–2. SFR, AEPs, and Tinnitus

Activity Compared to Control	Salicylate			Noise Trauma		
	SFR	Synchrony	AEP	SFR	Synchrony	AEP
ANF	(≈ ⇑)			⇓		
DCN			≈	⇑		≈
IC	⇑⇓			⇑		⇑
PAC	≈⇓	≈	⇑	⇑	⇑	⇑
SAC	⇑		⇑			⇑

(≈ ⇑): acute no change, chronic up; ≈: no change; ⇑⇓: up respectively down. Conflicting findings are shown for IC.

(Wang, Luo, Zhou, Xu, & Chen, 2006). This also interrupts the normal level of γ-amino-butyric acid (GABA)-ergic synaptic transmissions maintained by the serotonergic system (Wang, Luo, Huang, Zhou, & Chen, 2008).

In rats, a high salicylate dose resulted in decreased mean interspike intervals (suggestive for increased SFR and/or burst firing) in the central nucleus of IC (ICc) neurons (Jasterboff & Sasaki, 1986), and a lower dose did the same for neurons in the external nucleus of the IC (ICx) (Chen & Jastreboff, 1995). In the IC of guinea pigs, a low dose salicylate increased the mean SFR nearly 4-fold at 100 min. after application, firing rates then declined to baseline after 10 hours (Manabe et al., 1997). In contrast, an average dose decreased SFR significantly in mice ICc (Ma, Hidaka, & May, 2006). In cat, a low-dose of salicylate produced increased SFRs for high characteristic frequencies (CFs) in SAC, but not in PAC (Eggermont & Kenmochi, 1998). In awake rats, low-dose salicylate that induced behavioral signs of tinnitus decreased spontaneous firing rates in PAC significantly (Yang et al., 2006). It is clear that there are appreciable species differences for salicylate, and the combination of distinct peripheral and central effects suggests that it is not a general model for tinnitus.

The Noise Trauma Model for Central Tinnitus. After noise trauma, which generally decreased SFR in ANFs, enhancements of SFR were found in the central auditory nervous system: in vivo experiments in hamster DCN indicate massive increases in SFR of nonidentified superficial layer cells (i.e., fusiform, cartwheel or giant cells) 5 to 180 days after noise exposure, but not at 2 days (Kaltenbach, Zhang, & Afman, 2000). This SFR increase correlated significantly with the strength of the behavioral index of tinnitus in hamsters (Kaltenbach, Zacharek, Zhang, & Frederick, 2004). The cells responsible could be the fusiform cells that provide the output of the DCN to the IC (Brozoski, Bauer, & Caspary, 2002). However, Chang, Chen, Kaltenbach, Zhang, and Godfrey (2002) did not find increased SFR in fusiform or cartwheel cells after noise trauma. In addition, Ma and Young (2006) found, after noise trauma that induced a hearing loss of about 60 dB above 5 to 10 kHz one

month after the trauma in cat, that neurons in DCN did not show any indication of increased SFR compared to non-exposed control animals.

In IC of mice, noise trauma significantly increased SFR (Ma et al., 2006). In chinchillas there was increased burst firing in IC after a moderate noise exposure and also following carboplatin and cisplatin administration (Bauer et al., 2008). In cat PAC, a significant increase in SFR occurred after at least 2 hrs following the trauma, but not immediately (<15 min) following the noise exposure (Noreña & Eggermont, 2006; Noreña, Tomita, & Eggermont, 2003). At least 3 weeks after the trauma, the SFR was significantly larger than in controls at all CFs tested, not only in the region of the hearing loss, although the hearing-loss region showed more pronounced changes (Seki & Eggermont, 2003).

Neural Synchrony

The degree to which spikes from two different single units are time-locked or, alternatively, fire in synchrony can be quantified by the cross-correlation coefficient (Eggermont, 1992). The neural synchrony under spontaneous firing conditions studied in the same single-neuron pairs before and after application of salicylate (Ochi & Eggermont, 1996) showed no significant change as a function of time after salicylate administration. In contrast to the effects produced by salicylate, and despite the same average hearing loss produced by quinine and salicylate, the cross-correlation coefficient was increased significantly for a high quinine dose but not for a low dose (Ochi & Eggermont, 1997).

After a 1-hour exposure to a 5- or 6-kHz tone presented at a level of 115 to 120 dB SPL, the average hearing loss 6 hours after the trauma was about 40 dB in the range of 6 to 32 kHz. The acute recordings from the PAC in cats were performed using two multielectrode arrays of eight electrodes each, before and up to 6 hours after exposure to the trauma tone while leaving the electrodes in place. The increase in peak cross-correlation coefficients was significant within 15 minutes after the trauma, and increased to, on average, a 54% increase over the pre-exposure values, at 2 hours after the trauma (Noreña & Eggermont, 2003).

Chronic effects of noise trauma (Seki & Eggermont, 2002, 2003) showed that across the entire CF range, the peak cross-correlation coefficient values for neuron pairs in reorganized areas were significantly higher than for pairs in nonreorganized areas, and also significantly higher than for controls. Thus cortical tonotopic map reorganization and increase in peak cross-correlation coefficients are closely linked.

Because neural synchrony increase occurs before a detectable increase in SFR, it may be that the neural synchrony increase is a primary characteristic of the tinnitus that in humans usually occurs immediately after noise trauma. More chronic forms of tinnitus may require increased SFR as well.

BRAIN CHEMISTRY AND MOLECULAR BIOLOGY OF TINNITUS

Ion Channels

Ion channels in hair cells and neurons are the main cell structures where changes in the membrane potential are initiated, and result in transmitter release and/or action potential initiation and propagation. The ion channels at the top of the hair cells, also called transduction channels, are opened by mechanical deformation of the stereocilia and mainly conduct K^+ ions (because they are exposed to the K^+-rich endolymph). Ion channels at the base of the hair cells are involved in the initiation of transmitter release and conduct Ca^{2+} ions. Ion channels in neurons conduct Na^+, K^+, and Cl^- ions that are involved in action-potential generation and conduction. Ion channels can be opened and closed in response to voltage changes or are ligand mediated. Ion channels, especially K^+ and Ca^{2+}, come in many forms (Eggermont, 2005).

The IHCs in the cochlea are equipped with only one type of Ca^{2+} channels, namely the L-type. These calcium channels regulate the release of the neurotransmitter glutamate from the IHCs. Blocking these L-type channels with nimodipine results in a decrease in spontaneous and stimulus-driven firing rates in ANFs (Robertson & Paki, 2002). In tinnitus sufferers, nimodipine treatment was effective only in five out of 31 patients (Davies et al., 1994).

Lidocaine, which can relieve tinnitus temporarily, blocks voltage-sensitive Na^+ channels. Peripheral fast voltage-sensitive Na^+ channels are likely not involved either, since tinnitus could be suppressed with Lidocaine in patients with sectioned AN after vestibular schwannoma removal (Baguley et al., 2005). That means the suppressive effect is most likely to occur at levels more central than the auditory nerve.

Intracellular Ca^{2+} has a role in regulating the balance between inward and outward currents in neurons and hair cells. The function of the hair cells also depends on the Ca^{2+} signaling pathways governing the fast neurotransmitter release of IHCs and the slow motility changes of the OHCs. The effects of noise, salicylate, and quinine include a sustained increase in the Ca^{2+} concentration in hair cells (Fridberger, Flock, Ulfendahl, & Flock, 1998). Salicylates also cause a dose-dependent decrease in the free perilymphatic Ca^{2+} concentration (Cazals, 2000). During noise exposure, there is a very large transient increase in the endolymph Ca^{2+} concentration, similar to the sustained Ca^{2+} increase observed in animals with experimentally induced endolymphatic hydrops (the animal model for Ménière's disease) (Ikeda, Sunose, & Takasaka, 1994). Tinnitus, sustained as well as transient, is one of the defining characteristics of Ménière's disease. Caffeine, which is only weakly linked to tinnitus (see above), also increases intracellular calcium (Yoshimura, 2005).

Neurotransmitter Imbalance

Glutamate Neurotoxicity

Excess glutamate causes ANF-dendrite swelling followed by membrane disruption. Continuous release of glutamate from intact IHCs induces growth of new dendritic processes after noise trauma damage (Puel, 1995). This regrowth and synapse formation is probably the cause of a reduction in NIHL following recovery in an enriched acoustic environment compared with recovery in a quiet environment (Norena & Eggermont, 2003). Guitton et al. (2003)

and Guitton, Wang, and Puel (2004) suggested that salicylate-induced tinnitus results from inhibition of cyclooxygenase activity resulting in altered arachidonic acid metabolism, which potentiates NMDA receptor currents in the cochlea. The increased opening probability of NMDA receptors can result in burst-firing activity in ANFs, potentially leading to tinnitus. Such bursting activity has been found in some ANFs after noise trauma (Liberman & Kiang, 1978), suggesting that the NMDA receptors in ANF dendrites that normally are only activated at high intensity levels become hypersensitive (Table 5–3).

Glycine and GABA Downregulation and Glutamate Strengthening

Noise exposure lowers GABA-mediated inhibition in the IC (Szczepaniak & Moller, 1995). Glutamic acid decarboxylase (GAD) levels in the IC increased immediately after noise exposure but returned to lower than control values 30 days after exposure (Abbott et al., 1999). Because GAD is the rate-limiting enzyme in the formation of GABA, an increase in GAD concentration suggests an initial upregulation of the reservoir pool of GABA after the trauma (probably as a compensatory mechanism) but a downregulation later. In the first week after exposure to unilateral noise trauma (Muly et al., 2004), electrically evoked glutamatergic transmission in the ipsilateral ventral cochlear nucleus (VCN) slice increased, whereas its uptake was depressed. In the DCN, glutamate release was increased and uptake was unchanged. At 14 days after exposure,

glutamatergic release and uptake were lowered, probably because of the degeneration of ANFs. At 90 days after exposure, glutamatergic release and AMPA-receptor binding were sharply increased. This was attributed to neuroplastic mechanisms. The findings were consistent with a noise-induced strengthening of glutamatergic transmission in VCN and DCN, leading to hyperexcitability in the auditory pathways (Salvi et al., 2000). After salicylate application, an upregulation of GAD and a decrease in GABA$_A$-receptor affinity was observed in the IC of rats showing behavioral evidence for tinnitus (Bauer et al., 2000).

Age-related changes include significant decreases in glycine receptor sites in rat anteroventral CN (AVCN) and DCN (Milbrandt & Caspary, 1995). In old C57 mice, which exhibit progressive cochlear pathology with age, but not in middle age C57 and old CBA mice, the number of glycine receptors decreased significantly in DCN, suggesting that it is not only age that determines downregulation of glycine, but also the amount of hearing loss (Willott, Milbrandt, Bross, & Caspary, 1997). In aging animals, there was also an upregulation in the number of GABA$_A$ receptors, probably to compensate the significant loss of presynaptic GABA release (Caspary et al., 1999). The reduced GABA release might explain the increasing incidence of tinnitus in the elderly who have suffered moderate NIHL earlier in life. Drug treatments that purportedly increase GABA activity, for example, some anticonvulsant drugs, are frequently tested in clinical trials (see the therapy section in this chapter).

Table 5–3. Transmitter Systems

Activity Change	Salicylate				Noise Trauma			
	AMPA	NMDA	GABA	5-HT	AMPA	NMDA	GABA	ACh
ANF	≈	⇑						
DCN					⇓→⇑			⇑
IC				⇑			⇓→⇑	
AC				⇑		⇑→⇓		

(≈: no change; ⇑⇓: up respectively down; ⇓→⇑: initially down then recovers.)

Acetylcholine

Acetylcholine receptors (AChR) come in two flavors: muscarinic (mAChR) and nicotinic (nAChR). The latter are located on the cochlear hair cells and mediate the medial efferent olivocochlear bundle response. These nAChR's are ligand-mediated ion channels that regulate glutamate synapses (e.g., in AC to enhance learning and memory), and act as efferent system transmitters (Lustig, 2006). After noise trauma, choline-acetyl transferase, an enzyme involved in the production of ACh, increased by 74% in ipsilateral AVCN and by 55 to 74% in ipsilateral DCN at 8 days post-trauma. By 2 months posttrauma, the level was still increased by 53% in the deep layers of the DCN on the exposed side (Jin, Godfrey, Wang and Kaltenbach, 2006). AChRs play a role in homeostatic plasticity because they allow Ca^{2+} to enter through these channels (Morley & Happe, 2000). This could underlie the homeostatic changes proposed for the DCN following noise trauma that may undelie the increased SFR (Schaette & Kempter, 2006, 2008).

Serotonin (5-HT)

Serotonergic activity increases the perception of chronic pain and phantom limb pain and thus may play a role in the perception of tinnitus (Holgers, Zöger, & Svedlund, 2003; Simpson & Davies, 2000). The serotonin receptor agonist 1-(3-chlorophenyl) piperazine (mCPP) increases anxiety in humans and animals and exacerbates the behavioral perception of salicylate-induced tinnitus (Guitton, Pujol, & Puel, 2005). Salicylate by itself increases the serotonergic activity in the rat for up to 6 hours postinjection in IC and PAC (Liu et al., 2003). Serotonin has also been implicated in central hyperacusis (Marriage & Barnes, 1995). Serotonin activity is affected by the circadian rhythm (Thomas, 2006), suggesting that time of day could affect the tinnitus percept.

Hormones

Cortisol

Cortisol (a steroid-based hormone) is secreted from the adrenal cortex in response to stress, and acts through glucocorticoid receptors. A relation between tinnitus and stress levels has been demonstrated on the basis of cortisol levels (Hébert et al., 2004). Glucocorticoid receptors are present in the hair cells and supporting cells of the organ of Corti, and in the spiral ligament and stria vascularis, suggesting a possible role in homeostasis of inner ear fluids and in signal transduction (Horner, 2003). Glucocorticoids are also found in the brainstem nuclei, including the mesencephalic raphe nuclei and locus ceruleus, which contain serotonergic and noradrenergic neurons.

Catecholamines and Opioids

Catecholamines (adrenalin and noradrenalin) and endogenous opioids (such as endorphin, enkephalins, dynorphins) are released in response to stress from the adrenal medulla and act mainly through the nervous system. Catecholamines are the main neurotransmitters of the sympathetic nervous system, which is activated during stress. Under physiological conditions (70 dB SPL white noise stimulation), noradrenergic regulation of the processing of auditory information occurs dominantly in the DCN and posteroventral cochlear nucleus (PVCN) without changes in AVCN and IC (Cransac, Cottet-Emard, Hellström, & Peyrin, 1998).

Enkephalins and dynorphins are thought to act as neurotransmitters in the auditory system, while the noradrenergic fibers of the sympathetic innervation of the cochlea, that surrounds the labyrinthine artery and the modiolar branches, control cochlear blood flow. Sahley and Nodar (2001) have suggested that glutamate release by IHCs is enhanced in response to opioid dynorphins that are released into the synapses during stressful situations. This could lead to higher spontaneous firing rates and stress-related peripheral tinnitus.

Estrogen and Progesterone

Reproductive hormones may also have a role in the occurrence of tinnitus and hyperacusis. Estrogen has both an excitatory role and a neuroprotective effect, and there is a strong relationship between estrogen and serotoninergic pathways (Rubinow, Schmidt,

& Roca, 1998). Progesterone has a potent inhibitory effect, through the interaction with the GABA receptors. Therefore, alterations in these hormones, both physiologic and pathologic, may lead to increased susceptibility to developing tinnitus.

Immediate Early Eenes

Immediate early genes (IEG) are induced rapidly inside nerve cells by extracellular stimuli without the need of intermediate proteins.

c-Fos

c-Fos regulates the expression of the kainic acid receptor GluR6 and the brain-derived neurotrophic factor (BDNF), and c-Fos expression is linked to neuronal excitability.

Brain-Derived Neurotrophic Factor (BDNF)

BDNF is a small protein that acts by binding to its receptors such as tyrosine kinase TrkB. BDNF promotes survival through inactivation of components of the cell death machinery and also through activation of the transcription factor cAMP-response element binding protein (CREB), which drives expression of the prosurvival gene Bcl-2.

Calcium plays an important role in the regulation of neuronal gene expression. The first step in this calcium regulation is the influx of calcium into the cytoplasm. The transcription of BDNF is preferentially driven by calcium influx through L-type voltage-sensitive calcium channels (West et al., 2001). NMDA receptors as well as L-type Ca^{2+} channels are expressed in cochlear neurons (Niedzielski & Wenthold, 1995).

BDNF activates synaptic consolidation through transcription and rapid dendritic trafficking of messenger ribonucleic acid (mRNA) that is encoded by the immediate early gene Arc/Arg3.1 (Bramham & Messaoudi, 2005). BDNF is a key modulator of neuronal plasticity events. Spontaneous activity can also trigger BDNF trafficking to activated synapses and support its release from synapses.

Arc/Arg3.1

The activity-regulated cytoskeleton-associated protein/activity-regulated gene Arc/Arg3.1 is an IEG that is dynamically regulated by neuronal activity and is tightly coupled to behavioral encoding of information in neuronal circuits. Arg3.1/arc expression has been directly correlated with BDNF-induced plasticity changes. In particular, Arg3.1/arc expression is up-regulated, and transported to dendrites following synaptic stimulation. Arc/Arg3.1 mRNA accumulates there at sites of synaptic activity and is required together with BDNF for long-term potentiation (LTP) and long-term memory (Plath et al., 2006). Importantly, changes in Arc/Arg3.1 expression have been directly linked to information processing in the brain (Guzowski, McNaughton, Barnes, & Worley, 1999), and, correspondingly, Arc/Arg3.1-inducing stimuli trigger enduring changes in synaptic plasticity and behavior.

IEG Findings in Tinnitus

Table 5–4 shows findings following salicylate application and noise trauma. After salicylate injections, AC was the only auditory area with consistently increased numbers of c-fos immunoreactive neurons (IRN) (compared to controls). Exposure to impulse noise led to prolonged c-fos expression in AC and DCN. After both manipulations, c-fos expression was increased in the amygdala, in thalamic midline and intralaminar areas, in frontal cortex, as well as in hypothalamic and brainstem regions involved in behavioral and physiologic defensive reactions (Wallhäusser-Franke et al., 2003).

Mahlke and Wallhausser-Franke, (2004) found that in AC, Arc/Arg3.1 IRNs induced by sound were concentrated in regions corresponding to the stimulus frequency. Injections of salicylate led to accumulation of Arc/Arg3.1 IRN in the high-frequency areas. After both salicylate and nontraumatic auditory stimulation, c-fos IRN outnumbered Arc/Arg3.1 IRN in AC, and showed a broad distribution. In subcortical auditory structures, Arc/Arg3.1 IRN was absent in all but one brain. In VCN, c-fos IRN was always found after stimulation, whereas none was present when injecting salicylate. Simi-

Table 5–4. IEG and Tinnitus

Activity re Sound	Salicylate			Noise Trauma		
	c-fos	Arc/arg1.3	BDNF	c-fos	Arc/arg1.3	BDNF
ANF		≈	⇑	⇑		⇑
DCN	⇓	≈				
IC	⇓	≈				
AC	⇑	⇑⇓	⇓		⇓	⇓
Amygdala	⇑	⇑				

(≈: no change; ⇑⇓: up respectively down. Conflicting findings are shown for AC.)

larly, in IC, numbers of c-fos IRN were lowest after salicylate injections. In the amygdala, c-fos and Arc/Arg3.1 IRN were increased substantially after salicylate injections compared to nontraumatic auditory stimulation, suggesting that coactivation of the AC and the amygdala may by an essential feature of tinnitus-related activation.

Tan et al. (2007) monitored the expression of BDNF, Arg3.1/arc, and c-Fos in the peripheral and central auditory system hours and days following a traumatic acoustic stimulus that induced not only hearing loss but also tinnitus, according to their animal behavior model. A reciprocal responsiveness of activity-dependent genes became evident between the periphery and the PAC: c-Fos and BDNF expression were increased in spiral ganglion neurons, whereas Arg3.1/arc and (6 days posttrauma) BDNF expression was reduced in PAC. Since both c-Fos and BDNF are activity-dependent genes, their augmented transcription in the spiral ganglion could reflect enhanced glutamate release induced by traumatic noise and consequently NMDA/AMPA receptor activation (Puel, Ruel, Gervais d'Aldin, & Pujol, 1998; Duan et al., 2000). Reduced AMPA receptor trafficking is, for example, a direct molecular correlate of deprivation phenomena, and thus could likely be correlated with reduced Arc/Arg3.1 levels, increased AMPA responses, and increased firing rate.

The diminished levels of Arg3.1/arc and BDNF following acoustic trauma suggest reduced AMPA receptor trafficking and increased AMPA responses, and increased firing rates. Nontraumatic noise exposure increased Arg3.1/arc levels in AC, in agreement with the results of Mahlke and Wallhausser-Franke (2004).

Salicylate application (Panford-Walsh et al, 2008) induced an IEG expression pattern similar to that found after noise trauma (Tan et al., 2007): BDNF mRNA expression was increased in the spiral ganglion neurons of the cochlea and Arg3.1 expression was significantly reduced in AC. Local application of the $GABA_A$ receptor modulator midazolam resulted in the reversal of salicylate-induced changes in cochlear BDNF expression and cortical Arg3.1 expression, and reduced tinnitus perception in the animal model.

Thus the negative correlation between changes in SFR and those in BDNF and Arc/Arg 3.1 both for noise trauma and salicylate (compare Tables 5–2 and 5–4), correlates with the observed increased SFR.

IEGs can potentially be very powerful and sensitive mapping procedures in animal models to probe into the effects of tinnitus-inducing agents, but as shown here there is currently no clear agreement with putative electrophysiologic correlates of tinnitus. The effect of hearing loss on neurotransmitters and neuromodulators may document ways in which tinnitus manifests itself, and ultimately provide drugs specifically designed to alleviate tinnitus (see later in this chapter about the current status of drug treatment).

Question 4

Are there physiologic measures of tinnitus that could be used clinically?

Answer 4

Yes, but with great caution, because there are no physiologic methods that can unequivocally diagnose tinnitus in humans (or in animals). Physiologic methods can provide indications about the locus of the problem but are no substitute for asking the patient. For instance, otoacoustic emissions may be able to differentiate tinnitus related to hearing loss (emissions are of lower level or absent), from that resulting from head and neck injury (emissions may be increased because of reduced efferent input; see main text for details). Contralateral OAE suppression can also be used to indicate a less effective efferent system that some say could underlie tinnitus. The EEG spectrum when recorded with at least 20 electrodes could indicate certain central changes: look for excessive delta-frequency activity with superimposed gamma and reduced alpha-band activity (see again the main chapter text for more details). There are also strong indications that potential neural substrates of tinnitus (and hyperacusis) can be detected with cortical auditory evoked potentials. Among these are changes in tonotopic maps (use ASSR), and increased neural synchrony as reflected in increased AEP amplitudes. Functional MRI and PET can detect abnormal spontaneous neural activity, but these are hardly standard clinical tools.

NEURAL PLASTICITY

Even in adulthood the AC and thalamus remain highly plastic (see Chapter 6). This is most obvious in the tonotopic map changes that can be induced in animals by, for example, NIHL (Noreña & Egger-

mont, 2005), long exposure to nondamaging unusual sounds (Noreña et al., 2006), perceptual learning (Fritz, Elhilali, David, & Shamma, 2007) and day-to-day experience of environmental sounds (Kilgard, Vazquez, Engineer, & Pandya, 2007). Tonotopic map changes in animals after noise trauma that typically produces a partial, high-frequency, cochlear hearing loss, show an over representation in AC of the so called edge frequency of the audiogram, that is, the highest frequency that still has near-normal thresholds (Noreña & Eggermont, 2005). The region of AC that normally would represent the high frequencies (say 4–20 kHz) can, after noise trauma that affected the hearing at those frequencies, show its most sensitive responses at 4 kHz for the entire, previously high-frequency, region. It is also known that in such animals the AEPs locally recorded from the midbrain and cortex are greatly enhanced, suggesting increased neural synchrony (Salvi et al., 2000; Wang et al., 2002).

Tonotopic Maps in Animals

Local mechanical damage to the cochlea (Rajan, Irvine, Wise, & Heil, 1993; Robertson & Irvine, 1989), ototoxic-drug damage to the cochlea (Harrison, Nagasawa, Smith, Stanton, & Mount, 1991), and NIHL all cause tonotopic map changes in PAC (Eggermont & Komiya, 2000). The map changes (Figure 5–3) are not causally related to the hearing loss (Noreña & Eggermont, 2005) and can occur in the absence of hearing loss (Noreña et al., 2006), but are always accompanied by increased SFR and increased neural synchrony (Noreña & Eggermont, 2003, 2006; Seki & Eggermont, 2003).

Animal research, as reviewed above, has shown the response properties of neurons following ototoxic drugs and traumatic injuries, and pointed to changes that occur in the balance of excitation and inhibition at multiple levels of the auditory pathway. It is reasonable to assume that the effect of this change in transmitter level balance in the central nervous system contributes in some way to tinnitus. This points to a potential link between reorganization of the cortical tonotopic map, changes in neuron SFRs, changes in neural synchrony and tinnitus (Eggermont & Roberts, 2004).

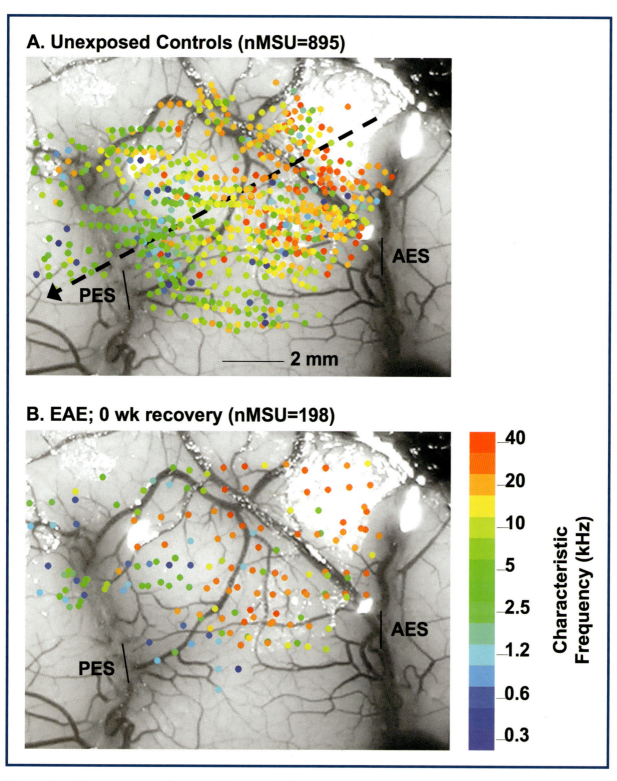

Figure 5–3. Tonotopic maps for control animals (**A**) and animals with lack of response to the 4 to 20 kHz area, which mimics a noise-induced hearing loss (**B**). Each dot represents a recording site and the color is according to the frequency scale in half-octave steps. Note that the gradual transition between low and high frequencies visible in the controls (*tonotopic gradient indicated by dotted arrow*) is replaced by an abrupt transition between the low and high frequencies. The paucity of recordings with very low CFs is due to the fact that these units are in the posterior ectosylvian sulcus (PES) and difficult to reach with our multielectrode arrays. AES indicates the anterior ectosylvian sulcus, which forms the border with the anterior auditory field. Based on data from Pienkowski and Eggermont (2009).

Map changes do not occur if, immediately after noise trauma, a compensatory complex sound that mimics in bandwidth and level of the expected hearing loss is presented for several weeks (Noreña & Eggermont, 2005). When this happens, the down-regulation of inhibition that usually follows noise-induced hearing loss likely does not occur and the unmasking of new excitatory inputs (Noreña et al., 2003) does not happen or, more likely, is reversed. When this "unmasking" trigger for tonotopic map reorganization is absent, map changes do not occur, despite a remaining hearing loss.

Tonotopic map changes can even occur in the absence of peripheral hearing loss. For instance, map changes can occur following a long and continuous presentation of a 4 to 20 kHz multifrequency sound (Noreña et al., 2006). This sound exposure, potentially by depressing the synapses of the lemniscal pathway in thalamus and cortex, creates a functional lesion that is very similar to that of a restricted cochlear lesion. For instance, the SFR and neural synchrony do increase significantly compared to normal-hearing controls and consequently one could speculate that this constitutes a model of tinnitus in the absence of a measurable hearing loss. However, if the animals are left in a quiet environment after the exposure, the cortical maps return to normal after several months (Pienkowski & Eggermont, 2009).

Tonotopic Map Changes in Humans?

Tinnitus seen as an auditory phantom sensation suggests similarities with the better-known phantom limb sensation. Phantom limb pain has been associated with changes in the body-surface map in sensorimotor cortex as deduced from MEG recordings and dipole source localization (Flor et al., 1995), and suggests that map changes in AC of individuals experiencing tinnitus (Mühlnickel, Elbert, Taub, & Flor, 1998) could underlie tinnitus. The source location for the edge-frequency dipole in the study of Weisz et al. (2005b) was also abnormal, but in contrast to their earlier (Muhlnickel et al., 1998) findings, the deviation from the control position was not related to tinnitus distress. This suggests that

map change in itself, albeit potentially related to the strength of the tinnitus percept, is not predictive of its annoyance.

One has to appreciate that unambiguous demonstration of auditory topographic map changes based on auditory evoked potentials (AEPs) or auditory-evoked magnetic fields (AEMFs) has been difficult. Most of the techniques used are based on recording the N_1 component in the MEG, and the tonotopic map is then constructed on the basis of equivalent dipole source locations for a series of tone frequencies. The equivalent dipole source location and strength is computed from the scalp distribution of activity in response to auditory stimulation. The AC in humans has at least five tonotopically organized areas in core and belt (Formisano et al., 2003), and the frequency gradient of these tonotopic maps reverses at their borders. The usual assumption of one dipole to summarize tonotopic map changes in all these cortical areas is therefore fraught with pitfalls (Lütkenhöner, Krumbholz, & Seither-Preisler, 2003a). However, mapping based on middle latency (between 15 and 50 ms) responses that originate in PAC, although there are still three tonotopically organized mirror-symmetric areas, may be more reliable (Lütkenhöner et al., 2003b).

Whereas AEPs and AEMFs can clearly indicate changes in the dipole moment and location of the equivalent dipoles, these changes could in fact reflect local changes in neural synchrony rather than in the size or change of the activated cortical region. These two effects cannot readily be separated, as they both change the amplitude of the AEP or AEMF, which are fundamental to dipole localization. Therefore, high-resolution tonotopic maps using fMRI are needed to provide independent information about potential changes in human auditory cortical activity maps.

Tinnitus and Pain

Chronic tinnitus and chronic pain display considerable similarities, including plastic changes in the central nervous system leading to hypersensitivity to sensory stimuli and a change in the way those stimuli are perceived. Involvement of the sympathetic nervous system has been postulated both in chronic pain and tinnitus (Møller, 1997). Tinnitus has been classified among the positive symptoms that arise after lesions of the nervous system (Jeanmonod et al., 1996), sharing with neurogenic pain the phenomenon of low-threshold calcium spike-burst firing in the medial thalamus.

WHERE IN THE BRAIN?

Tinnitus sensations often persist even when input from the ear is removed by section of the AN in humans (House and Brackman, 1981) or animals (Zacharek, Kaltenbach, Mathog, & Zhang, 2002). Thus, it is likely that most tinnitus has a central origin. But where this is located in the brain is hard to elucidate. My hypothesis is that it will be more central than the DCN, simply because changes in SFR after noise trauma occur in AC within 2 hrs after the trauma, whereas it takes more than 2 days in the DCN. I speculate that the thalamocortical system is most important for chronic tinnitus.

It is fair to state that the thalamocortical system is more a representational system than a bottom-up information processing system that is driven by sensory information. The cortex represents a view of the world that can be changed whenever the input from the outside world (i.e., from the auditory periphery) violates its expectations (as an old and trusted learning rule states: Rescorla, & Wagner, 1972). This is also reflected in the various event-related potentials that are generated by such violations. One has only to think about the mismatch negativity (MMN) and the P_3 as deviance-signaling components.

A consequence of the "learning by violation" rule may be that the cortex tries to adjust the output of subcortical structures by its corticofugal feedback activity (Yan & Suga, 1998). In this way increased activity at a particular cortical site can, for instance, change the representation of frequency in the auditory midbrain, brainstem (Luo et al., 2008) and even affects the activity of hair cells in the cochlea (Suga et al., 2000). We elaborate on this and derive from it the potential importance of subcortical structures in the generation of tinnitus.

Efferent connections make the auditory system a reentrant system characterized by multiple, loosely interconnected, regional feedback loops (Figure 5–4). The intra- and intercortical loops comprise both the interaction within a given cortical area and between cortical areas. A reflection of these interactive loops is found in the various oscillatory brain rhythms; for instance, the gamma-band oscillation with its frequency in the 40 to 60 Hz range relies on connections producing delays of 15 to 25 ms that comprises conduction times between cells and synaptic integration times. This is a purely cortical rhythm, whereby each cortical area generates its own frequency.

The rhythms in the 8 to 14 Hz range (delays of about 100 ms required) likely are all dependent on the thalamus, where the interplay between the reticular nucleus and the thalamic projection cells can generate rhythmic bursting with long delays caused by the duration of inhibition and/or hyperpolarization. Disturbances in that rhythm have been implicated in various positive syndromes, and specifically in tinnitus (Llinas et al., 2005). As mentioned before, Weisz et al. (2007) examined gamma-band activity during slow wave activity and showed that it was more prominent in tinnitus subjects than in controls. The hemispheric lateralization of the gamma-band activity did correlate with the lateralization of the perceived tinnitus.

The amygdala, the fear center of the brain, receives two inputs from the auditory system, a fast one via the thalamus and a slower one via the SAC (Farb & LeDoux, 1999; Woodson, Farb, & Ledoux, 2000). This also constitutes a recurrent loop as the amygdala feeds back on the AC. This integration of the limbic system and the thalamocortical complex is involved in emotional aspects of tinnitus.

The corticofugal connections from layer V in AC affect both the thalamus and IC, and cortical response properties. The IC is subsequently involved in a loop that includes the DCN. The CN is also directly affected by corticofugal fibers (Schofield & Coomes, 2005) as is the superior olivary complex (Coomes & Schofield, 2004). The olivocochlear bundle in turn connects the brainstem with the cochlea.

Feedback loops are intended to stabilize systems and as such they are used in countless engineering systems. It may well be that these temporal

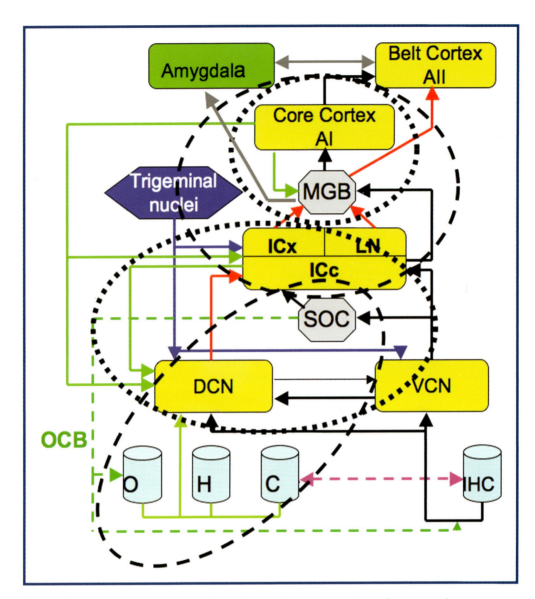

Figure 5–4. Schematic representation of the auditory system. Nested recurrent loops execute a cortical influence on the entire auditory system. Feedback patterns are schematized in green; the olivocochlear bundle is shown in dashed green lines. Auditory tonotopic (lemniscal) projections are shown in black, trigeminal input is shown in blue. The extralemniscal pathway is indicated in red. The dashed or dotted ellipsoids show various feedback loop systems that are all interconnected. The connections with the amygdala are shown with gray lines. Yellow boxes indicate areas where recordings have been made in the central auditory system in animal models of tinnitus.

feedback loops also stabilize tinnitus that either originates at more peripheral sites such as the ANFs or DCN, or at more central sites such as IC and AC. In the long run, peripheral and central activity may enhance each other and the result will be that there is no particular site in the central auditory system that can be held solely responsible for chronic tinnitus.

Typically opening the feedback loops by blocking connections (e.g., by using drugs such a lidocaine (Baguley et al., 2005), or desynchronizing the activity

(Eggermont & Roberts, 2004) of the nested loops (e.g., by stimulation via a hearing aid, through a cochlear implant (Quaranta, Wagstaff, & Baguley, 2004), or by direct electrical (De Ridder et al., 2008) or transcranial magnetic stimulation (Plewnia et al., 2007) of the AC will likely be an important aspect in successful treatments of long-standing chronic tinnitus.

TREATMENT OF TINNITUS

Drug Treatments

I only report here on results of prospective, placebo-controlled, single- or double-blind clinical trials. Potential tinnitus-alleviating drugs are often selected from those used in treating a putative transmitter imbalance in the CNS, as occurring in epilepsy, neuropathic pain and depression. This is largely because designing a new drug is a costly business. There are similarities between the neural mechanisms underlying epilepsy and central tinnitus in their animal models (Eggermont, 2005a). Anticonvulsants therefore theoretically have the potential for relieving tinnitus distress, as their mode of action is to reduce central excitation and/or increase inhibition. However, the success has been minimal as the following examples show (more in Davies (2004) and Dobie (2004) and Eggermont (2005b)). The effective anticonvulsant lamotrigine is ineffective for tinnitus relief (Simpson, Gilbert, Weiner, & Davies, 1999). In some individuals, gabapentin is effective in reducing subjective and objective aspects of tinnitus, with the best therapeutic response when tinnitus was associated with acoustic trauma (Bauer & Brozoski, 2007). There is also little evidence to recommend memantine for the treatment of tinnitus (Figueiredo, Langguth, Mello de Oliveira, & Aparecida de Azevedo, 2008).

Tinnitus is often accompanied by some degree of depression and it is almost impossible to separate the aetiology of the two conditions (Zöger, Svedlund, & Holgers, 2006). Typically, controlled studies were unable to show any influence of such drugs (e.g., nortryptyline) on the tinnitus severity, although nortryptyline improved the depressive state

of the patients (Dobie, 2004; Dobie, Sakai, Sullivan, Katon, & Russo, 1993).

Cognitive Behavioral Therapy and Tinnitus Retraining Therapy

I base this section largely on the comparison study by McKenna (2004). There are currently two main behavioral approaches to tinnitus management. They are the psychological approach that treats tinnitus within a cognitive-behavioral model (Hallam, Rachman, & Hinchcliffe, 1984), and the neurophysiological approach (Jastreboff, 1990) that gives rise to Tinnitus Retraining Therapy (TRT).

The cognitive-behavioral approach assumes that the process of habituation to tinnitus is fundamentally similar to that to external stimuli. Tolerance to tinnitus will be facilitated in the cognitive-behavioral approach by reducing levels of autonomic nervous system arousal, changing the emotional meaning of the tinnitus, and reducing other stresses.

The main components of TRT are directive counseling and use of sound generators. TRT proposes that the process of increased auditory gain within the auditory system during periods of restricted sound input, or as a consequence of cochlear damage, may account for the emergence of tinnitus. The key assumption in TRT is that tinnitus becomes problematic because of the improper activation of the brain's limbic system, which plays a role in emotion, memory and learning.

The cognitive-behavioral approach and TRT have much in common. They both consider the emotional, that is, limbic system, processing of tinnitus as the key factor in determining distress. Both approaches see habituation as the essential process involved in resolving the problem. One potentially important difference is that cognitive-behavioral therapy is provided by psychologists, whereas TRT is provided by trained audiologists.

Kroener-Herwig et al. (2000) evaluated 10 clinical studies in TRT research and found methodological shortcomings such as a lack of controlled randomized group studies. As no comparative studies had been conducted, there was no support for the assumption that TRT was superior to the cognitive-behavioral approach. Even at the time of this writing, comparative studies are not available. Martinez Devesa, Waddell, Perera, and Theodoulou (2007) found in a meta-analysis of six randomized control trials that cognitive-behavioral therapy did not result in significant changes in the subjective loudness of tinnitus, or in the associated depression. However there was a significant improvement in the quality of life (decrease of global tinnitus severity) of the participants, thus suggesting that cognitive-behavioral therapy has an effect on the qualitative aspects of tinnitus and contributes positively to the management of tinnitus.

Sound Therapy

Hearing aids, after first being proposed for the alleviation of tinnitus more than 60 years ago (Saltzmann and Ersner, 1947), were considered as a viable option for relief of tinnitus from the late seventies on (Roeser & Price, 1980; Surr, Montgomery, & Mueller, 1985; Vernon et al., 1977). Amplification provides masking in the frequency range of tinnitus, especially if the hearing aids have a good high-frequency response, and in addition it allows brain plasticity to play a role as our previous discussion has indicated. It is important that the amplification in this high-frequency range is high enough to balance the output of the ANFs across frequency. The central auditory system has a gain regulation that depends on the level of ANF input. Formby, Sherlock, and Gold (2003) showed that after continuous earplugging for two weeks, listeners rated the loudness of sounds higher than before the earplugging, whereas after an equal continuous period of exposure to low-level noise they rated the sound's loudness lower. This indicates that when there is less sound coming in, the gain of the auditory system is turned up, with the possible consequence that the spontaneous activity is also amplified, potentially leading to tinnitus. When sound is provided, for example, by a hearing aid or a sound-generating device, the benefit is that the central gain, which works on both spontaneous and stimulus-driven activity, is turned down and amelioration of the tinnitus may result.

Electrophysiologic support for the potential of sound therapy, at least in preventing tinnitus to occur following noise trauma, was provided in animal studies by Noreña and Eggermont (2005, 2006)

and reviewed in several places in this chapter. Other evidence that acoustic stimulation in the frequency range of the hearing loss is better than overall broadband noise masking comes from the residual inhibition studies of Roberts (2007) and Roberts et al. (2008), that found longer-lasting residual inhibition for sounds matched to the hearing loss.

This method is likely not applicable in persons with normal hearing and tinnitus. However, provided that despite normal thresholds the ANF output is less in a certain frequency range than in the remainder, sound therapy may still prove to be a viable clinical treatment. The main therapeutic aspect of sound is that it balances the firing rate of the ANFs across frequency. If the output is already balanced, as likely in normal-hearing persons without tinnitus, the sound would provide an imbalance and be more harmful than beneficial.

The same objective of balancing the output of the cochlea has been implicitly promoted by the Neuromonics Tinnitus Treatment that combines acoustic stimulation in the frequency range of the hearing loss with counseling, and this approach appears effective (Davis et al., 2007). In a sense, TRT also uses sound as part of the treatment in combination with counseling. Here, however, the sound is used to help the patient habituate to the emotional aspects of tinnitus, and subsequently to the perceptual aspects of tinnitus, and is somewhat subservient to the counseling aspects of the procedure (Henry, Schechter, Nagler, & Fausti, 2002; Jastreboff et al., 1994).

Cochlear Implants

All currently available cochlear implants (CI) can provide effective and similar levels of tinnitus suppression. Ruckenstein, Hedgepeth, Rafter, Montes, and Bigelow (2001) found a significant reduction for 35 of 38 patients (92%) in tinnitus intensity using cochlear implants. More recently, a comparison between pre- and postimplantation THI scores showed a decreased score in 13 of 20 patients with preimplantation tinnitus, an unchanged score in six and increased score in one (Di Nardo et al., 2007).

Twenty-one unilaterally deaf subjects who complained of severe intractable tinnitus that was unresponsive to treatment received a CI. Electrical stimulation via the CI resulted in a significant reduction in tinnitus loudness, as measured by the Visual Analog Scale, from 8.5 ± 1.3 to about 2.4 ± 1.8 at 1 and 2 years year after implantation. The Tinnitus Questionnaire also revealed a significant positive effect of CI stimulation (van de Heyning et al., 2008). In this particular study, the tinnitus had to be unilateral and confined to the deaf ear, existed for more than two years and had to be stable. The patients were all unresponsive to drug treatment, to cognitive therapy or TRT. The authors suggested that severe tinnitus could be an indication for CI.

It may also be feasible to implant a partially deaf ear with useful hearing in the low frequencies but no hearing in the high frequencies, where amplification cannot be used to treat tinnitus. Special short electrodes have been developed for such cases, and it is reported that they do not affect the low-frequency acoustic hearing whereas they reduce the tinnitus (Gantz et al., 2006). For a general discussion on the use of cochlear implants in persons with tinnitus, see Baguley and Atlas (2007).

The beneficial effect of a CI on tinnitus, reported by a majority of patients, could be due to a masking effect and above all to a possible CI stimulation-dependent reorganization of the central auditory pathways and cortex. In the context of the latter suggestion, it would be interesting to look at these effects over time following implantation.

Transcranial Magnetic Stimulation

Transcranial magnetic stimulation (TMS) is a technique for noninvasive stimulation of the human brain. For that purpose, a brief high-intensity magnetic field is generated that can reach up to about 2 tesla (comparable to the standard MRI static magnetic fields of 1.5 to 3 tesla) and typically lasts for about 100 ms. The field can excite or inhibit a small area of cortex below the coil. Repetitive TMS (rTMS) can produce effects that outlast the period of stimulation; inhibition is obtained with stimulation at about 1 Hz, and excitation with stimulation at 5 Hz and higher (Hallett, 2007).

The problem in any clinical trial is to come up with a good placebo or sham stimulus. This is specifically difficult for TMS. During TMS of the temporo-

parietal region, peripheral activation of the ipsilateral facial nerve and trigeminal afferents can occur and this is easily detected. The use of low concurrent peripheral stimulation during both sham and active rTMS is an easy way to minimize this possible bias and to reduce behavioral differences between the two stimulation conditions (Rossi et al., 2007).

I present here only two examples of TMS use in tinnitus, but many more are and will be published (see Langguth, Hajak, Kleinjung, Cacace, & Møller, 2007 in the further reading section). Rossi et al (2007) found daily application of high intensity 1 Hz rTMS to the left temporoparietal region an efficient strategy to transiently alleviate chronic tinnitus, independent of tinnitus lateralisation or bilaterality and of eventual concurrent changes in mood. Plewnia et al (2007) found that tinnitus loudness was reduced after temporoparietal, PET-guided low-frequency rTMS. This reduction, lasting up to 30 min, was dependent on the number of stimuli applied, and was negatively correlated with the length of the medical history of tinnitus in our patients. These effects were related to stimulation of cortical association areas, not PAC.

So, TMS application suggests that tinnitus is a central phenomenon, located only partially in the AC. It also suggests that tinnitus is only transiently suppressed with the various rTMS paradigms currently in use.

Alternative Medicine

Herbal Treatments

Extracts from the *Ginkgo biloba* tree have been used in Chinese medicine for thousands of years. Standardised extracts from the leaves of the tree purportedly have a significant therapeutic effect on the symptoms of cerebral insufficiency, including memory disturbances and other cognitive deficits (but see Birks & Grimley Evans [2007] who concluded that this is still inconsistent and inconclusive). EGb-761 is a standardized *Ginkgo biloba* extract containing 24% flavonoids, which have antioxidant properties (Smith, Zheng, & Darlington, 2005).

Systematic clinical trials, which are double-blind and placebo-controlled and included a large number of tinnitus sufferers, concluded that "50 mg Ginkgo biloba extract given 3 times daily for 12 weeks is no more effective than placebo in treating tinnitus" (Drew & Davies, 2001, p. 1) and "Ginkgo biloba does not benefit patients with tinnitus" (p. 6). (Rejai, Sivakumar, & Balaji, 2004). Hilton and Stuart (2004) concluded similarly, based on a meta-analysis of controlled clinical trials.

It is interesting that there is only one animal study (Jastreboff et al., 1997) that investigated the effects of *Ginkgo biloba* extract on salicylate-induced tinnitus using a conditioned behavior paradigm in rats. Daily oral administration of 25, 50 and 100 mg/kg EGb 761 was found to reduce tinnitus. Smith et al. (2005, p. 79) remarked, "It should be noted, however, that these are very high doses (even the lowest dose of 25 mg/kg equates to 1750 mg for a 70 kg human) and it is unlikely that such high doses could be used in humans without adverse side effects."

This likely will not close the door on the use of *Ginkgo biloba* to alleviate tinnitus, but as low doses are safe it serves as an acceptable placebo, but not more than that.

Acupuncture

In one of the first tinnitus studies performed, there was no significant difference between traditional Chinese acupuncture and a placebo needle placement (Hansen, Hansen and Bentzen, 1982). Nilsson, Axelsson, and Li (1992) studied 56 patients with continuous and severe tinnitus that were treated with traditional Chinese acupuncture. While there was some individual improvement, statistical analysis of the whole group did not show any significant general treatment effects. A meta analysis of several studies (Park, White, & Ernst, 2000) found that two unblinded studies showed a positive result, whereas four blinded studies showed no significant effect of acupuncture. They concluded that "acupuncture has not been demonstrated to be efficacious as a treatment for tinnitus on the evidence of rigorous randomized controlled trials" (p. 489).

Homeopathy

Simpson, Donaldson, & Davies (1998) reported on the assessment of a homeopathic preparation "Tin-

nitus" in tablet form by a double-blind, placebo-controlled clinical trial. Although questionnaire responses indicated that the homeopathic preparation was preferred to the placebo by 14 of 28 subjects, an analysis of variance indicated that neither the VAS scores nor the audiological measures showed significant improvement in tinnitus symptoms in response to "Tinnitus" versus the placebo. It was concluded that "Tinnitus" could not be shown to be more effective than the matched placebo.

Ear Canal Magnets

A double-blind placebo-controlled trial of a proposed treatment of tinnitus by placing rare earth magnets close to the tympanic membrane was carried out on 50 patients. The same material but unmagnetized and cut to the same shape and size was used for placebo magnets. The trial failed to show significant benefit (Coles et al., 1991).

Treatment Summary

It must be evident that there is currently no general cure for tinnitus, certainly not using prescription drugs, herbal or alternative treatments. This does not rule out that some individuals can greatly benefit from such therapy, as has in fact been documented, but it cannot be promised or advertised to the general tinnitus sufferer with any confidence. The best way to alleviate tinnitus is, in my opinion, sound therapy provided by well-fitted open-vented hearing aids, by providing sound that mimics the tinnitus spectrum, and by cochlear implants. Cognitive-behavioral therapy (including TRT) and medical treatment of comorbid depression may be needed in debilitating tinnitus, potentially combined with sound therapy.

Acknowledgments. The author was supported by the Alberta Heritage Foundation for Medical Research, by the Natural Sciences and Engineering Research Council of Canada, by a Canadian Institutes of Health Research New Emerging Team Grant, and by the Campbell McLaurin Chair of Hearing Deficiencies.

FURTHER READINGS

Handbooks

Tyler, R. S. (Ed.). (2000). *Tinnitus handbook*. San Diego, CA: Singular.

Snow, J. B. (Ed.) (2004). *Tinnitus: Theory and management*. Hamilton, Ontario: B. C. Decker.

Langguth, B., Hajak, G., Kleinjung, T., Cacace, A., & Møller, A. (Eds.). (2007). Tinnitus: pathophysiology and treatment. *Progress in Brain Research, 166,* 1–543.

Review Papers

Al-Mana, D., Ceranic, B., Djahanbakhch, O., & Luxon, L. M. (2008) Hormones and the auditory system: A review of physiology and pathophysiology. *Neuroscience, 153,* 881–900.

Davies, E. (2004) The pharmacological management of tinnitus. *Audiological Medicine, 2,* 26–28.

Eggermont, J. J. (2005b). Tinnitus: Neurobiological substrates. *Drug Discovery Today, 10,* 1283–1290.

McKenna, L. (2004) Models of tinnitus suffering and treatment compared and contrasted. *Audiological Medicine, 2,* 41–53.

Shore, S. E., & Zhou, J. (2006) Somatosensory influence on the cochlear nucleus and beyond. *Hearing Research, 216–217,* 90–99.

REFERENCES

Abbott, S. D., Hughes, L. F., Bauer, C. A., Salvi, R., & Caspary, D. M. (1999). Detection of glutamate decarboxylase isoforms in rat inferior colliculus following acoustic exposure. *Neuroscience, 93,* 1375–1381.

Andersson, G. (2003). Tinnitus loudness matchings in relation to annoyance and grading of severity. *Auris Nasus Larynx, 30,* 129–133.

Anderson, J. E., Teitel, D., & Wu, Y. W. (2008). Venous hum causing tinnitus: Case report and review of the literature. *Clinical Pediatrics.* Published online before print July 14, 2008. doi: 10.1177/0009922808321113

Attias, J., Urbach, D., Gold, S., & Shemesh, Z. (1993) Auditory event related potentials in chronic tinnitus patients with noise induced hearing loss. *Hearing Research, 71,* 106–113.

Baguley, D. M. (2003). Hyperacusis. *Journal of the Royal Society of Medicine, 96,* 582–585.

Baguley, D. M., & Atlas, M. D. (2007). Cochlear implants and tinnitus. *Progress in Brain Research, 166,* 347–355.

Baguley, D. M., Jones, S., Wilkins, I., Axon, P. R., & Moffat, D. A. (2005). The inhibitory effect of intravenous lidocaine infusion on tinnitus after translabyrinthine removal of vestibular schwannoma: A double-blind, placebo-controlled, crossover study. *Otology and Neurotology, 26,* 169–176.

Baguley, D. M., Phillips, J., Humphriss, R. L., Jones, S., Axon, P. R., & Moffat, D. A. (2006). The prevalence and onset of gaze modulation of tinnitus and increased sensitivity to noise after translabyrinthine vestibular schwannoma excision. *Otology and Neurotology, 27,* 220–224.

Barnea, G., Attias, J., Gold, S., & Shahar, A. (1990). Tinnitus with normal hearing sensitivity: Extended high-frequency audiometry and auditory-nerve brain-stem-evoked responses. *Audiology, 29,* 36–45.

Bauer, C. A., & Brozoski, T. J. (2001). Assessing tinnitus and prospective tinnitus therapeutics using a psychophysical animal model. *Journal of the Association for Research in Otolaryngology, 2,* 54–64.

Bauer, C. A., & Brozoski, T. J. (2007). Gabapentin. *Progress in Brain Research, 166,* 287–301.

Bauer, C. A., Brozoski, T. J., Holder, T. M., & Caspary, D. M. (2000). Effects of chronic salicylate on GABAergic activity in rat inferior colliculus. *Hearing Research, 147,* 175–182.

Bauer, C. A., Turner, J. G., Caspary, D. M., Myers, K. S., & Brozoski, T. J. (2008). Tinnitus and inferior colliculus activity in chinchillas related to three distinct patterns of cochlear trauma. *Journal of Neuroscience Research, 86,* 2564–2578.

Birks, J., & Grimley Evans, J. (2007). Ginkgo biloba for cognitive impairment and dementia. *Cochrane Database Systematic Reviews, 18,* CD003120.

Bramham, C. R., & Messaoudi, E. (2005). BDNF function in adult synaptic plasticity: The synaptic consolidation hypothesis. *Progress in Neurobiology, 76,* 99–125.

Brozoski, T. J., Bauer, C. A., & Caspary, D. M. (2002). Elevated fusiform cell activity in the dorsal cochlear nucleus of chinchillas with psychophysical evidence of tinnitus. *Journal of Neuroscience, 22,* 2383–2390.

Burns, E. M. (1984). A comparison of variability among measurements of subjective tinnitus and objective stimuli. *Audiology, 23,* 426–440.

Burns, E. M., & Keefe, D. H. (1992). Intermittent tinnitus resulting from unstable otoacoustic emissions. In J.-M. Aran, & R. Dauman (Eds.), *Tinnitus 91* (pp. 89–94). Amsterdam, NL: Kugler.

Cacace, A. T. (2003). Expanding the biological basis of tinnitus: crossmodal origins and the role of neuroplasticity. *Hearing Research, 175,* 112–132.

Cacace, A. T., Cousins, J. P., Parnes, S. M., Semenoff, D., Holmes, T., McFarland, D. J., . . . Lovely, T. J. (1999). Cutaneous-evoked tinnitus. I. Phenomenology, psychophysics and functional imaging. *Audiology and Neurotology, 4,* 247–257.

Caspary, D. M., Holder, T. M., Hughes, L. F., Milbrandt, J. C., McKernan, R. M., & Naritoku, D. K. (1999). Age-related changes in GABA(A) receptor subunit composition and function in rat auditory system. *Neuroscience, 93,* 307–312.

Cazals, Y. (2000). Auditory sensori-neural alterations induced by salicylate. *Progress in Neurobiology, 62*, 583–631.

Ceranic, B. J., Prasher, D. K., Raglan, E., & Luxon, L. M. (1998). Tinnitus after head injury: Evidence from oto-acoustic emissions. *Journal of Neurology, Neurosurgery and Psychiatry, 65*, 523–529.

Chang, H., Chen, K., Kaltenbach, J. A., Zhang, J., & Godfrey, D. A. (2002). Effects of acoustic trauma on dorsal cochlear nucleus neuron activity in slices. *Hearing Research, 164*, 59–68.

Chen, G. D., & Jastreboff, P. J. (1995). Salicylate-induced abnormal activity in the inferior colliculus of rats. *Hearing Research, 82*, 158–178.

Colding-Jørgensen, E., Lauritzen, M., Johnsen, N. J., Mikkelsen, K. B., & Saermark, K. (1992). On the evidence of auditory evoked magnetic fields as an objective measure of tinnitus. *Electroencephalography and Clinical Neurophysiology, 83*, 322–327.

Coles, R., Bradley, P., Donaldson, I., & Dingle, A. (1991). A trial of tinnitus therapy with ear canal magnets. *Clinical Otolaryngology and Allied Sciences, 16*, 371–372.

Coomes, D. L., & Schofield, B. R. (2004). Projections from the auditory cortex to the superior olivary complex in guinea pigs. *European Journal of Neuroscience, 19*, 2188–2200.

Coupland, S. G., Ponton, C. W., Eggermont, J. J., Bowen, T., & Grant, R. M. (1991). Assessment of cisplatin-induced oto-toxicity using derived-band ABRs. *International Journal of Pediatric Otorhinolaryngology, 22*, 237–248.

Cransac, H., Cottet-Emard, J. M., Hellström, S., & Peyrin, L. (1988). Specific sound-induced noradrenergic and seroto-nergic activation in central auditory structures. *Hearing Research, 118*, 151–156.

Davies, E. (2004). The pharmacological management of tinnitus. *Audiological Medicine, 2*, 26–28.

Davies, E., Knox, E., & Donaldson, I. (1994). The usefulness of nimodipine, an L-calcium channel antagonist, in the treatment of tinnitus. *British Journal of Audiology, 28*, 125–129.

Davis, P. B., Paki, B., & Hanley, P. J. (2007). Neuromonics Tinnitus Treatment: Third clinical trial. *Ear and Hearing, 28*, 242–259.

Day, R.O., Graham, G.G., Bieri, D., Brown, M., Cairns, D., Harris, G., . . . Smith, J. (1989). Concentration-response relationships for salicylate-induced ototoxicity in normal volunteers. *British Journal of Clinical Pharmacology, 28*, 695–702.

Del Bo. L., Forti. S., Ambrosetti, U., Costanzo, S., Mauro, D., Ugazio, G., Langguth, B., & Mancuso, A. (2008). Tinnitus aurium in persons with normal hearing: 55 years later. *Otolaryngology-Head and Neck Surgery, 139*, 391–394.

Delgutte, B. (1990). Physiological mechanisms of psychophysical masking: Observations from auditory-nerve fibers. *Journal of the Acoustical Society of America, 87*, 791–809

De Ridder, D., De Mulder, G., Verstraeten, E., Van der Kelen, K., Sunaert, S., Smits, M., . . . Moller, A. R. (2008). Primary and secondary auditory cortex stimulation for intractable tinnitus. *ORL Journal of Otorhinolaryngology and Related Specialties, 68*, 48–54;

Di Nardo, W., Cantore, I., Cianfrone, F., Melillo, P., Scorpecci, A., & Paludetti, G. (2007). Tinnitus modifications after cochlear implantation. *European Archives of Otorhinolaryngology, 264*, 1145–1149.

Dineen, R., Doyle, J., & Bench, J. (1997). Audiological and psychological characteristics of a group of tinnitus sufferers, prior to tinnitus management training. *British Journal of Audiology, 31*, 27–38.

Dobie, R. A. (2004) Clinical trials and drug therapy for tinnitus. In J. B. Snow Jr, (Ed.), *Tinnitus: Theory and management* (pp. 266–277). Hamilton, Ontario: B. C. Decker.

Dobie, R. A., Sakai, C. S., Sullivan, M. D., Katon, W. J., & Russo, J. (1993). Antidepressant treatment of tinnitus patients: Report of a randomized clinical trial and clinical prediction of benefit. *American Journal of Otology, 14*(1), 18–23.

Drew, S., & Davies, E. (2001). Effectiveness of Ginkgo biloba in treating tinnitus: Double blind, placebo controlled trial. *British Medical Journal, 322.* doi:10.1136/bmj.322.7278.73

Duan, M., Agerman, K., Ernfors, P., & Canlon, B. (2000). Complementary roles of neurotrophin 3 and a N-methyl-D-aspartate antagonist in the protection of noise and aminoglycoside-induced ototoxicity. *Proceedings of the National Academy of Sciences of the United States of America, 97*, 7597–7602.

Eggermont, J. J. (1984). Tinnitus: Some thoughts about its origin. *Journal of Laryngology and Otology, 9*(Suppl.), 31–37.

Eggermont, J. J. (1990). On the pathophysiology of tinnitus; a review and a peripheral model. *Hearing Research, 48*, 111–124.

Eggermont, J. J. (1992). Neural interaction in cat primary auditory cortex. Dependence on recording depth, electrode separation, and age. *Journal of Neurophysiology, 68*, 1216–1228.

Eggermont, J. J. (2003). Central tinnitus. *Auris Nasus Larynx, 30*(Suppl.), S7–S12.

Eggermont, J. J. (2004). The cortex and tinnitus. In J. B. Snow (Ed.), *Tinnitus: Theory and management* (pp. 171–188). Hamilton, Ontario: B. C. Decker.

Eggermont, J J. (2005a). Plasticity of tonotopic and correlation maps in cat primary auditory cortex. In J. Syka, & M. Merzenich (Eds.), *Plasticity and signal representation in the auditory system* (pp. 139–151). New York, NY: Springer Science.

Eggermont, J. J. (2005b). Tinnitus: Neurobiological substrates. *Drug Discovery Today, 10*, 1283–1290.

Eggermont, J. J. (2006). Electric and magnetic fields of synchronous neural activity propagated to the surface of the head: Peripheral and central origins of AEPs. In R. R. Burkard, M. Don, & J. J. Eggermont (Eds.), *Auditory evoked potentials* (pp. 2–21). Baltimore, MD: Lippincott Williams & Wilkins.

Eggermont, J. J., & Kenmochi, M. (1998). Salicylate and quinine selectively increase spontaneous firing rates in secondary auditory cortex. *Hearing Research, 117*, 149–160.

Eggermont, J. J., & Komiya, H. (2000). Moderate noise trauma in juvenile cats results in profound cortical topographic map changes in adulthood. *Hearing Research, 142*, 89–101.

Eggermont, J. J., & Roberts, L. E. (2004). The neuroscience of tinnitus. *Trends in Neuroscience, 27,* 676–682.

Erlandsson, S. I. (2000). Psychological profiles of tinnitus patients. In R. S. Tyler (Ed.), *Tinnitus handbook* (pp. 25–57). San Diego, CA: Singular.

Evans, E. F., Wilson, J. P., & Borerwe, T. A. (1981). Animal models of tinnitus. *Ciba Foundation Symposium, 85,* 108–138.

Farb, C. R., & Ledoux, J. E. (1999). Afferents from rat temporal cortex synapse on lateral amygdala neurons that express NMDA and AMPA receptors. *Synapse, 33,* 218–229.

Feldmann. H. (1971). Homolateral and contralateral masking of tinnitus by noise-bands and by pure tones. *Audiology, 10,* 138–144.

Figueiredo, R. R., Langguth, B., Mello de Oliveira, P., & Aparecida de Azevedo, A. (2008). Tinnitus treatment with memantine. *Otolaryngology-Head and Neck Surgery, 138,* 492–496.

Flor, H., Elbert, T., Knecht, S., Wienbruch, C., Pantev, C., Birbaumer, N., . . . Taub, E. (1995) Phantom-limb pain as a perceptual correlate of cortical reorganization following arm amputation. *Nature, 375,* 482–484.

Folmer, R. L., & Griest, S. E. (2003). Chronic tinnitus resulting from head or neck injuries. *Laryngoscope, 113,* 821–827.

Folmer, R. L., Griest, S. E., Meikle, M. B., & Martin, W. H. (1999). Tinnitus severity, loudness, and depression. *Otolaryngology-Head and Neck Surgery, 121,* 48–51.

Formby, C, Sherlock, L. P., & Gold, S. L. (2003). Adaptive plasticity of loudness induced by chronic attenuation and enhancement of the acoustic background. *Journal of the Acoustical Society of America, 114,* 55–58.

Formisano, E., Kim, D. S., Di Salle, F., van de Moortele, P. F., Ugurbil, K., & Goebel, R. (2003). Mirror-symmetric tonotopic maps in human primary auditory cortex. *Neuron, 40,* 859–869.

Fowler, E. P. (1944). Head noises in normal and disordered ears. Significance, measurement, differentiation and treatment. *Archives of Otolaryngology, 39,* 498–503.

Fridberger, A., Flock, A., Ulfendahl, M., & Flock, B. (1998). Acoustic overstimulation increases outer hair cell Ca2+ concentrations and causes dynamic contractions of the hearing organ. *Proceedings of the National Academy of Sciences of the United States of America, 95,* 7127–7132.

Fritz, J. B., Elhilali, M., David, S. V., & Shamma, S. A. (2007). Auditory attention—focusing the searchlight on sound. *Current Opinion in Neurobiology, 17,* 437–455.

Gantz, B. J., Turner, C., & Gfeller, K. E. (2006). Acoustic plus electric speech processing: Preliminary results from a multicenter clinical trial of the Iowa/Nucleus hybrid implant. *Audiolology and Neurotology, 11*(Suppl. 1), 63–68.

Giraud, A. L., Chery-Croze, S., Fischer, G., Fischer, C., Vighetto, A., Gregoire, M. C., . . . Collet, L. (1999). A selective imaging of tinnitus. *NeuroReport, 10,* 1–5.

Guitton, M. J., Caston, J., Ruel, J., Johnson, R. M., Pujol, R., & Puel, J. L. (2003). Salicylate induces tinnitus through activation of cochlear NMDA receptors. *Journal of Neuroscience, 23,* 3944–3952.

Guitton, M. J., Pujol, R., & Puel, J. L. (2005). m-Chlorophenylpiperazine exacerbates perception of salicylate-induced tinnitus in rats. *European Journal of Neuroscience, 22,* 2675–2678.

Guitton, M. J., Wang, J., & Puel, J. L. (2004). New pharmacological strategies to restore hearing and treat tinnitus. *Acta Otolaryngologica, 124,* 411–415.

Guzowski, J. F., McNaughton, B. L., Barnes, C. A., & Worley, P. F. (1999). Environment-specific expression of the immediate-early gene Arc in hippocampal neuronal ensembles. *Nature Neuroscience, 2,* 1120–1124.

Halla, J. T., Atchison, S. L., & Hardin, J. G. (1991). Symptomatic salicylate ototoxicity: A useful indicator of serum salicylate concentration? *Annals of the Rheumatic Diseases, 50,* 682–684.

Hallam, R. S., Rachman, S., & Hinchcliffe, R. (1984). Psychological aspects of tinnitus. In S. Rachman (Ed.), *Contributions to medical psychology 3.* Oxford, UK: Pergamon.

Hallberg, L. R., & Erlandsson, S. I. (1993). Tinnitus characteristics in tinnitus complainers and noncomplainers. *British Journal of Audiology, 27,* 19–27.

Haller, S., Wetzel, S. G., Radue, E. W., & Bilecen D. (2006). Mapping continuous neuronal activation without an ON-OFF paradigm: Initial results of BOLD ceiling fMRI. *European Journal of Neuroscience, 24,* 2672–2678.

Hallett, M. (2007). Transcranial magnetic stimulation: A primer. *Neuron, 55,* 187–199.

Hansen, P. E., Hansen, J. H., & Bentzen, O. (1982). Acupuncture treatment of chronic unilateral tinnitus—a double-blind cross-over trial. *Clinical Otolaryngology and Allied Sciences, 7,* 325–329.

Harrison, R. V., Nagasawa, A., Smith, D. W., Stanton S., & Mount, R. J. (1991). Reorganization of auditory cortex after neonatal high frequency cochlear hearing loss. *Hearing Research, 54,* 11–19.

Hébert, S., Paiement, P., & Lupien, S. J. (2004). A physiological correlate for the intolerance to both internal and external sounds. *Hearing Research, 190,* 1–9.

Heffner, H. E., & Harrington, I. A. (2002). Tinnitus in hamsters following exposure to intense sound. *Hearing Research, 170,* 83–95.

Henry, J. A., Dennis, K. C., & Schechter, M. A. (2005). General review of tinnitus: Prevalence, mechanisms, effects, and management. *Journal of Speech, Language and Hearing Research, 48,* 1204–1235.

Henry, J. A., Schechter, M. A., Nagler, S. M., & Fausti, S. A. (2002). Comparison of tinnitus masking and tinnitus retraining therapy. *Journal of the American Academy of Audiology, 13,* 559–581.

Hiller, W., & Goebel, G. (2006). Factors influencing tinnitus loudness and annoyance. *Archives of Otolaryngology-Head and Neck Surgery, 132,* 1323–1330

Hilton, M., & Stuart, E. (2004). Ginkgo biloba for tinnitus. *Cochrane Database Systematic Reviews, 2,* CD003852.

Hoffman, H. J., & Reed, G. W. (2004). Epidemiology of tinnitus. In J. B. Snow Jr. (Ed.), *Tinnitus: theory and management* (pp. 16–41). Hamilton, Ontario: B. C. Decker.

Hoke, M., Feldmann, H., Pantev, C., Lütkenhöner, B., & Lehnertz, K. (1989). Objective evidence of tinnitus in auditory evoked magnetic fields. *Hearing Research, 37,* 281–216.

Holgers, K. M., Erlandsson, S. I., & Barrenäs, M. L. (2000). Predictive factors for the severity of tinnitus. *Audiology, 39,* 284–291.

Holgers, K. M., Zöger, S., & Svedlund, K. (2003). Tinnitus suffering: A marker for a vulnerability in the serotonergic system? *Audiological Medicine, 2,* 138–143.

Holgers, K. M., Zöger, S., & Svedlund, K. (2005). Predictive factors for development of severe tinnitus suffering—further characterisation. *International Journal of Audiology, 44,* 584–592.

Horner, K. C. (2003). The emotional ear in stress. *Neuroscience Biobehavioral Reviews, 27,* 437–446.

House, J. W., & Brackmann, D. E. (1981). Tinnitus: Surgical treatment. *Ciba Foundation Symposium, 85,* 204–216.

Huang, Z. W., Luo, Y., Wu, Z., Tao, Z., Jones, R. O., & Zhao, H. B. (2005). Paradoxical enhancement of active cochlear mechanics in long-term administration of salicylate. *Journal of Neurophysiology, 93,* 2053–2061.

Ikeda, K., Sunose, H., & Takasaka, T. (1994). Ion transport mechanisms in the outer hair cell of the mammalian cochlea. *Progress in Neurobiology, 42,* 703–717.

Irvine, D. R., Rajan, R., & McDermott, H. J. (2000). Injury-induced reorganization in adult auditory cortex and its perceptual consequences. *Hearing Research, 147,* 188–199.

Jacobson, G. P., Ahmad, B. K., Moran, J., Newman, C. W., Tepley, N., & Wharton, J. (1991). Auditory evoked cortical magnetic field (M100-M200) measurements in tinnitus and normal groups. *Hearing Research, 56,* 44–52.

Jastreboff, P. J. (1990). Phantom auditory perception (tinnitus): Mechanisms of generation and perception. *Neuroscience Research, 8,* 221–254.

Jastreboff, P. J., Brennan, J. F., Coleman, J. K., & Sasaki, C. T. (1988). Phantom auditory sensation in rats: An animal model for tinnitus. *Behavioral Neuroscience, 102,* 811–822.

Jastreboff, P. J., Gray W. C., & Gold S. L. (1996). Neurophysiological approach to tinnitus patients. *American Journal of Otology, 17,* 236–240.

Jastreboff, P. J., Hazell, J. W., & Graham, R. L. (1994). Neurophysiological model of tinnitus: Dependence of the minimal masking level on treatment outcome. *Hearing Research, 80,* 216–232.

Jastreboff, P. J., & Sasaki, C. T. (1986). Salicylate-induced changes in spontaneous activity of single units in the inferior colliculus of the guinea pig. *Journal of the Acoustical Society of America, 80,* 1384–1391.

Jastreboff, P. J., Zhou, S., Jastreboff, M. M., Kwapisz, U., & Gryczynska, U. (1997). Attenuation of salicylate-induced tinnitus by Ginkgo biloba extract in rats. *Audiology and Neurotology, 2,* 197–212.

Jeanmonod, D., Magnin, M., & Morel, A. (1996). Low-threshold calcium spike bursts in the human thalamus. Common physiopathology for sensory, motor and limbic positive symptoms. *Brain, 119,* 363–375.

Jin, Y. M., Godfrey, D. A., Wang, J., & Kaltenbach, J. A. (2006). Effects of intense tone exposure on choline acetyltransferase activity in the hamster cochlear nucleus. *Hearing Research, 216–217,* 168–175.

Juliano, L. M., & Griffiths, R. R.. (2004). A critical review of caffeine withdrawal: Empirical validation of symptoms and signs, incidence, severity, and associated features. *Psychopharmacology (Berl), 176,* 1–29.

Kaltenbach, J. A., Zacharek, M. A., Zhang, J., & Frederick, S. (2004). Activity in the dorsal cochlear nucleus of hamsters previously tested for tinnitus following intense tone exposure. *Neuroscience Letters, 355,* 121–125.

Kaltenbach, J. A., Zhang, J., & Afman, C. E. (2000). Plasticity of spontaneous neural activity in the dorsal cochlear nucleus after intense sound exposure. *Hearing Research, 147,* 282–292.

Kemp, S. & George, R. N., (1992) Diaries of tinnitus sufferers. *British Journal of Audiology, 26,* 381–386

Kiang, N. Y., Moxon, E. C., & Levine, R. A. (1970). Auditory-nerve activity in cats with normal and abnormal cochleas. *Ciba Foundation Symposium, 85,* 241–273.

Kilgard, M. P., Vazquez, J. L., Engineer, N. D., & Pandya, P. K. (2007). Experience dependent plasticity alters cortical synchronization. *Hearing Research, 229,* 171–179.

Kroener-Herwig, B., Biesinger, E., Gerhards, F., Goebel, G., Verena Greimel, K., & Hiller, W. (2000). Retraining therapy for chronic tinnitus. A critical analysis of its status. *Scandinavian Audiology, 29,* 67–78.

Kuk, F. K., Tyler, R. S., Russell, D., & Jordan, H. (1990). The psychometric properties of a tinnitus handicap questionnaire. *Ear and Hearing, 11,* 434–445.

Lanting, C. P., De Kleine, E., Bartels, H., & Van Dijk, P. (2008). Functional imaging of unilateral tinnitus using fMRI. *Acta Otolaryngology, 128,* 415–421.

Levine, R. A. (1999). Somatic (craniocervical) tinnitus and the dorsal cochlear nucleus hypothesis. *American Journal of Otolaryngology, 20,* 351–362.

Liberman, M. C., & Kiang, N. Y. (1978). Acoustic trauma in cats. Cochlear pathology and auditory-nerve activity. *Acta Otolaryngologica Supplement, 358,* 1–63.

Lin, X., Chen, S., & Tee, D. (1998). Effect of quinine on the excitability and voltage-dependent currents of isolated spiral ganglion neurons in culture. *Journal of Neurophysiology, 79,* 2503–2512.

Liu, J., Li, X., Wang, L., Dong, Y., Han, H., & Liu, G. (2003). Effects of salicylate on serotoninergic activities in rat inferior colliculus and auditory cortex. *Hearing Research, 175,* 45–53.

Liyanage, S. H., Singh, A., Savundra, P., & Kalan, A. (2006). Pulsatile tinnitus. *Journal of Laryngology and Otology, 120,* 93–97.

Llinás, R., Urbano, F. J., Leznik, E., Ramírez, R. R., & van Marle, H. J. (2005). Rhythmic and dysrhythmic thalamocortical dynamics: GABA systems and the edge effect. *Trends in Neuroscience, 28,* 325–333.

Lobarinas, E., Sun, W., Cushing, R., & Salvi, R. (2004). A novel behavioral paradigm for assessing tinnitus using schedule-induced polydipsia avoidance conditioning (SIP-AC). *Hearing Research, 190,* 109–114.

Lockwood, A. H., Wack, D. S., Burkard, R. F., Coad, M. L., Reyes, S. A., Arnold, S.A., & Salvi, R. J. (2001). The functional anatomy of gaze-evoked tinnitus and sustained lateral gaze. *Neurology, 56,* 472–480.

Luo, F., Wang, Q., Kashani, A., & Yan, J. (2008). Corticofugal modulation of initial sound processing in the brain. *Journal of Neuroscience, 28,* 11615–11621.

Lustig, L. R. (2006). Nicotinic acetylcholine receptor structure and function in the efferent auditory system. *Anatomical Record Part A: Discoveries in Molecular, Cellular, and Evolutionary Biology, 288,* 424–434.

Lütkenhöner, B., Krumbholz, K., Lammertmann, C., Seither-Preisler, A., Steinsträter, O., & Patterson, R. D. (2003b). Localization of primary auditory cortex in humans by magnetoencephalography. *NeuroImage, 18,* 58–66.

Lütkenhöner, B., Krumbholz, K., & Seither-Preisler, A. (2003a). Studies of tonotopy based on wave N100 of the auditory evoked field are problematic. *Neuroimage, 19,* 935–949.

Ma, W. L., Hidaka, H., & May, B. J. (2006). Spontaneous activity in the inferior colliculus of CBA/J mice after manipulations that induce tinnitus. *Hearing Research, 212,* 9–21.

Ma, W. L., & Young, E. D. (2006). Dorsal cochlear nucleus response properties following acoustic trauma: Response maps and spontaneous activity. *Hearing Research, 216–217,* 176–188.

Maffei, G., & Miani, P. (1962). Experimental tobacco poisoning. Resultant structural modifications of the cochlea and tuba acustica. *Archives of Otolaryngology, 75,* 386–396.

Mahlke, C., & Wallhäusser-Franke, E. (2004). Evidence for tinnitus-related plasticity in the auditory and limbic system, demonstrated by arg3.1 and c-fos immunocytochemistry. *Hearing Research, 195,* 17–34.

Manabe, Y., Yoshida, S., Saito, H., & Oka, H. (1997). Effects of lidocaine on saliylate-induced discharge of neurons in the inferior colliculus of the guinea pig. *Hearing Research, 103,* 192–198.

Marriage, J., & Barnes, N. M. (1995). Is central hyperacusis a symptom of 5-hydroxytryptamine (5-HT) dysfunction? *Journal of Laryngology and Otology, 109,* 915–921.

Martinez Devesa, P., Waddell, A., Perera, R., & Theodoulou, M. (2007). Cognitive behavioural therapy for tinnitus. *Cochrane Database Systematic Reviews.* CD005233.

McKenna, L. (2004). Models of tinnitus suffering and treatment compared and contrasted. *Audiological Medicine, 2,* 41–53.

Meikle, M. B. (1992). Methods for evaluation of tinnitus relief procedures. In J. M. Aran & R. Dauman (Eds.), *Tinnitus 91* (pp. 555–562). Amsterdam, NL: Kugler.

Meikle, M. B. (1995). The interaction of central and peripheral mechanisms in tinnitus. In J. A. Vernon & A. R. Møller (Eds.), *Mechanisms of tinnitus* (pp. 181–206). Needham Heights, MA: Allyn & Bacon.

Meikle, M. B., & Griest, S. E. (1989). Gender-based differences in characteristics of tinnitus. *Hearing Journal, 42,* 68–76.

Meikle, M., & Taylor-Walsh, E. (1984). Characteristics of tinnitus and related observations in over 1800 tinnitus clinic patients. *Journal of Laryngology and Otology* (Suppl. 9), pp. 17–21.

Melcher, J. R., Sigalovsky, I. S., Guinan, J. J. Jr., & Levine, R. A. (2000). Lateralized tinnitus studied with functional magnetic resonance imaging: abnormal inferior colliculus activation. *Journal of Neurophysiology, 83,* 1058–1072.

Milbrandt, J. C., & Caspary, D. M. (1995). Age-related reduction of [3H]strychnine binding sites in the cochlear nucleus of the Fischer 344 rat. *Neuroscience, 67,* 713–719.

Mills, R. P., Albert, D. M., & Brain, C. E. (1986). Tinnitus in childhood. *Clinical Otolaryngology and Allied Sciences, 11,* 431–434.

Møller, A. R. (1997). Similarities between chronic pain and tinnitus. *American Journal of Otology, 18*(5), 577–585.

Moody, D. B. (2004). Animal models of tinnitus. In J. B. Snow (Ed.), *Tinnitus: Theory and management* (pp. 80–95). Hamilton, Ontario: B. C. Decker.

Moore, B. C., Huss, M., Vickers, D. A., Glasberg, B. R., & Alcántara, J. I. (2000). A test for the diagnosis of dead regions in the cochlea. *British Journal of Audiology, 34,* 205–224.

Morley, B. J., & Happe, H. K. (2000). Cholinergic receptors: dual roles in transduction and plasticity. *Hearing Research, 147,* 104–112.

Muhlnickel, W., Elbert, T., Taub, E., & Flor, H. (1998). Reorganization of auditory cortex in tinnitus. *Proceedings of the National Academy of Sciences of the United States of America, 95,* 10340–10343.

Mulheran, M. (1999). The effects of quinine on cochlear nerve fibre activity in the guinea pig. *Hearing Research, 134,* 145–152.

Müller, M., Klinke, R., Arnold, W., & Oestreicher, E. (2003). Auditory nerve fibre responses to salicylate revisited. *Hearing Research, 183,* 37–43.

Muly, S. M., Gross, J. S., & Potashner, S. J. (2004). Noise trauma alters D-[3H]aspartate release and AMPA binding in chinchilla cochlear nucleus. *Journal of Neuroscience Research, 75,* 585–596.

Newman, C. W., & Sandridge, S. A. (2004). Tinnitus Questionnaires. In J. B. Snow Jr. (Ed.), *Tinnitus: Theory and management* (pp. 237–254). Hamilton, Ontario: B. C. Decker.

Newman, C. W., Sandridge, S. A., & Jacobson, G. P. (1998). Psychometric adequacy of the Tinnitus Handicap Inventory (THI) for evaluating treatment outcome. *Journal of the American Academy of Audiology, 9,* 153–160.

Niedzielski, A. S., & Wenthold, R. J. (1985). Expression of AMPA, kainate, and NMDA receptor subunits in cochlear and vestibular ganglia. *Journal of Neuroscience, 15,* 2338–2353.

Nilsson, S., Axelsson, A., & Li, D. G. (1992). Acupuncture for tinnitus management. *Scandinavian Audiology, 21,* 245–251.

Noreña, A. J., & Eggermont, J. J. (2003). Changes in spontaneous neural activity immediately after an acoustic trauma: Implications for neural correlates of tinnitus. *Hearing Research, 183,* 137–153.

Noreña, A. J., & Eggermont, J. J. (2005). Enriched acoustic environment after noise trauma reduces hearing loss and prevents cortical map reorganization. *Journal of Neuroscience, 25,* 699–705.

Noreña, A. J., & Eggermont, J. J. (2006). Enriched acoustic environment after noise trauma abolishes neural signs of tinnitus. *NeuroReport, 17,* 559–563.

Noreña, A. J., Gourévitch, B., Aizawa, N., & Eggermont, J. J. (2006). Spectrally enhanced acoustic environment disrupts frequency representation in cat auditory cortex. *Nature Neuroscience, 9,* 932–939.

Norena, A., Micheyl, C., Chéry-Croze, S., & Collet, L. (2002). Psychoacoustic characterization of the tinnitus spectrum: Implications for the underlying mechanisms of tinnitus. *Audiology and Neurotology, 7,* 358–369.

Noreña, A. J., Tomita, M., & Eggermont, J. J. (2003). Neural changes in cat auditory cortex after a transient pure-tone trauma. *Journal of Neurophysiology, 90,* 2387–2401.

Norton, S. J., Schmidt, A. R., & Stover, L. J. (1990). Tinnitus and otoacoustic emissions: Is there a link? *Ear and Hearing, 11,* 159–166.

Nottet, J. B., Moulin, A., Brossard, N., Suc, B., & Job, A. (2006). Otoacoustic emissions and persistent tinnitus after acute acoustic trauma. *Laryngoscope, 116,* 970–975.

Ochi, K., & Eggermont, J. J. (1995). Effects of salicylate and quinine on spontaneous activity in cat auditory cortex. In G. A. Reich & J. A. Vernon (Eds.), *Proceedings of the fifth international tinnitus seminar* (pp. 455–456). Portland, OR: American Tinnitus Association.

Ochi, K., & Eggermont, J. J. (1996). Effects of salicylate on neural activity in cat primary auditory cortex. *Hearing Research, 95,* 63–76.

Ochi, K., & Eggermont, J.J. (1997). Effects of quinine on neural activity in cat primary auditory cortex. *Hearing Research, 97,* 105–118.

Panford-Walsh, R., Singer, W., Rüttiger, L., Hadjab, S., Tan, J., Geisler, H. S., . . . Knipper, M. (2008). Midazolam reverses salicylate-induced changes in brain-derived neurotrophic factor and arg3.1 expression: Implications for tinnitus perception and auditory plasticity. *Molecular Pharmacology, 74,* 595–604.

Park, J., White, A. R., & Ernst, E. (2000). Efficacy of acupuncture as a treatment for tinnitus: A systematic review. *Archives of Otolaryngology-Head and Neck Surgery, 126,* 489–492.

Penner, M. J. (1980). Two-tone forward masking patterns and tinnitus. *Journal of Speech and Hearing Research, 23,* 779–786.

Penner, M. J. (1992). Linking spontaneous otoacoustic emissions and tinnitus. *Audiology, 26,* 115–123.

Penner, M. J. (1993). Synthesizing tinnitus from sine waves. *Journal of Speech and Hearing Research, 36,* 1300–1305.

Penner, M. J. (2000). Spontaneous otoacoustic emissions and tinnitus. In R. S. Tyler (Ed.), *Tinnitus handbook* (pp. 203–220). San Diego, CA: Singular.

Penner, M. J., & Burns, E. M. (1987). The dissociation of SOAEs and tinnitus. *Journal of Speech and Hearing Research, 30,* 396–403.

Penner, M. J., & Coles, R. R. (1992). Indications for aspirin as a palliative for tinnitus caused by SOAEs: A case study. *British Journal of Audiology, 26,* 91–96.

Penner, M. J., & Jastreboff, P. J. (1996). Tinnitus: Psychophysical observations in humans and an animal model. In T. R. Van De Water, A. N. Popper, & R. R. Fay (Eds.), *Clinical aspects of hearing* (pp. 258–304). New York, NY: Springer- Verlag.

Pienkowski, M., & Eggermont, J. J. (2009). Recovery from reorganization induced in adult cat primary auditory cortex by a band-limited spectrally enhanced acoustic environment. *Hearing Research, 257,* 24–40.

Pienkowski, M., & Eggermont, J. J. (2010). Intermittent exposure of mature animals to moderate-level, bandlimited sound can impair central auditory function without producing peripheral hearing loss. *Hearing Research, 261,* 30–35.

Plath, N., Ohana, O., Dammermann, B., Errington, M.L., Schmitz, D., Gross, C., . . . Kuhl. D. (2006). Arc/Arg3.1 is essential for the consolidation of synaptic plasticity and memories. *Neuron, 52,* 437–444.

Plewnia, C., Reimold, M., Najib, A., Brehm, B., Reischl, G., Plontke, S. K., & Gerloff, C. (2007). Dose-dependent attenuation of auditory phantom perception (tinnitus) by PET-guided repetitive transcranial magnetic stimulation. *Human Brain Mapping, 28,* 238–246.

Prosen, C. A., & May, B. J. (2005). Behavioral and electrophysiological assessment of tinnitus in a mouse model. *Abstracts of the Association for Research in Otolaryngology, 28,* 410.

Puel, J. L. (1995). Chemical synaptic transmission in the cochlea. *Progress in Neurobiology, 47,* 449–476.

Puel, J. L., Ruel, J., Gervais d'Aldin, C., & Pujol, R. (1998). Excitotoxicity and repair of cochlear synapses after noise-trauma induced hearing loss. *NeuroReport, 9,* 2109–2114.

Quaranta, N., Wagstaff, S., & Baguley, D. M. (2004). Tinnitus and cochlear implantation. *International Journal of Audiology, 43,* 245–251.

Rabinowitz, P. M., Slade, M. D., Galusha, D., Dixon-Ernst, C., & Cullen, M. R. (2006). Trends in the prevalence of hearing loss among young adults entering an industrial workforce 1985 to 2004. *Ear and Hearing, 27,* 369–375.

Rajan, R., Irvine, D. R., Wise, L. Z., & Heil, P. (1993). Effect of unilateral partial cochlear lesions in adult cats on the representation of lesioned and unlesioned cochleas in primary auditory cortex. *Journal of Comparative Neurology, 338,* 17–49.

Rejai, D., Sivakumar, A., & Balaji, N., (2004). Ginkgo biloba does not benefit patients with tinnitus: A randomized placebo-controlled double-blind trial and meta-analysis of randomized trials. *Clinical Otolaryngology and Allied Sciences, 29,* 226–231.

Rescorla, R., & Wagner, A. (1972). A theory of Pavlovian conditioning: Variations in the effectiveness of reinforcement and nonreinforcement. In A. Black & W. Prokasy (Eds.), *Classical conditioning II: Current research and theory* (pp. 64–99). New York, NY: Appleton-Century-Crofts.

Riga, M., Papadas, T., Werner, J. A., & Dalchow, C. V. (2007). A clinical study of the efferent auditory system in patients with normal hearing who have acute tinnitus. *Otology and Neurotology, 28*, 185–190.

Roberts, L. E. (2007). Residual inhibition. *Progress in Brain Research, 166*, 487–495.

Roberts, L. E., Moffat, G., Baumann, M., Ward, L. M., & Bosnyak, D. J. (2008). Residual inhibition functions overlap tinnitus spectra and the region of auditory threshold shift. *Journal of the Association for Research in Otolaryngology, 9*, 417–435.

Robertson, D., & Irvine, D. R. (1989). Plasticity of frequency organization in auditory cortex of guinea pigs with partial unilateral deafness. *Journal of Comparative Neurology, 282*, 456–471.

Robertson, D., & Paki, B. (2002). Role of L-type Ca2+ channels in transmitter release from mammalian inner hair cells. II. Single-neuron activity. *Journal of Neurophysiology, 87*, 2734–2740.

Roeser, R. J., & Price, D. R. (1980). Clinical experience with tinnitus maskers. *Ear and Hearing, 1*, 63–68.

Rossi, S., Ferro, M., Cincotta, M., Ulivelli, M., Bartalini, S., Miniussi, C., . . . Passero, S. (2007). A real electro-magnetic placebo (REMP) device for sham transcranial magnetic stimulation (TMS). *Clinical Neurophysiology, 118*, 709–716.

Rubinow, D. R., Schmidt, P. J., & Roca, C. A. (1998). Estrogen-serotonin interactions: Implications for affective regulation. *Biological Psychiatry, 44*, 839–850.

Ruckenstein, M. J., Hedgepeth, C., Rafter, K. O., Montes, M. L., & Bigelow, D. C. (2001). Tinnitus suppression in patients with cochlear implants. *Otology and Neurotology, 22*, 200–204.

Ruel, J., Chabbert, C., Nouvian, R., Bendris, R., Eybalin, M., Leger, C. L., . . . Puel, J. L. (2008). Salicylate enables cochlear arachidonic-acid-sensitive NMDA receptor responses. *Journal of Neuroscience, 28*, 7313–7323.

Rüttiger, L., Ciuffani, J., Zenner, H. P., & Knipper, M. (2003). A behavioral paradigm to judge acute sodium salicylate-induced sound experience in rats: A new approach for an animal model on tinnitus. *Hearing Research, 180*, 39–50.

Sahley, T. L., & Nodar, R. H. (2001). A biochemical model of peripheral tinnitus. *Hearing Research, 152*, 43–54.

Saltzmann, M., & Ersner, M. S. (1947). A hearing aid for the relief of tinnitus aurum. *Laryngoscope, 48*, 358–366.

Salvi, R. J., Hamernik, R. P., Henderson, D., & Ahroon, W. A. (1983) Neural correlates of sensorineural hearing loss. *Ear and Hearing, 4*, 115–129.

Salvi, R. J., Wang, J. & Ding, D. (2000). Auditory plasticity and hyperactivity following cochlear damage. *Hearing Research, 147*, 261–274.

Savastano, M. (2007). Characteristics of tinnitus in childhood. *European Journal of Pediatrics, 166*, 797–801.

Schaette, R., & Kempter, R. (2006). Development of tinnitus-related neuronal hyperactivity through homeostatic plasticity after hearing loss: A computational model. *European Journal of Neuroscience, 23*, 3124–3138.

Schaette, R., & Kempter, R. (2008). Development of hyperactivity after hearing loss in a computational model of the dorsal cochlear nucleus depends on neuron response type. *Hearing Research, 240*, 57–72.

Schofield, B. R., & Coomes, D. L. (2005). Projections from auditory cortex contact cells in the cochlear nucleus that project to the inferior colliculus. *Hearing Research, 206*, 3–11.

Seki, S., & Eggermont, J. J. (2002). Changes in cat primary auditory cortex after minor-to-moderate pure-tone induced hearing loss. *Hearing Research, 173*, 172–186.

Seki, S., & Eggermont, J. J. (2003). Changes in spontaneous firing rate and neural synchrony in cat primary auditory cortex after localized tone-induced hearing loss. *Hearing Research, 180*, 28–38.

Shoham, S., O'Connor, D. H., & Segev, R. (2006). How silent is the brain: Is there a "dark matter" problem in neuroscience? *Journal of Comparative Physiology Part A: Neuroethology, Sensory, Neural, and Behavioral Physiology, 192*, 777–784.

Shore, S. E., & Zhou. J. (2006). Somatosensory influence on the cochlear nucleus and beyond. *Hearing Research, 216–217*, 90–99.

Simpson, J. J., & Davies, W. E. (2000). A review of evidence in support of a role for 5-HT in the perception of tinnitus. *Hearing Research, 145*, 1–7.

Simpson, J. J., Donaldson, I., & Davies, W. E. (1998). Use of homeopathy in the treatment of tinnitus. *British Journal of Audiology, 32*, 227–233.

Simpson, J. J., Gilbert, A. M., Weiner, G. M., & Davies, W. E. (1999). The assessment of lamotrigine, an antiepileptic drug, in the treatment of tinnitus. *American Journal of Otology, 20*, 627–631.

Sindhusake, D., Golding, M., Newall, P., Rubin, G., Jakobsen, K., & Mitchell, P. (2003). Risk factors for tinnitus in a population of older adults: The blue mountains hearing study. *Ear and Hearing, 24*, 501–507.

Sininger, Y. S., Eggermont, J. J., & King, A. J. (1992). Spontaneous activity from the peripheral auditory system in tinnitus. In J.-M. Aran & R. Dauman (Eds.), *Tinnitus 91* (pp. 341–345). Amsterdam, NL: Kugler.

Smith, P. F., Zheng, Y., & Darlington, C. L. (2005). Ginkgo biloba extracts for tinnitus: More hype than hope? *Journal of Ethnopharmacology, 100*, 95–99.

Smits, M., Kovacs, S., de Ridder, D., Peeters, R. R., van Hecke, P., & Sunaert, S. (2007). Lateralization of functional magnetic resonance imaging (fMRI) activation in the auditory pathway of patients with lateralized tinnitus. *Neuroradiology, 49*, 669–679.

Stypulkowski, P. H. (1990). Mechanisms of salicylate ototoxicity. *Hearing Research, 46*, 113–146.

Stouffer, J. L., & Tyler, R. S. (1990). Characterization of tinnitus by tinnitus patients. *Journal of Speech and Hearing Disorders, 55*, 439–453.

Suga, N., Gao, E., Zhang, Y., Ma, X., & Olsen, J. F. (2000). The corticofugal system for hearing: Recent progress. *Proceedings of the National Academy of Sciences of the United States of America, 97*, 11807–11814.

Surr, R. K., Montgomery, A. A., & Mueller, H. G. (1985). Effect of amplification on tinnitus among new hearing aid users. *Ear and Hearing, 6*, 71–75.

Szczepaniak, W. S., & Møller, A. R. (1995). Evidence of decreased GABAergic influence on temporal integration in the inferior colliculus following acute noise exposure: A study of evoked potentials in the rat. *Neuroscience Letters, 196*, 77–80.

Tan, J., Rüttiger, L., Panford-Walsh, R., Singer, W., Schulze, H., Kilian, S.B., . . . Knipper, M. (2007). Tinnitus behavior and hearing function correlate with the reciprocal expression patterns of BDNF and Arg3.1/arc in auditory neurons following acoustic trauma. *Neuroscience, 145*, 715–726.

Takeno, S., Harrison, R. V., Mount, R. J., Wake, M., & Harada, Y. (1994). Induction of selective inner hair cell damage by carboplatin. *Scanning Microscopy, 8*, 97–106.

Thai-Van, H., Micheyl, C., Moore, B. C., & Collet, L. (2003). Enhanced frequency discrimination near the hearing loss cut-off: A consequence of central auditory plasticity induced by cochlear damage? *Brain, 126*, 2235–2245.

Thomas, D. R. (2006). 5-HT5A receptors as a therapeutic target. *Pharmacology and Therapeutics, 111*, 707–714.

Turner, J. G., Brozoski, T. J., Bauer, C. A., Parrish, J. L,, Myers, K., Hughes, L.F., & Caspary, D.M. (2006). Gap detection deficits in rats with tinnitus: A potential novel screening tool. *Behavioral Neuroscience, 120*, 188–195.

Tyler, R. S., & Conrad-Armes, D. (1983). The determination of tinnitus loudness considering the effects of recruitment. *Journal of Speech and Hearing Research, 26*, 59–72.

Tyler, R. S., & Conrad-Armes, D. (1984). Masking of tinnitus compared to masking of pure tones. *Journal of Speech and Hearing Research, 27*, 106–111.

Van de Heyning, P., Vermeire, K., Diebl, M., Nopp, P., Anderson, I., & De Ridder, D. (2008). Incapacitating unilateral tinnitus in single-sided deafness treated by cochlear implantation. *Annals of Otology, Rhinology and Laryngology, 117*, 645–652.

Vernon, J., Schleuning, A., Well, I., & Hughes, F. (1977). A tinnitus clinic. *Ear, Nose, and Throat Journal, 56*, 58–71.

Wahlström, B., & Axelsson, A. (1995). The description of tinnitus sounds. In G. E. Reich, & J. A. Vernon (Eds.), *Proceedings of the Fifth International Tinnitus Seminar* (pp. 298–301). Portland, OR: American Tinnitus Association.

Waldvogel, D., Mattle, H. P., Sturzenegger, M., & Schroth, G. (1998). Pulsatile tinnitus—a review of 84 patients. *Journal of Neurology, 245*, 137–142.

Wallhausser-Franke, E., Mahlke, C., Oliva, R., Braun, S., Wenz, G., & Langner, G. (2003). Expression of c-fos in auditory and non-auditory brain regions of the gerbil after manipulations that induce tinnitus. *Experimental Brain Research, 153*, 649–654.

Wang, J., Ding, D., & Salvi, R. J. (2002). Functional reorganization in chinchilla inferior colliculus associated with chronic and acute cochlear damage. *Hearing Research, 168*, 238–249.

Wang, H. T., Luo, B., Zhou, K. Q., & Chen. L. (2008). Sodium salicylate suppresses serotonin-induced enhancement of GABAergic spontaneous inhibitory postsynaptic currents in rat inferior colliculus in vitro. *Hearing Research, 236*, 42–51.

Wang, H. T., Luo, B., Zhou, K. Q., Xu, T. L., & Chen, L. (2006). Sodium salicylate reduces inhibitory postsynaptic currents in neurons of rat auditory cortex. *Hearing Research, 215*, 77–83.

Weisz, N., Hartmann, T., Dohrmann, K., Schlee, W., & Norena, A. (2006). High-frequency tinnitus without hearing loss does not mean absence of deafferentation. *Hearing Research, 222*, 108–114.

Weisz, N., Moratti, S., Meinzer, M., Dohrmann, K., & Elbert, T. (2005a). Tinnitus perception and distress is related to abnormal spontaneous brain activity as measured by magnetoencephalography. *PLoS Medicine, 2*, e153.

Weisz, N., Müller, S., Schlee, W., Dohrmann, K., Hartmann, T., & Elbert, T. (2007). The neural code of auditory phantom perception. *Journal of Neuroscience, 27*, 1479–1484.

Weisz, N., Voss, S., Berg, P., & Elbert, T. (2004). Abnormal auditory mismatch response in tinnitus sufferers with high-frequency hearing loss is associated with subjective distress level. *BMC Neuroscience, 5*, 8.

Weisz, N., Wienbruch, C., Dohrmann, K., & Elbert, T. (2005b). Neuromagnetic indicators of auditory cortical reorganization of tinnitus. *Brain, 128*, 2722–2731.

West, A. E., Chen, W. G., Dalva, M. B., Dolmetsch, R. E., Kornhauser, J. M., Shaywitz, A. J., . . . Greenberg, M. E. (2001). Calcium regulation of neuronal gene expression. *Proceedings of the National Academy of Sciences of the United States of America, 98*, 11024–11031.

Wienbruch, C., Paul, I., Weisz, N., Elbert, T., & Roberts, L. E. (2006). Frequency organization of the 40-Hz auditory steady-state response in normal hearing and in tinnitus. *NeuroImage, 33*, 180–194.

Willott, J. F., Milbrandt, J. C., Bross, L. S., & Caspary, D. M. (1997). Glycine immunoreactivity and receptor binding in the cochlear nucleus of C57BL/6J and CBA/CaJ mice: Effects of cochlear impairment and aging. *Journal of Comparative Neurology, 385*, 405–414.

Woodson, W., Farb, C. R., & Ledoux, J. E. (2000). Afferents from the auditory thalamus synapse on inhibitory interneurons in the lateral nucleus of the amygdala. *Synapse, 38*, 124–137.

Yan, J., & Ehret, G. (2002). Corticofugal modulation of midbrain sound processing in the house mouse. *European Journal of Neuroscience, 16*, 119–128.

Yan, W., & Suga, N. (1998). Corticofugal modulation of the midbrain frequency map in the bat auditory system. *Nature Neuroscience, 1*, 54–58.

Yang, G., Lobarinas, E., Zhang, L., Turner, J., Stolzberg, D., Salvi, R., & Sun, W. (2007). Salicylate induced tinnitus: Behavioral measures and neural activity in auditory cortex of awake rats. *Hearing Research, 226*, 244–253.

Yoshimura, H. (2005). The potential of caffeine for functional modification from cortical synapses to neuron networks in the brain. *Current Neuropharmacology, 3*, 309–316.

Zacharek, M. A., Kaltenbach, J. A., Mathog, T. A., & Zhang, J. (2002). Effects of cochlear ablation on noise induced hyperactivity in the hamster dorsal cochlear nucleus: Implications for the origin of noise induced tinnitus. *Hearing Research, 172*, 137–143.

Zelman, S. (1973). Correlation of smoking history with hearing loss. *Journal of the American Medical Association, 223*, 920.

Zöger, S., Svedlund, J., & Holgers, K. M. (2006). The effects of sertraline on severe tinnitus suffering—a randomized, double-blind, placebo-controlled study. *Journal of Clinical Psychopharmacology, 26*, 32–39.

6

Current Issues in Auditory Plasticity and Auditory Training

Kelly Tremblay and David Moore

LEARNING OBJECTIVES

- To understand the concept and use of the term "plasticity," from a historical perspective.
- To understand why the term "plasticity" is defined in many ways and used differently in many different areas of science.
- To understand how plasticity is a part of everyday learning.
- To understand how a person with hearing loss has experienced many different neuroplastic processes as a result of auditory deprivation and stimulation.
- To understand why auditory training is only a subcomponent of auditory rehabilitation

Key Words. Auditory learning, auditory rehabilitation, listening training, neuroplastic, hearing aids, cochlear implants

INTRODUCTION

Almost everyone knows an older person who has had a stroke. If the stroke was mild, behavioral recovery begins rapidly and can be apparently complete within a matter of days. Even moderate or severe deficits typically result in some spontaneous behavioral recovery within a week or so (Cramer, 2008a) and, because of the brain's plasticity, "task-oriented and repetitive training" following a stroke is "well established as having a major influence on behavioral outcome" (Cramer, 2008b, p. 549).

The potential generalization of these observations to the topic of hearing loss and auditory plasticity might not be obvious, but there are close parallels. Almost everyone knows an older person with age-related hearing loss. Hair cell loss, like necrosis of brain tissue, is permanent. There currently is no known way to regenerate hair cells in the human cochlea, so rehabilitation is in part dependent on the brain's capacity to change. The first step is to compensate for the cochlear damage by finding alternative ways (e.g., hearing aid) to get an audible signal from the ear to the auditory brain. The second goal is to try and improve what the person is able to do with the amplified sounds through "task-oriented and repetitive training." Hearing health care providers around the world practice the first step every day, fitting millions of people with hearing aids each year. But the concept of brain plasticity is not a matter of common knowledge, so the second stage of rehabilitation is not always provided by clinicians. For this reason, we share our definition of plasticity as it relates to people with communication disorders. With an emphasis on audition, it is hoped that readers will connect neuroscience theory to practice so that advancement can take place in both directions.

BRAIN PLASTICITY — DEFINITION AND HISTORY

The term "plasticity" has received many and various definitions in the context of neuroscience research (Parks et al., 2004). Here, we take it to mean a capacity for change in the structure and/or function of the nervous system, as a result of sensory experience (Eggermont, 1990). The term is typically reserved for reactive, or secondary, effects in response to a change in the otherwise normal system (e.g., Kolb, 1995; Pascual-Leone et al., 2005). In the situation of a stroke, for example, the capacity for change would not be defined by the brain injury per se, but by the compensatory reactions to the insult (Brion, Demeurisse, & Capon, 1989; Buckner, Corbetta, Schatz, Raichle, & Petersen, 1996; Liepert, Storch, Fritsch, & Weiller, 2000; Ward & Cohen, 2004) and the therapy (Taube, 2011). Neuroplastic and behavioral changes can also take place in the absence of injury. Physiologic and behavioral changes associated with repetitive behaviors, such as musical instrument training (Kraus et al., 2009), would therefore also fall under our definition of plasticity.

Establishing brain-behavior relationships has been a longstanding goal of both basic and applied scientists, with the hope that evidence at the cellular or molecular level will manifest itself into rehabilitation treatments, and observed behavioral changes might better define biological processes. But at both ends of the research continuum, a challenge is to link cause and effect. An important example of this in neuroplasticity is that behavioral changes, especially in humans, cannot usually be associated with a known neural mechanism. They can only be indirectly linked to physiologic changes, since cellular processes are currently accessible only by using invasive recording methods. Instead, noninvasive tools such as electroencephalography (EEG), magnetoencephalography (MEG), functional magnetic resonance imaging (fMRI), and near-infrared spectroscopy are being used to measure changes in brain-generated voltage, magnetic fields, blood oxygen levels, and blood oxy- and deoxy-hemoglobin concentrations, respectively. Despite their limitations when trying to identify known neural mechanisms, a strength of these noninvasive approaches is that it is possible to obtain both physiological and perceptual measures from the same person so that brain-behavior relationships can be established. In turn, presumed cause and effects can be further explored using animal models so that contributing neural mechanisms can be further defined.

It goes without saying that there are also limitations when using animals to study neuroplastic processes associated with the perception of signals relevant to human communication. It is simply not possible to ask a mouse to judge the quality of a sound. Invasive methods are however used to identify candidate mechanisms in nonhumans and there is increasing hope for understanding their involvement in human behavioral change. Two examples are relevant here: First is the work of J. Willott and colleagues who have documented that age-related hearing loss at the periphery has secondary neuroplastic effects along central auditory nuclei. Another example is the work by E. W. Rubel and his colleagues (e.g., Harris et al., 2008) who have made a number of important observations of the afferent influences (i.e., auditory nerve input) on intracellular molecular signaling pathways in the cochlear nucleus. The observations of Rubel and colleagues have not yet been related directly either to reduced (through hearing loss) or enhanced (through sound stimulation) neural activity in the human auditory system. However, by means such as measurement of gene and protein expression, mechanisms which are closely shared between humans and laboratory animals, linking physiology to function will, we predict, eventually become possible. In the meantime, we assume that such mechanisms, and a multitude of others at the mechanical, molecular, cellular, and systems levels of ear and brain function underlie everything we hear. Prior to the advance of technologic tools, since ancient times, clinical observations following various forms of irreversible damage to the nervous system, and its sense organs, were used to model human systems, even if they were not always attributed to neural mechanisms. But the typically more subtle effects of sensory experience on brain and behavior have not begun to be understood experimentally until relatively recently. Again, we can assume that clinical practice led the way. For example, eye patching was found, more than 100 years ago, to result in improved vision in a "lazy" (turned or unfocussed) eye (Levi & Li, 2009a). But it has been only in the last 30 to 40 years that this phenomenon (amblyopia) has been studied scientifically, and only in the last 5 to 15 years that visual training has been found to be an alternative, effective treatment (Levi & Li, 2009b).

In some instances, the demonstration of brain plasticity by neuroscientists has had unexpected (and unwanted) negative consequences for behavioural and clinical thinking. Wiesel and Hubel's Nobel Prize–winning work on the effect of monocular deprivation (closing one eye) on the physiology of single neurons in the visual cortex (Wiesel, 1982) is a case in point. They showed that, in both immature and adult animals with a history of normal vision, most cortical neurons respond to appropriate visual stimulation of either eye. If one eye was sutured closed early in postnatal life, thus depriving the animal of form vision in that eye, most cortical neurons would subsequently respond only to stimulation of the open eye, even after many months of normal vision following opening of the previously sutured eye. However, an equivalent period of monocular deprivation in an adult did not change the proportion of cortical neurons responding to the two eyes. This ground-breaking work, conducted in the early 1960s, led to a flurry of other findings of developmental "sensitive periods" in the brain resulting, over the next 20 to 30 years, in a belief among many neuroscientists that brain plasticity existed only during early development. This belief permeated and influenced clinical culture so that it was thought, for instance, that eye patching could not have any therapeutic effect beyond the critical period (Barry, 2009). Subsequent single neuron research in the somatosensory cortex (Kaas et al., 1983) confirmed earlier, but largely unrecognized subcortical observations (Wall and Egger, 1971), that the representation of the body surface in the *adult* central nervous system underwent functional reorganization following lesions of the sensory periphery. These findings were later extended to the adult auditory (Robertson & Irvine, 1989) and visual (Kaas et al., 1990) cortex. More recent work has shown that sensory experience in adulthood can also influence both the response properties of single neurons in the cortex and the map of the sensory receptor sheet across the cortical surface (Li et al., 2004). Even the gross structural properties of cortical gray matter in humans can be changed by training (Draganski et al., 2004). Consequently, the view has gradually re-emerged that long-term and neurologically explicable behavioral changes based on experience can occur in adults and, to bring the story full circle, the effects of stroke on the motor cortex are now seen as a model system for studying the mechanisms underlying such plasticity (*Developmental Psychobiology*, special issue, 2011).

Following this general pattern, earlier auditory research focused on the effects of manipulations of auditory stimulation in immature animals on the subsequent development of brain structure and function. This grew out of two influences. One was neurobiological studies in birds (Levi-Montalcini, 1949; Rubel, 1981) showing the dependence of normal embryonic hindbrain development on input from the otocyst (developing inner ear). The second was, in many cases literally, "copy cat" studies of visual system plasticity. In these studies the hypothesis was that neonatal ear occlusion (Brugge et al. 1985; Clopton & Silverman, 1977; Moore and Irvine, 1981) or controlled environmental rearing (Moore & Aitkin, 1975; Sanes & Constantive-Paton, 1985) would steer the response of neurons toward the experienced stimuli. Subsequently, much research has been devoted to the understanding, mostly at a cellular or molecular level, of the "afferent influences" of auditory nerve activity on the brain in general, but especially on the cochlear nucleus (e.g. Harris et al., 2008). Recent studies of "environmental influences" have continued to prefer single- or multiunit recording methods and have focused on the mammalian cortex (Dahmen & King, 2007).

Other early studies, however, demonstrated peripheral auditory system plasticity and were primarily concerned with the effects of noise exposure (for more information on noise exposure see Chapter 1). One example was the mechanisms of "temporary threshold shift" (TTS), in which exposure to a moderately high level of noise was found to produce reversible changes in the fine structure of the cochlea (see Nordmann et al., 2000). Recently, changes in the function of the descending, olivocochlear system have been demonstrated following experimentally controlled auditory experience in humans (auditory training; de Boer & Thornton, 2008) and ferrets (altered localization cues, Irving et al., 2011). In an earlier study (Liberman, 1975), it was shown that rearing in a very low noise environment could reduce (i.e., sensitize) what is considered the "normal" response threshold of auditory nerve fibers. Recent research has demonstrated loss of auditory nerve fibers following exposure to only moderately high sound levels causing functional TTS (Kujawa & Liberman , 2009). It was noteworthy in this work that no change in the threshold sensitivity of the cochlea was observed. Permanent hearing loss, resulting in tinnitus, has also now been clearly associated with a cascade of neural plasticity (see Eggermont, Chapter 5). In this instance, as in stroke and in phantom limb sensations following amputation, the plasticity appears to be based on disinhibition, sometimes called "unmasking," of central excitation.

Question 1

Has the MMN been used to test CI users and could it be used as a clinical tool?

Answer 1

There was tremendous interest in using the MMN to assess CI users for both research and clinical interests beginning in the 1990s. Possible applications included using the MMN response to help guide clinicians when mapping the device, or understanding neuroplasticity in individuals following implantation. However, as the tool evolved it became increasingly obvious that the likelihood of implementing the MMN into clinical protocols was small. The MMN can be difficult to quantify in individuals and requires a great deal of signal averaging, and thus more time, compared to other, more robust, cortical potential options (e.g., P1-N1-P2).

PLASTICITY IN RELATION TO COMMUNICATION DISORDERS

The concept of physiologic plasticity in relation to people with speech and hearing disorders is only beginning to be explored, again in part because of recent technological advances that permit the ability to record physiologic changes in the human brain in noninvasive ways. Animal research has provided a platform for exploring neural mechanisms underlying some of the disorders and to some degree the physiologic effects of remediation, but so too have clinical observations. Interacting with a person who is being fit with a hearing aid allows one to: (1) learn what specific auditory experiences are challenging for the individual; and equally important, which are not, (2) connect a medical history to their symptoms, and (3) receive feedback to determine what intervention approaches may or may not be helpful. Because this type of information cannot be obtained from a mouse, it can be advantageous to investigators to use such information when developing testable hypotheses that can be carried out in humans and in animals so that evidence based practice can result. What follows are a few examples of how bench and applied sciences have contributed to our understanding of the different types of disorders that impact human communication.

Disorders Involving Auditory Deprivation

Otitis Media

Otitis media can be defined as an inflammation of the middle ear and is what is commonly referred to as an ear infection. Acute otitis media, in which the infection is usually painful, is the most frequently diagnosed disease in infants and young children, but otitis media with effusion (OME), where middle ear fluid usually goes unnoticed, is even more common, with at least 75% of children experiencing at least one episode by their third birthday (Dhooge, 2003; Hogan & Moore, 2003; NIH, 2002). Children are more prone to ear infections because their eustachian tubes are shorter and aligned more horizontally compared to the adult ear. Inflammation in the middle ear space, for which interesting mouse models have recently been reported (Rye et al., 2011), is often associated with the buildup of fluid, sometimes resulting in a slight to moderate conductive hearing loss. OME can be especially problematic because the age of peak incidence coincides with that of typical speech and language development. For this reason, there is interest in determining if periods of auditory deprivation, resulting from OME, impact the physiologic representation of sound in the central auditory system as well as speech-language development. In this example, physiological plasticity could be viewed as being reactive to the acute (or chronic) change in audibility in an otherwise normal system.

There is ample evidence in animal experiments to show that the central auditory system (CAS) changes as a function of sound attenuation brought on by a conductive hearing loss, as introduced above. Occluding the ears of developing ferrets, induces an acute conductive hearing loss that is similar to that of otitis media and alters binaural sound input into the brain (Moore et al., 1989), including sound localization (Irving et al., 2011; Kacelnik et al., 2006). Parallel studies in adult humans have also shown physiologic (Formby et al., 2003) and behavioral (Irving et al., 2011; Kumpnik et al., 2010) effects of unilateral conductive hearing loss using ear plugs.

There is evidence that links OME to communication disorders among environmentally deprived children (Roberts et al., 2004). These children have often been subject to poor child care (Vernon-Feagans et al., 2002) and other social circumstances involving excess environmental noise that prevented adequate listening experiences. So even though there might be physiological effects of auditory deprivation, they do not appear to be substantial enough to interfere with typical speech and language development for children who are being raised in enriched communication environments. For the typically developing child it might be that: (1) the affected mechanisms are not be critical to speech and language, (2) redundancy in the auditory system compensates for the disruptions imposed by periods of deprivation, or (3) deprivation-related plasticity is supplanted with stimulation-related changes arising from a child's interaction with sound in their everyday auditory environment.

Unilateral Sensorineural Hearing Loss

The ability to understand speech in the presence of background noise is a challenge for most individuals. Humans evolved with two ears presumably because they aid in the ability to localize sound sources, separate ecologically important sound sources from background noise, and extract acoustic information important for speech sound discrimination. With that said, humans experience a wide variety of auditory disorders that can impact the benefits that come with symmetrical hearing. Conductive hearing loss such as OME, for example, is often bilaterally asymmetric (Halliday & Moore, 2010) but tumors can affect the conduction of sound in a way that disrupts the binaural balance between ears. Vestibular schwannomas, for example, typically affect just one ear, resulting in a progressive asymmetric sensorineural hearing loss. A person's exposure to noise, as is the case with a violin player or rifle hunter, might also result in asymmetric sensorineural damage. Unlike conductive losses, where the central effects of deprivation can be temporary and reversible, sensorineural hearing losses are usually associated with permanent deficits. Although this is certainly true of the cochlear aspects of the hearing loss, central concomitants of a sensorineural loss (including cognitive factors [e.g., Pichora-Fuller], may well be partly or wholly reversed by appropriate experience. It is therefore important to understand how attenuated input in one or both ears impacts the ability to neurally encode binaural cues and if perceptual impairments result. Knowing a patient's lifestyle and professional demands (e.g., taxi driver or viola player) informs the clinician about the possible consequences posed by the hearing loss as well as the perceptual and remedial needs of the patient. A taxi driver, for instance, will have great difficulty following orders if the hearing loss affects the ear that is used to listen to customers.

Even though the certain aspects of profound sensorineural hearing loss are not reversible, asymmetrical patterns of neural activation do appear to adjust to continued monaural input. When Ponton et al. (2001) compared the scalp topography of brain activation in normal hearing teens and adults to that of people who had experienced profound unilateral hearing loss following 8th nerve acoustic tumor removal; they found that the typical asymmetric topography seen in normal hearing adults was more symmetrical, with more synchronous activation occurring between hemispheres for the unilaterally deaf. To understand these changes it is important to know that many studies have shown that CAS activity evoked by monaural presentation is stronger and has lower activation thresholds in auditory pathways contralateral to the ear of stimulation at levels above the superior olivary complex (Kitzes, 1984; Popelar et al., 1994; Reale et al., 1987). When sound is presented monaurally to the human ear, for example, evoked potentials (EEG) and magnetic fields (MEG) measured over the hemisphere contralateral to the stimulated ear are much larger in amplitude and earlier in latency (Pantev et al., 1986; Vaughan & Ritter, 1970). These neural activation patterns suggest sound is traveling from the ear to the contralateral hemisphere of the brain at a faster rate, and with greater synchrony, than ipsilateral pathways. Data from fMRI reinforce this notion showing asymmetric patterns following monaurally elicited cortical activation (Scheffler et al., 1998).

Data from Ponton et al. show that the topography of EEG responses changes depend on the duration of unilateral hearing loss (Figure 6–1). P1-N1-P2 peaks reflect synchronous neural activity of structures in the thalamocortical segment of the central auditory system in response to acoustic

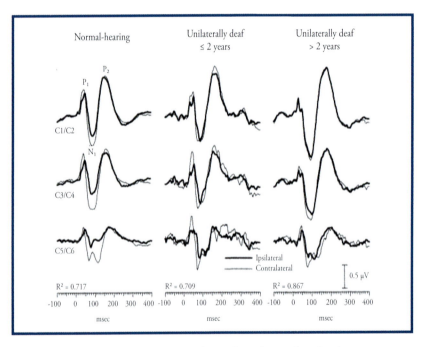

Figure 6–1. Ipsilateral and contralateral peak amplitudes become more equal as the time since onset of unilateral deafness increases from ≤2 years to >2 years. This is apparent for all electrode pairs. Odd numbered electrode sites (C1, C3, C5) record activity over the left hemisphere whereas even numbered electrode sites (C2,C4,C6) are placed over the right hemisphere. Electrode pairs C1-C2 and C3-C4 also show that interhemispheric timing and amplitude differences are smaller in the unilaterally deaf than in the normal-hearing group for the P1 and N1 peaks, respectively. Reprinted with permission from Ponton et al. 2001.

changes (Naatanen & Picton, 1987; Vaughan & Ritter, 1970; Wolpaw & Penry, 1975). In normal hearing adults, P1-N1-P2 responses are larger in amplitude and shorter in latency (reflecting neural conduction time) contralateral to the ear of stimulation. In contrast, latencies and amplitudes become more symmetrical across hemispheres (e.g., C3/C4 comparison) among people who have experienced 2 or more years of unilateral auditory deprivation. Even though the perceptual consequences of such physiologic changes were not documented by Ponton and colleagues, their results provide an example of how the human auditory system is dynamic, capable of change, even in adulthood. In this respect, neural plasticity could be described as reactive, to the loss of sound input, and then adaptive to the use of the intact monaural system. A limitation of this study is that perceptual measures were not obtained so the relationship between these brain responses and specific binaural functions is not known. However, one interpretation is that with continued interaction in various auditory environments, the intact ear sends signals more efficiently through the ipsilateral pathways to help compensate for the impaired ear. This dynamic aspect of the central auditory system might also explain why people with unilateral hearing loss do not always report a significant hearing handicap and do not always seek audiologic rehabilitation.

Patients with unilateral hearing loss often describe themselves as being able to adapt to their auditory environment and do not seek out audiologic assistance. When this is not the case, a person might choose to wear a contralateral routing of signals (CROS) type hearing aid where a microphone fit over the impaired ear redirects sound to the intact ear. Patients can do remarkably well while wearing CROS type prostheses, suggesting that individuals are able to learn how to use the information from the deaf ear that is provided to them.

With that said, when rehabilitation is sought, wearing a hearing prosthesis does not fully replace the two ears nature provided. Wearing a CROS aid does not necessarily result in a reduced hearing handicap score for all people (Charles, Bishop, & Eby, 2010). It might be that a person's reaction to wearing a CROS type hearing aid relates to each person's own biological reaction to the period of audi-

tory deprivation, as well as the effects of stimulation associated with the modified input that is now entering the intact ear. These possibilities have motivated scientists to question, what happens when sound is reintroduced to a previously deprived system? Examples include people who are fitted with hearing aids and/or cochlear implants.

Question 2

If being exposed to sounds changes your brain, is there any scientific evidence to support the idea of subliminal learning?

Answer 2

There is an extensive literature on subliminal learning and attention. Some aspects of subliminal perception are a matter of everyday experience (for example, your name being "heard" in an otherwise unattended speech stream). For any study of learning, an appropriate control group is essential, to measure test-retest effects, but a major issue is what you do with this control group while the experimental group is training. "Doing nothing" isn't really an option, because we are always "doing something," even when asleep. On the other hand, giving more active exposure to, for example, arcade-style computer games has been shown to enhance visual spatial attention which could, in turn, result in or from general arousal that will have an impact on (or may even be necessary for) auditory learning. Coming back to subliminal learning, it is likely that the same cues that trigger subliminal perception will have an effect on learning. But a fundamental premise of effective learning is task engagement. Doing an easy task that you get correct 100% of the time is much less effective than trying to do a very difficult (or even impossibly difficult) task. As they say, "no gain without pain."

Disorders Involving Auditory Deprivation and Remediated with Auditory Stimulation

Hearing Aid Amplification and Cochlear Implantation

Clinical knowledge of the effectiveness of eye patching might have preceded its scientific study by at least 100 years, but hearing aids have an even longer clinical history, going back to ancient times. However, despite the obvious benefits that come from amplifying sound levels, little is known about the effects of amplification on the CAS. Based on the animal literature, a couple of things are presumed to take place in reaction to sensorineural hearing losses. First, without sound input, auditory nerve and ventral cochlear nucleus (VCN) neurons responsible for establishing sound frequency and intensity coding in the CAS become inactive (Willot, 1996). The result is what Irvine and Rajan (1996) describe as "deprivation or injury-related" plasticity. In the case of a person with age-related hearing loss (presbycusis), a gradual decline in hearing might mean that the CAS has reacted to years of continued sound attenuation and distortion in a way that has altered the biological coding of intensity, timing and frequency information contained in the auditory signal. For example, we know that long-term deafening results in the atrophy of neuron cell bodies (Born & Rubel, 1985; Moore, 1990) and synaptic changes (Ryugo et al., 2010) at various levels of the auditory brainstem that are certain to affect sound coding. Second, introducing sound to a previously deprived auditory system is also presumed to alter the way spectral and temporal speech cues are being represented. In the above example, some synaptic changes in the VCN resulting from ototoxic deafening were found to be reversed by electrical stimulation of the cochlea (Ryugo et al., 2010). Irvine and Rajan (1996) refer to this process as "stimulation-induced" or "use-related" neural plasticity. In rehabilitation, hearing aids and cochlear implants, through their signal processing circuitry, modify the content of the incoming sound (Figure 6–2). Processed signals are thus presumed to stimulate novel neural response patterns. Sometimes described within the context of perceptual learning (McGraw, Webb, & Moore, 2009;

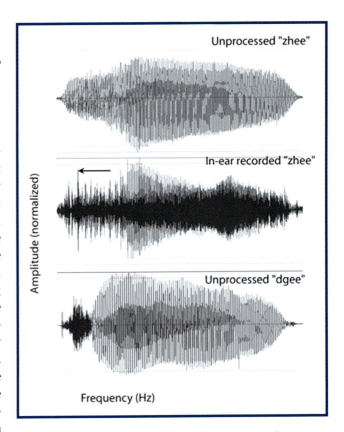

Figure 6–2. The top panel of the figure shows the unprocessed time waveform for the affricate vowel syllable /ʒi/ (zhee). The middle panel shows the same signal, recorded in the subject's ear at the output of the hearing aid. When compared to the input signal, the amplified version shows a large amplitude spike close to the onset of the consonant (*identified by the arrow*). The subject misidentified this syllable as the affricate /dʒi/ (dgee). The unprocessed (dgee) is shown for comparison in the lower panel. Note the overshoot in the consonant onset of the amplified (zhee), is similar to the abrupt onset of the unprocessed affricate (dgee). Reprinted from Souza and Tremblay (2006) with permission of *Trends in Amplification*. The final, definitive version of this paper has been published in Trends in Amplification, Vol 10/Sept./2011 by SAGE Publications Ltd. All rights reserved. © http://tia.sagepub.com/content/10/3.toc

Watson, 1991), it is also presumed that people *learn* how to relate the modified auditory signal, and the altered neural spectral and temporal codes, to an existing memory of sound.

Relatively little is known about how hearing aid amplification affects the spectral and temporal coding of sound in the human CAS. There are many reasons for the void of information, starting with the fact that few people have the expertise in both basic and applied sciences to approach the rehabilitation of hearing aid users within a combined theoretical framework. Neuroscientists often use cellular/molecular approaches to define normal CAS function and rarely work with humans who have communication disorders. Even fewer have the skills to translate statistical significance in the laboratory into life-impacting functional significance. In contrast, hearing health care providers are not always scientists, so the concept of plasticity is not typically integrated into their training and its scientific principles are not routinely integrated into their practice of auditory rehabilitation. Instead, emphasis is placed on improving sound audibility (by means of hearing aids, cochlear implant, or assistive listening devices). Obviously, this is a necessary first step, but it alone is not enough.

As shown in Figure 6–2, hearing aids distort speech sounds in a way that could lead to much perceptual confusion. The effect of signal processing in cochlear implants is even more obvious because the user is now extracting meaning from electrical pulse trains. The ability to sort out phonetic confusions at the word and sentence levels involves much more than just the ear; it also involves attention, cognition, and memory (Pichora-Fuller, 2006). It is no surprise then that increasing sound audibility, through the use of hearing aids, does not automatically resolve perceptual problems. Kochkin (2002) reports that over 16% of people receiving hearing aids completely reject them altogether and only 60% report being satisfied with their aids. Even when hearing aids are provided free, as they are in the United Kingdom, the rejection rate approximates 15 to 25% (Davis et al., 2007). These statistics are surprising when you think of all of the technological advances that have improved signal quality over the past generation. It suggests that there is more to successful rehabilitation than the engineered aspects of the signal.

So why is it that two individuals with the same configuration of hearing loss demonstrate significantly different improvements in speech understanding while wearing similar prosthetic devices? The answers involve more than just the ear or the prosthesis (Ramirez-Inscoe & Moore, 2011; Souza & Tremblay, 2006; Willott, 1996). It is likely that the degree of benefit a particular person receives from a hearing prosthesis depends in part on the patient's age as well as their own biological response to auditory deprivation and stimulation. People who do not experience significant benefits from hearing aids or cochlear implants may have auditory systems that are less plastic, that is, less capable of representing new acoustic cues. Poor speech perceivers might also have difficulty "learning" how to relate new neural patterns to an existing memory of the sounds of speech. There is evidence for these forms of reduced plasticity and that they are due to both genetic and environmental influences (Moore & Shannon, 2009). An alternative hypothesis would be that good perceivers have systems that are less plastic in some important respects, with their CAS being less disrupted by the loss of auditory input. An example is the age-dependence of language acquisition following profound deafness and cochlear implantation (for a review see Gordon et al., 2011). Prelingual deafness is associated with good outcomes only following implantation within the first few years of life, whereas those deafened postlingually often have excellent outcomes when implanted many years later (Moore & Shannon, 2009). One can think of many other scenarios to explore, but at present little is known about the mechanisms underlying these forms of plasticity.

Another reason why little is known about the impact hearing aid amplification and cochlear implantation has on the human CAS is because it can be difficult to quantify central auditory function in people who wear a prosthetic device. The limitations of functional imaging become apparent when the hearing prosthesis and its interactions with the magnet and noise of the powerful imaging scanner are considered. What's more, it is becoming increasingly apparent that the basic principles of EEG/MEG do not apply when stimuli are delivered through a hearing prosthesis. Hearing aids and cochlear implants introduce artifact and distortion into the ongoing EEG/MEG, making it difficult to separate biology from technology (Campos Viola et al. 2009; Castaneada-Villa, 2010; Debener et al. 2008; Friesen & Picton, 2010; Gilley et al. 2006; Martin, 2007; Wong & Gordon 2009). Hearing instruments also alter the acoustic properties of the incoming stimulus, and these modified signals contribute to neural response patterns in ways that are not yet fully understood (Marywinich et al., 2010; Billings, Tremblay, & Miller, 2011). Therefore, before stimulation-related effects on the CAS can be interpreted, it is necessary to understand the interaction between the signal processor and the CAS. Scientists who are cross-trained in these areas are able to recognize where interactions between the basic and applied sciences create breakthroughs and where they create pitfalls. What follow are descriptions of experiments that are of interest to clinicians and neuroscientists.

Hearing Aids and the CAS. Even though the concept of auditory plasticity was not readily considered back in the 1980's, clinician scientists sought out ways to quantify the effects of hearing aid amplification on the CAS. Motivation for this type of research was aimed at defining the integrity of the afferent pathway and determining if the amplified signal was being detected at the levels of the brainstem and cortex, in spite of auditory deprivation. Great potential was seen for using auditory brainstem responses (ABR) to assure the amplified signal was reaching the brainstem, and also to estimate the aided hearing sensitivity of people (especially babies) who needed hearing aids but could not reliably participate in behavioral testing (Beauchaine, Gorga, Reiland, & Larson, 1986; Davidson, Wall, & Goodman, 1990; Hecox, 1983; Kiessling, 1982; Kileny, 1982; Mahoney, 1985). To do this, ABRs would be recorded in response to sounds presented in sound field while the patient wore their hearing aid. Despite the initial enthusiasm, recording ABRs in response to amplified sound proved to be problematic because the necessary stimuli (clicks or tone-bursts) needed to evoke the ABR were too brief in duration to activate the hearing aid circuitry. There were also other confounding variables, such as stimulus rate, as well as the compression characteristics of the hearing aid (Gorga, Beauchaine, & Reiland 1987). In digital hearing aids, for example, the delay characteristics of the digital processor can interfere with the onset response of the ABR. This is further complicated by the fact that the delay in digital hearing aids varies across frequency (Kates, 2005; Stone & Moore, 1999). Even for normal-hearing, unaided listeners, subtle manipulations in the rise time or presentation rate of the stimulus used to evoke the ABR can greatly alter

the evoked response pattern (for a review, see Hall 1992). Because latency and amplitude of the ABR peaks are greatly affected by the hearing aid signal processing circuitry, making it difficult to separate effects of biology from technology, the ABR has not been used to examine the effects of amplification on the CAS.

Scientists therefore turned to cortical auditory evoked potentials (CAEPs). The P1-N1-P2 complex is a widely studied CAEP measure because it too is highly sensitive to the acoustic content of the stimulating signal and could be used clinically to estimate audiometric thresholds (Hyde, 1997; Lightfoot & Kennedy, 2006). It can be recorded relatively quickly in cooperative individuals, and is highly repeatable from one test-session to another (Tremblay, Billings, Friesen, & Souza, 2006). Two additional strengths of the P1-N1-P2 are: (1) it provides information about the neural encoding of sound beyond the brainstem. Based on animal and human experiments, P1 and N1 responses reflect voltage changes in the auditory cortex (Ross & Tremblay, 2009; Steinschneider et al., 1994), and (2) it can be elicited by more ecologically relevant stimuli than clicks (e.g., temporal envelope of words) (for a review see Martin, Korczak, & Tremblay, 2008). For these reasons, CAEPs such as the P1-N1-P2 have been used to study the effects of hearing aid amplification on the neural representation of different speech sounds within the human CAS, and many investigators have documented that it is possible to deliver stimuli in sound field and reliably record the P1-N1-P2 complex while wearing a hearing aid (Billings et al., 2007; Tremblay et al., 2006a, 2006b). However, just as the ABR is highly influenced by the stimulus level, rise-time, rate, and duration, so too is the P1-N1-P2 response. This means unintended variables can become present when the sounds used to evoke neural activity are processed through hearing aid or implant devices.

P1-N1-P2 evoked potentials have been recorded in children and adults with varying degrees of hearing loss (Gravel, Kurtzberg, Stapells, Vaughan, & Wallace, 1989; Korczak, Kurtzberg, & Stapells, 2005; Rapin & Graziani, 1967; Stapells & Kurtzberg, 1991). Without amplification, the evoked neural response pattern is typically delayed or absent. With amplification, an aided neural response pattern can sometimes be seen but results have been inconsistent.

Why the inconsistency? One option is to interpret these results within the realm of plasticity, with absent responses indicating insufficient transmission of sound to the cortex resulting from inadequate audibility, or impaired neural processing. Another option is to examine the contribution of the hearing aid device to the recordings. Once again, hearing aids modify the physical characteristics of sound, and hearing aids introduce noise, compress signals, and alter the frequency content of the signal. When evoked potentials are generated by sound delivered through a hearing aid, the effects of hearing aid processing on the physical characteristics of the sound also affects the evoked neural response pattern. Recent evidence by Billings and colleagues shows why it is important to consider the interaction between the device and CAEPS and how erroneous conclusions about CAS function can result (Figure 6–3).

In a series of experiments, Billings et al. examined the effects of hearing aid amplification on CAEPs and found that P1-N1-P2 responses do not reliably reflect hearing aid gain (Billings et al., 2007, 2009, 2011; Tremblay et al., 2006). Peak latencies and amplitudes of the P1-N1-P2 response are, in the unaided and normally hearing ear, earlier and larger with increasing stimulus level (see Figure 6–3). Shorter latencies imply faster conduction time and larger amplitudes imply increased neural synchrony or the recruitment of additional neural tissue responding to the stimulus. Such latency-intensity functions are evident even with small intensity steps (e.g., 2 dB). But when Billings et al. (2007) increased the signal level by 20 dB, through the gain of the hearing aid, peak latencies and amplitudes were unaffected. Similar phenomena are reported by Marynewich, Small, and Stapells (2010). One explanation for the lack of amplification effect comes from the information obtained from acoustic recordings made at the output of the hearing aid, in the ear canal. Not only did these probe microphone recordings verify that the hearing aid was in fact amplifying the level of the signal by approximately 20 dB, it also showed an increase in the level of noise floor (presumably generated by the microphone and other internal circuitry). This means the signal-to-noise ratio (SNR) was similar with and without amplification. Cortical neurons in cats have been shown to be driven more by SNR than absolute signal level (Phillips, 1985; Phillips & Kelly, 1992), and follow up studies by Billings et al. (2009, 2010, 2011) confirm this also to be true in humans. So while the absence of change (in peak latencies or amplitudes) could be interpreted to mean a lack of neuroplasticity related to sound transmission, from the ear to the brain, an alternative explanation is that the pattern of evoked neural activity reflects the individual signal processing strategies of the device (e.g., changes in SNR) rather than brain plasticity. Here we have described the known effects of SNR, but there are other potential interactions to consider. For example, little is known about how the effects of automatic gain controls on the rise time of the signal or the stability of the acoustic content over time can influence evoked neural patterns.

Taken together, the ABR and CAEP studies described above demonstrate some of the pitfalls that can take place when one records these brain responses when sound is processed by a hearing aid. Inferences drawn from peak latencies and amplitudes

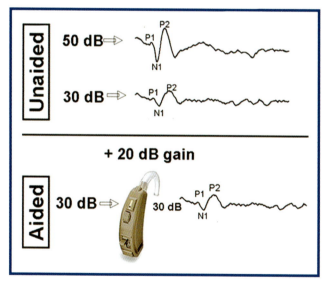

Figure 6–3. P1-N1-P2 peaks are earlier in latency and larger in amplitude when evoked by a 50 dB SPL signal compared to a 30 dB SPL signal (*top panel*). But when a 30 dB signal is processed through a hearing aid, and 20 dB of gain is provided, the resultant waveform does not reflect the increase in signal level (*bottom panel*). Despite the fact that a 50 dB signal is being transmitted to the cochlea, the aided waveform still appears similar in morphology to the response elicited by the 30 dB signal.

are heavily influenced by device settings, rather than independent neural processes. Shifts in latency, or changes in response amplitude could therefore be mistaken for enhanced neuroplastic activity if device variables are not controlled for. It is for this reason little is directly known about the CAS plasticity in relation to hearing aid amplification in humans, and the use of ABR or CAEPs to estimate aided hearing sensitivity is discouraged. Clinicians need be aware of these cautions because evoked potential systems are being marketed for specifically this purpose, to estimate aided thresholds using the P1-N1-P2 response (Munro et al., 2011). One emerging direction is the use of auditory steady state responses (Picton et al., 1998) as well as frequency following responses (see Skoe & Kraus, 2010 for a review). It is too early to speculate how these evoked responses might be used in the clinic, or to examine neuroplastic effects associated with amplification, but an encouraging note is that the brainstem appears to be driven less by SNR than absolute noise level (Burkard & Hecox, 1983).

Cochlear Implants and the CAS. Similar recording problems can occur when stimuli are delivered in sound field and processed by a cochlear implant. Like hearing aids, cochlear implants have a microphone and automatic gain controls. After going through the speech processor, the signal is directed to selected locations (channels) along an electrode array that differ both in place-pitch mapping as well as current intensity. Although SNR is likely not to be as problematic when testing implant users if the level of noise is not audible to the listener, CAEP latency and amplitude values are known to be affected by the number of channels that are active (Friesen et al., 2009), the electrode location being stimulated (Brown et al., 2008), as well as the stimulus type, level and rate (Davids, Papsin, Valero, & Gordon, 2008a, 2008b; Firszt, 2002a, 2002b; Kim, Brown, et al., 2009; Xiaxio, 2010). This means interpretation of CAEP results become complicated because speech processor settings influence waveform morphology and these settings vary widely from one cochlear implant user to the next. Moreover, all cochlear implant speech processors are inherently nonlinear. An increase in the level of an acoustic signal presented in the sound field may or may not translate into a change

in the amount of current provided by the cochlear implant. As a result, latencies and amplitudes may be expected to vary significantly from patient to patient in response to the same set of stimuli, regardless of speech intelligibility or neuroplastic status. These problems are more manageable during longitudinal studies if implant settings are accounted for and/or held constant. However, cross-sectional designs are more cumbersome because CAEPs are averaged across individuals who are wearing different devices. Each individual wears and implant that is programmed differently and these implant settings influence CAEP latencies and amplitudes regardless of intended variable under investigation.

One way to minimize the influence of individual cochlear implant speech processor settings is to bypass the speech processor and use programs (e.g., Nucleus Implant Communicator) to control the output of the implant directly. An advantage of this approach is that the evoking pulse train is so short that overlapping artifacts contaminating the ABR and CAEP can be avoided. With that said, saturation of the recording amplifier, and hence stimulus artifact can still often remain a problem, even with fast-recovery amplifiers. A limitation of direct stimulation is the limited types of stimuli that can be used. Nevertheless, there is convincing evidence to suggest stimulation-related plasticity takes place following implantation (Ponton et al., 1996; see Gordon et al., 2011, for a review). There is converging evidence that neural response patterns change over time, following implantation. The outcomes of hearing aid amplification are less clear.

Acclimatization or Auditory Learning?

In separate but eventually converging discussions, audiologists, neuroscientists and hearing aid experts joined together to talk about the concepts of neuroplasticity, and how they might relate to people with hearing loss. It was in 1995 that the 1st Eriksholm Workshop on Auditory Deprivation and Acclimatization was held in Copenhagen. As the title of the conference would suggest, clinicians and scientists came together to consider the impact of auditory deprivation and acclimatization for clinical practice and research design and the conference proceedings were published in *Ear and Hearing* (Arlinger et al.,

1996). It was then that the concepts of auditory deprivation were discussed on a global scale, crossing disciplines to facilitate a consensus. One definition that came out of the meeting was the meaning of "acclimatization," the notion that systematic changes in auditory performance take place as a result of changes in acoustic information available to the listener (for reviews see Neuman, 2005; Palmer, Nelson, & Lindley, 1998; Turner, Humes, Bentler, & Cox, 1996). In the case of hearing aid users, this would involve an improvement in performance that could not be attributed purely to task, procedural, or training effects (Arlinger et al., 1996). A presumption was that auditory stimulation, through the use of a hearing aid, was contributing to perceptual changes that could not merely be attributed to increased experience with testing materials. Inferences linking improved perception to stimulation-related plasticity were needed. This line of research became popular for two reasons: First, if perceptual and physiologic changes took place over time, clinicians wanted to know if there was an ideal time window to determine hearing aid benefit (Gatehouse & Killion, 1993). Manufacturers provide 30-day trial periods and there was concern that this time window might not be sufficient for some people to realize their full potential with a hearing aid. A second motivating factor had to do with the emerging concept of auditory plasticity. Was there evidence of acclimatization and, if so, what physiologic mechanisms might underlie any observed perceptual gains (Willott, 1996)?

Incidental reports have been made of changes in real-life gain preferences and comfortable loudness levels across time after being fit with a new hearing aid (Keidser et al. 2008), as well as changes in acoustic reflex thresholds thought to reflect brainstem neuroplasticity (Munro, 2007a, 2007b ; Philibert, 2005). However, for the most part, the reported effects of hearing aid acclimatization originally presented by Gatehouse and colleagues in the early 1990s have not been replicated (Bentler, Neibuhr, Getta, & Anderson, 1993; Humes, Halling, & Coughlin, 1996; Humes, Wilson, Barlow, & Garner, 2002; Munro & Lutman, 2000; Saunders & Cienkowski, 1997; Surr, Cord, & Walden, 1998; Taylor, 1993). The concept of acclimatization among hearing aid users was finally put to rest by a series of a studies by Humes et al. (2002) when they tracked perceptual measures

among hearing aid users following 1, 2, and 3 years of hearing aid use (Humes & Wilson, 2003). They used several objective tests of speech recognition, as well as self-assessment measures, to evaluate hearing aid benefit over time. In short, there was no overwhelming evidence of hearing aid acclimatization. The greatest gains appeared to come from the immediate change of making previously inaudible signals audible. Taken together, these results suggest that even if stimulation-related plasticity is taking place in the CAS following hearing aid amplification, it does not appear to manifest itself as functionally significant gains in performance (e.g., speech in noise measures, self-assessment measures). This means, in the absence of targeted therapy (e.g., auditory training), fitting people with hearing aids and sending them out to interact in the real auditory world does not appear to result in gradual benefit over time. For this reason the concept of hearing aid acclimatization is generally accepted to be nonexistent or too small to measure in hearing aid users (Turner & Bentler, 1998).

In contrast to the hearing aid literature, there is support in favor of acclimatization among implant users. It might be that the impact of going from hearing something, to something different (as is the case for hearing aid users), is less drastic a change, making it more difficult to measure, than going from nothing to something (as is the case of implant users). Longitudinal studies suggest it can take up to 30 to 40 months following cochlear implantation for some individuals to make maximal use of their hearing prosthesis (Ruffin et al., 2007; Tye-Murray et al., 1992; Tyler et al.,1997). Physiologic changes have been documented in the CAS of implanted humans and animals and they can take place quite rapidly following implantation (see Eggermont, 2008, and Gordon, Wong, et al., 2011, for reviews). For example, when cortical evoked potentials (P1 and N1) are used to quantify neural conduction time in CI users of different ages, a hallmark finding is that "time in sound" drives changes in the central auditory system (Ponton et al., 1996). When CI users, regardless of their chronological age, wore their implant for 1 year (1-year time in sound), P1 latencies resembled those of a normal hearing 1-year-old infant. This finding suggests that the parts of the auditory system generating the long-latency CAEP components, the planum temporale, are arrested in development when deafness occurs (Kral & Eggermont, 2007). When the CI is activated the maturation starts up again and continues from where it was at the time of onset of deafness. There do appear to be limits, however. According to the longitudinal data of Ponton and Eggermont (2001), a 3-year deprivation of sound under the age of 6 appears to be too long to develop the appropriate CAEPs even in young adulthood.

The idea that there might be "limits" to physiologic changes raises many questions relevant to the rehabilitation of people who wear implants. First, does the absence of a response, or delayed peak latencies, mean *abnormal perception* will result? Second, do other intervention methods (e.g., auditory training) reduce or remove these limits and so promote those methods? To answer the first question, the predictive relation between human communication and the presence and latency of P1 and N1 needs to be known. But, unfortunately, the sensitivity and specificity of P1 and N1 responses to speech and language performance are not known. Sensitivity and specificity are part of a statistical classification system that is used when considering the implementation of diagnostic tools into clinical medicine. In this case, a sensitive measure would mean delayed peak latencies are effective markers of people with abnormal speech and language function. Specificity would mean these same peak latencies do not erroneously identify people with normal speech and language function as being disordered. In adults, there are ample examples of abnormal P1's in populations (e.g., alcoholics) who do not have perceptual problems (Kathmann et al., 1996; Maurage et al., 2008, 2009), and normal P1 and N1 responses in older adults who do have speech perception difficulties (Tremblay et al., 2002, 2003). These isolated examples are used to emphasize the point that the clinical sensitivity and specificity of P1, N1, and P2 responses have not yet been established. Therefore, any clinical judgment that involves these particular CAEPs must be made with caution, knowing full well that a person's individual results depend on the stimulus type being used, the rate of presentation, as well as the means of presentation.

With that said, the previously discussed Ponton et al. (1996, 2001) studies serve as exemplars in implant research. The stimuli were delivered directly to the electrode array, bypassing the implant processor, so implant settings did not likely confound the latency and amplitude of the described CAEPs. With these controls in mind, it can be confidently stated that (re)introducing sound to a previously deprived auditory system has neuroplastic effects in the human auditory system. What's more, there is emerging evidence of cross-modal plasticity whereby the introduction of sound, via the implant, affects visual processing as well (Buckley, 2011; Meredith et al., 2011). However, when auditory stimuli are presented in sound field, and processor controls affecting stimulus level and location are not reported or held constant (Purdy et al., 2001; Sharma et al., 2002), it is very well possible that neural response patterns reflect device- rather than experience-related changes in brain activity.

To summarize, despite the number of experiments aimed to address issues of acclimatization and learning among people who wear hearing aids and cochlear implants, few have taken into the account the effect of the device. When sounds are presented in sound field, and processed by a device, device settings should be described and accounted for. With these points in mind, arguments in support of behavioral and physiologic evidence of "acclimatization" can be made. For hearing aids, this is not the case. Many of the perceptual changes previously thought to reflect neuroplastic processes resulting from hearing aid use have since been attributed to changes in audibility related to hearing aid gain.

Question 3

How do the concepts of sound exposure relate to second language learning? Can you learn another language by merely listening to language training tapes?

Answer 3

The key word here is "listening." Auditory scientists distinguish between *passive* "hearing" and *active* "listening." Even under anesthesia, the auditory system responds to sounds, but the responses become progressively more sluggish as the system is ascended, from the cochlea to the cortex. Without arousal, attention and memory the cortex, the "listening brain," doesn't work. Effective listening and learning require engagement with the task. Little wonder then that people make the most dramatic advances with second language (L2) learning when they are forced to use L2 continuously in their daily lives, both in and outside their home, in order to have any social communication.

TRAINING AND THE BRAIN

Hearing Loss

If there is no evidence of acclimatization among hearing aid users, and the satisfaction rate among users is little more than half, this means that the auditory needs of many people are not being met. For some patients, simply providing appropriate hearing aids and sending them out into the real world might be sufficient; others, however, could benefit from rehabilitation sessions that include auditory training.

The concept of auditory training as a means of auditory rehabilitation is not new. Focused listening training involving auditory and/or visual cues was a foundation of the audiologic profession back in the 1950s (Kricos & McCarthy, 2007) but the cost effectiveness of auditory listening therapy was scrutinized and the reliance on emerging technology as a form of intervention gave way. As a result, the focus of many clinicians shifted away from one-on-one rehabilitation/counseling sessions to simply dispensing hearing aid devices. According to Kricos, in 1980 the number of audiologists who reported providing auditory training services in the United States was 31%. By 1990, the number decreased to 16% (Schow, Balsara, Smedley, & Whitcomb, 1993).

Although the practice and interest in auditory training waned, the concept of plasticity became a hot topic among neuroscientists. As briefly described in the earlier section describing history and definition of plasticity, what was previously thought to be a hardwired system was shown to exhibit changes as a function of experience. Bakin and Weinberger (1990), for example, were among the first to show that classical conditioning induced specific receptive field plasticity in the auditory cortex of the guinea pig. With a new perspective, scientists began to question the role of plasticity in relation to hearing loss and if it would be possible to exploit neuroplastic properties of the brain in a way that could improve perception. One possibility would be to stimulate changes in the brain that would promote learning (Robinson & Summerfield, 1996).

Since that time, there has been a resurgence of auditory training programs in audiology clinics. Some are designed intentionally for hearing aid users, others for implants. Regardless of the intended population, training programs typically emphasize bottom-up (analytical) processing and/or synthetic (top-down) strategies (Sweetow & Palmer, 2005). Analytic training emphasizes the acoustic content (spectral, temporal, and intensity cues) of the signal, and involves tasks aimed at identifying or discriminating sounds that differ acoustically. A premise of this type of training is that training alters the physiologic representation of the acoustic content of the signal in a way that enhances perception. Synthetic training is designed to improve perception by enhancing a person's ability to attend, integrate, and use contextual information. Both approaches have been used extensively in the audiology community and a special issue on this topic can be found in the journal *Seminars in Hearing* (2006). A more recent example includes the work Burk and Humes (2008) who have shown that laboratory-based auditory training exercises can improve the perception of older hearing aid users and that these gains can be retained for months.

Decades ago, auditory training programs consisted of face-to-face interactions between the clinician and patient. The listening tasks often involved auditory-visual interaction exercises and practice sessions expanded beyond typical clinical environments to real world noisy situations. As computers became available, there was a shift to designing home-based, self-directed training programs. An assumption was that home-based programs could reach a broader population. They would be less expensive to the patient and health care systems because neither clinicians nor insurance or government reimbursement would be involved. Moreover, home-based training programs were thought to promote greater patient compliance, because people could exercise their hearing at their own convenience. Two examples of training programs that have made their way into the U.S. clinical market are: (1) Listening and Communication Enhancement (LACE—manufactured by Neurotone Inc.), and (2) Computer Assisted Speech Testing (CAST) and its more recent offspring, SEAT (Sound Express Auditory Training), both produced by Tiger Speech Technology. LACE was designed with hearing aid users in mind and includes both synthetic and analytic components. The computer based version features training sessions involving speech in noise, rapid speech, competing speech, and auditory memory in a sentence-based context. Sweetow and Sabes (2006) have reported behavioral improvements in ability to understand speech in noise, as well as a small but significant reduction in perception of handicap after one month of training. Remarkable gains have also been seen for implant users who have participated in CAST training programs (Fu & Galvin, 2007). A strength of these two sample training approaches is that the investigators attempt to examine an association between statistically significant gains in performance on the training task to significant reductions in hearing handicap. Moreover, unlike the many published training experiments, CAST and LACE investigators go beyond traditional group comparisons to further understand who, on an individual basis, benefits from training and who does not. They also recognize through their science the importance of developing a clinical treatment that should generalize to situations outside the laboratory in a way that positively impacts a patient's quality of life. However, a remaining weakness of most training science is defining the effective component of training. Do analytical-type training programs really alter the physiologic representation of the trained acoustic cue? Or is it that focused attention on any type of auditory material is sufficient to alter neural function and perception? Taking this point even further, there is almost no effectiveness research to guide clinicians. Boothroyd (2010) defines even more gaps in knowledge when assessing the current status of auditory training programs as they relate to rehabilitating people with hearing loss.

To answer these questions, a collective effort among scientists and clinicians is to characterize the components of training programs (e.g., stimulus exposure, task and procedural learning, attention, memory and intelligence) as they relate to perceptual learning. In the case of implants, physiological correlates of auditory learning are being explored using vocoded speech, so that magnets need not enter the fMRI scanners (Eisner et al., 2010). Three seminal papers demonstrate the ways in which presumptions are being challenged. First are the findings of Preminger and Ziegler (2008) who used group-based training sessions to improve auditory-only and auditory-visual speech perception. Despite no statistically significant changes in performance on speech measures following training, participants did report a statistically significant improvement on a quality of life measure. These results suggest that hearing handicap can be improved from group training sessions but they are not necessarily the result of the intended analytical and synthetic components aimed at improving speech perception. Second are the findings of Amitay, Irwin, and Moore (2006) who reported improved discrimination ability among normal hearing adults when the stimuli being "learned" were identical to one another. Their results highlight the contribution of nonauditory and nonanalytic components to the perception of auditory stimuli and raise many provocative questions about the role of attention, and decision-making (Micheyl, McDermott, & Oxenham, 2009) associated with auditory learning. A third paradigm shift comes from a series of human physiological studies that show mere stimulus exposure, as well as interacting with the stimuli through the use of a task, alters the way sound is represented in the brain (Tremblay et al., 2010). These physiological changes appear not to reflect the sensory (analytic) aspects of sound, as initially intended, and do not coincide with improved perception. Instead, perceptual gains appear to require the combination of stimulus exposure, goal directed instructions, task execution, and feedback (Tremblay et al. 2011). Collectively, these sorts of information are not only helping to define normal aspects involved in auditory perceptual learning, but also raising new questions about hearing disorders. One such example involves the diagnosis of "auditory processing disorders" (APD). There is new evidence that the roots of communication problems in children diagnosed with this disorder might not be entirely "auditory." They might involve attention, cognition, (Moore et al., 2010) or a host of neurologically deficient sound consolidation processes in the absence of goal directed learning.

Question 4

If musical training helps with so many aspects of perception, would you suggest children diagnosed with APD receive musical training?

Answer 4

This seems a very sensible suggestion. Current APD management strategies highlight environmental optimization and some form of auditory training. Improving the listening environment is a "no brainer"—we need good signal-to-noise to hear. Auditory training is much more controversial. But across the whole spectrum of "brain training," opinion is coming around to the view that, first, it can be very effective (e.g., stroke rehabilitation) and, second, it is mainly or solely due to "top-down" influences of cognitive processes on the traditional auditory system. Improving sensorimotor-related cognition in general appears to be critically dependent on large amounts of highly engaging and challenging training. The focus and dedication of sports stars honing their amazing skills is testimony to this. Musical training has also long been associated with protracted effort that, like sports training, offers rewards in terms of mastery of an inherently satisfying activity, and even a livelihood. If children with APD, listening difficulties, can be encouraged from a young age to embrace musical training, current scientific evidence strongly suggests the benefits both for listening and general cognitive skills could extend beyond those offered by any other form of "intervention."

Disorders That Do Not Involve Compromised Stimulus Audibility

Children who are diagnosed with APD present an array of different symptoms and can be labeled in various ways. Sometimes the symptoms are considered to be part of a central auditory processing disorder (CAPD). According to the National Institutes of Health (http://www.nidcd.nih.gov/health/voice/auditory.html), other frequently used terms include auditory perception problems, auditory comprehension deficits, central auditory dysfunction, central deafness, and "word deafness." Auditory processing difficulties are also closely associated with conditions such as dyslexia, attention deficit disorder, autism spectrum disorder, specific language impairment, pervasive developmental disorder, or developmental delay (Ferguson et al., 2011; Sharma et al., 2009, making it difficult to disentangle causes and effects. For this reason the term APD has been misapplied to children who have no hearing or language disorder but have challenges in learning.

Descriptions of APD vary from country to country and from profession to profession. According to the National Institutes of Health, children with APD are described as being unable to recognize subtle differences between sounds in words, even though the sounds themselves are loud and clear. There is no known peripheral pathology to account for these difficulties, and no known treatment. Instead clinicians try to manage the symptoms, including problems remembering information presented orally, difficulty carrying out multistep directions, and poor listening skills in general. One such approach is the use of auditory training exercises. Auditory processing difficulties underlying language impairments have been suggested to be primarily a temporal processing disorder (Merzenich et al., 1996). Subsequently, training programs were designed to enhance the neural representation of the rapidly changing acoustic cues contained in speech (Merzenich, Jenkins et al., 1996) to help remediate the auditory difficulties thought to underlie speech and language disorders. However, the "temporal processing hypothesis" has been challenged (for a review see Moore, Halliday, & Amitay, 2009) and emerging evidence shows that multimodal and cognitive factors including attention, motivation, and intelligence are more likely to underpin APD (Moore et al., 2010).

There is, nevertheless, a plethora of evidence to suggest that auditory training, in various forms, can change the neural encoding of sound (for reviews see Kraus & Skoe, 2010; Tremblay, 2006). Perceptual gains following training are sometimes seen in children diagnosed with APD (Moncrieff & Wertz, 2008). However, precisely what is being altered with training remains a topic of debate. To address this issue it is necessary to revisit the topic of perceptual learning in general, beyond children with learning and language disorders.

Auditory perceptual learning has long been examined in populations of normally hearing people. Examples include second language learning, musician training, as well as auditory memory training in aging adults. In all instances, perceptual gains associated with training have been observed. Shahin et al. (2005) for example showed enhanced electrophysiologic responses in musicians when evoked by sounds (e.g., piano) that the musicians were trained on. More surprising, however, are findings that music training benefits auditory processing not only in the musical domain, but also in the processing of speech stimuli (Musacchia et al., 2007; Schon, Magne, & Besson, 2004; Wong, Skoe, Russo, Dees, & Kraus, 2007). Relative to nonmusicians, musicians also show more robust encoding of timing and pitch features in speech signals at the level of the brainstem (for a review, see Chandrasekaran & Kraus, 2010). Music training also has been shown to improve working memory (Forgeard, Winner, et al., 2008; Jakobson, Lewycky, Kilgour, & Stoesz, 2008; Parbery-Clark, Skoe, Lam, et al., 2009), attention (Strait et al., 2010; Tervaniemi et al., 2009), and executive function (Bialystok & DePape, 2009) abilities. Collectively, these findings could be used to argue that speech stimuli need not be used to enhance speech communication, and that interacting with sound can result in perceptual gains that involve more than just audition.

In the human auditory system, speech sound training experiments have been used to show that neural response patterns can change quite rapidly (Alain, 2010; Ben-David et al., 2009; Ross & Tremblay, 2009; Tremblay et al., 1998), precede changes in perception, and are retained for months (Trem-

blay et al., 2010). Even more impressive, Skoe and Kraus (2010) have been able to show that incoming stimuli are constantly being monitored, even when the stimulus is physically invariant and attention is directed elsewhere. These real-time transformations are thought to subserve humans' strong disposition for grouping auditory objects, and likely reflect corticofugal modulations.

Question 5

Is it appropriate to use the term "plasticity" for purely behavioral observations of learning or compensation to injury, in the absence of evidence that structural brain changes occurred that clearly underlie these behavioral changes?

Answer 5

The answer depends on how the reader chooses to define plasticity. If the assumed definition is simply the "capacity for change," then the term plasticity is relevant to all aspects of behavioral changes given that all aspects of behavior are presumed to be mediated by structural and/or chemical changes in the brain. If there is no evidence of brain change, null effects might be explained by the tool being insensitive or inappropriate for the neural processes involved.

CONCLUSIONS

The adult brain used to be considered a hard-wired neural network, at least by neuroscientists, but is now widely accepted to be a malleable computing system. The infant brain is even more malleable, and even prenatal auditory experience is thought to influence the way in which it will develop. As neuroscientists attempt to define how, where, and why neuroplasticity takes place, clinicians exploit these principles in ways that can improve perception. At the same time, they encounter every day in their clinics unique examples of neuroplasticity at work. Sometimes, but all too infrequently, those examples inform discovery science in a process of reverse translation. Whether it is to define normal processes associated with perceptual learning, or to remediate disorders, bench and clinical sciences are part of the same research continuum.

FURTHER READINGS

Chen, Z., Haykin, S., Eggermont, J. J., & Becker, S. (2007). *Correlative learning: A basis for brain and adaptive systems.* Wiley series on adaptive and learning systems for signal processing, communications, and control. Hoboken, NJ: John Wiley & Sons.

Irvine, D. E. F. (2010). Plasticity of the auditory pathway. In Adrian Rees and Alan Palmer (Eds.), *The Oxford handbook of auditory science — the auditory brain.* Oxford, UK: Oxford University Press.

REFERENCES

Alain, C., Campeanu, S., & Tremblay, K. (2010). Changes in sensory evoked responses coincide with rapid improvement in speech identification performance. *Journal of Cognitive Neuroscience, 22,* 392–403.

Amitay, S., Irwin, A., & Moore, D. (2006). Discrimination learning induced by training with identical stimuli. *Nature Neuroscience, 9,* 1446–1448.

Arlinger, S., Gatehouse, S., Bentler, R. A., Byrne, R. A., Cox, D., & Dirks, R. M .(1996). Report of the Eriksholm Workshop on auditory deprivation and acclimatization. *Ear and Hearing, 17,* 87S–98S.

Bakin, J. S., & Weinberger, N. M. (1990). Classical conditioning induces CS-specific receptive field plasticity in the auditory cortex of the guinea pig. *Brain Research, 536,* 271–286.

Barry, S. R. (2009). *Fixing my gaze.* New York, NY: Basic Books.

Beauchaine, K. A., Gorga, M. P., Reiland, J. K., & Larson, L. L. (1986). Application of ABRs to the hearing aid selection process: Preliminary data. *Journal of Speech and Hearing Research, 29,* 120–128.

Ben-David, B. M., Campeanu, S., Tremblay, K.L., & Alain, C. (2009). Auditory evoked potentials dissociate rapid perceptual learning from task repetition without learning. *Psychophysiology, 48,* 797–807.

Bentler, R. A., Niebuhr, D. P., Getta, J. P., & Anderson, C. V. (1993). Longitudinal study of hearing aid effectiveness II: Subjective measures. *Journal of Speech and Hearing Research, 36,* 820–831.

Bialystok, E., & DePape, A. M. (2009). Musical expertise, bilingualism, and executive functioning. *Journal of Experimental Psychology: Human Perception and Performance, 35,* 565–574.

Billings, C. J., Tremblay, K. L., & Miller, C. W. (2011). Aided cortical auditory evoked potentials in response to changes in hearing aid gain. *International Journal of Audiology, 50,* 459–467.

Billings, C. J., Tremblay, K. L., Souza, P. E., & Binns, M. A. (2007). Effects of hearing aid amplification and stimulus intensity on cortical auditory evoked potentials. *Audiology and Neurotology, 12,* 234–246.

Billings, C. J., Tremblay, K. L., Stecker, G. C., & Tolin, W. M. (2009). Human evoked cortical activity to signal-to-noise ratio and absolute signal level. *Hearing Research, 254,* 15–24.

Bishop, C. E., & Eby, T. L. (2010). The current status of audiologic rehabilitation for profound unilateral sensorineural hearing loss. *Laryngoscope, 120,* 552–556.

Boothroyd, A. (2010). Adapting to changed hearing. The potential role of formal training. *Journal of the American Academy of Audiology, 9,* 601–611.

Born, D. E., & Rubel, E. W. (1985). Afferent influences on brain stem auditory nuclei of the chicken: Neuron number and size following cochlea removal. *Journal of Comparative Neurology, 231,* 435–445.

Burk, M. H., & Humes, L. E. (2008). Effects of long-term training on aided speech-recognition performance in noise in older adults. *Journal of Speech Language and Hearing Research. 51,* 759–771.

Brion, J. P., Demeurisse, G., & Capon, A. (1989). Evidence of cortical reorganization in hemiparetic patients. *Journal of the American Heart Association, 20,* 1079–1084.

Brown, C. J., Etler, C S., He, S., O'Brien, S., Erenberg, J. R., Kim, A., Dhuldhoya, N. &, Abbas, P. J. (2008). The electrically evoked auditory change complex: Preliminary results from nucleus cochlear implant users. *Ear and Hearing, 29,* 704–717.

Brugge, J. F. Orman, S. S., Coleman, J. R., Chan, J. C. K., & Phillips, D. P. (1985). Binaural interactions in cortical area AI of cats reared with unilateral atresia of the external ear canal. *Hearing Research, 20,* 275–287.

Buckley, K. A., & Tobey, E. A. (2011). Cross-modal plasticity and speech perception in pre- and postlingually deaf cochlear implant users. *Ear and Hearing, 32,* 2–15.

Buckner, R. L., Corbetta, M., Schatz, J., Raichle, M. E., & Petersen, S. E. (1996). Preserved speech abilities and compensation following prefrontal damage. *Proceedings of the National Academy of Sciences of the United States of America, 93,* 1249–1253.

Burkard, R., & Hecox, K. (1983). The effect of broadband noise on the human brainstem auditory evoked response. I. Rate and intensity effects. *Journal of the Acoustical Society of America, 74,* 1204–1213.

Campos Viola, F., Thorne, J., Edmonds, B., Schneider, T., Eichele, T., & Debener, S. (2009). Semi-automatic identification of independent components representing EEG artifact. *Clinical Neurophysiology, 120,* 868–877.

Castañeda-Villa, N., Manuel Cornejo-Cruz, J., & James, C. (2010). Independent component analysis for robust assessment of auditory system maturation in children with cochlear implants. *Cochlear Implants International, 11*(2), 71–83.

Chandrasekaran, B., & Kraus, N. (2010). Music, noise-exclusion, and learning. *Music Perception, 27,* 297–306.

Charles, E., Bishop, AuD., & Eby, T. L. (2010). The current status of audiologic rehabilitation for profound unilateral sensorineural hearing loss. *Laryngoscope, 120,* 552–556.

Clopton, B. M., & Silverman, M. S. (1977). Plasticity of binaural interaction II. Critical period and changes in midline response. *Journal of Neurophysiology, 40,* 1275–1280.

Cramer, S. C. (2008a). Repairing the human brain after stroke: I. Mechanisms of spontaneous recovery. *Annals of Neurology, 63,* 272–287.

Cramer, S. C. (2008b). Repairing the human brain after stroke. II. Restorative therapies. *Annals of Neurology, 63,* 549–560.

Dahmen, J. C., & King, A. J. (2007). Learning to hear: Plasticity of auditory cortical processing. *Current Opinion in Neurobiology, 17,* 456–464.

Davids, T., Valero, J., Papsin, B. C., Harrison, R. V., & Gordon, K. A. (2008a). Effects of stimulus manipulation on electrophysiological responses of pediatric cochlear implant users. Part II: Rate effects. *Ear and Hearing, 244,* 15–24.

Davids, T., Valero, J., Papsin, B. C., Harrison, R. V., & Gordon, K. A. (2008b). Effects of stimulus manipulation on electrophysiological responses of pediatric cochlear implant users. Part I: Duration effects. *Ear and Hearing, 244,* 7–14.

Davidson, S. A., Wall, L. G., & Goodman, C. M. 1990. Preliminary studies on the use of an ABR amplitude projection procedure for hearing aid selection. *Ear and Hearing, 11,* 332–339.

Davis, A., Smith, P., Ferguson, M., Stephens, D., & Gianopoulos, I. (2007). Acceptability, benefit and costs of early screening for hearing disability: A study of potential screening tests and models. *Health Technology Assessment, 11,* 1–294.

de Boer, J., & Thornton, A. R. D. (2008). Neural correlates of perceptual learning in the auditory brainstem: Efferent activity predicts and reflects improvement at a speech-in-noise discrimination task. *Journal of Neuroscience, 28,* 4929–4937.

Debener, S., Mullinger, K. J., Niazy, R. K., & Bowtell, R. W. (2008). Properties of the ballistocardiogram artefact as revealed by EEG recordings at 1.5, 3 and 7 T static magnetic field strength. *Journal of Psychophysiology, 67,* 189–199.

Dhooge, I. J. (2003). Risk factors for the development of otitis media. *Current Allergy and Asthma Reports, 3,* 321–325.

Draganski, B., Gaser, C., Busch, V., Schuierer, G., Bogdahn, U., & May, A. (2004). Neuroplasticity: Changes in grey matter induced by training. *Nature, 427,* 311–312.

Eggermont, J. J. (1990). *The correlative brain.* Berlin, Heidelberg: Springer-Verlag.

Eggermont, J. J. (2008). The role of sound in adult and developmental auditory cortical plasticity. *Ear and Hearing. 29,* 819–829.

Eisner, F., McGettigan, C., Faulkner, A., Rosen, S., Scott, S. K. (2010). Inferior frontal gyrus activation predicts individual differences in perceptual learning of cochlear-implant simulations. *Journal of Neuroscience, 30,* 7179–7186.

Ferguson, M. A., Hall, R. L., Riley, A., & Moore, D. R. (2011). Communication, listening, speech and cognition in children diagnosed with auditory processing disorder (APD) or specific language impairment (SLI). *Journal of Speech, Language and Hearing Research, 54,* 211–227.

Firszt, J. B., Chambers, R. D., & Kraus, N. (2002b). Neurophysiology of cochlear implant users II: Comparison among speech perception, dynamic range, and physiological measures. *Ear and Hearing, 6,* 516–531.

Firszt, J. B., Chambers, R. D., & Kraus, N., & Reeder, R. M. (2002a). Neurophysiology of cochlear implant users I: effects of stimulus current level and electrode site on the electrical ABR, MLR, and N1-P2 response. *Ear and Hearing, 23,* 502–515.

Forgeard, M., Winner, E., Norton, A., & Schlaug, G. (2008). Practicing a musical instrument in childhood is associated with enhanced verbal ability and nonverbal reasoning. *PLoS One, 3,* e3566.

Formby, C., Sherlock, L. P., & Gold, S. L. (2003). Adaptive plasticity of loudness induced by chronic attenuation and enhancement of the acoustic background. *Journal of the Acoustical Society of America, 114,* 55–58.

Friesen, L. M., & Picton, T. W. (2010). A method for removing cochlear implant artifact. *Hearing Research, 259,* 95–106.

Friesen, L. M., Tremblay, K. L., Rohila, N., Wright, R. A., Shannon, R. V. Baskent, D., & Rubinstein, J. T. (2009). Evoked cortical activity and speech recognition as a function of the number of simulated cochlear implant channels. *Clinical Neurophysiology, 120,* 776–782.

Fu, Q. J., & Galvin, J. J., III. (2007). Perceptual learning and auditory training in cochlear implant recipients. *Trends in Amplification, 11,* 193–205.

Gatehouse, S. (1993). Role of perceptual acclimatization in the selection of frequency responses for hearing aids. *Journal of the American Academy of Audiology, 4,* 296–306. Retrieved from http://www.ncbi.nlm.nih.gov/entrez/query.fcgi?cmd=Retrieve&db=pubmed&dopt=Abstract&list_uids=8219296

Gatehouse, S., & Killion, M. C. (1993). HABRAT: Hearing aid benefit accommodation time. *Hearing Journal, 44,* 10.

Gilley, P. M., Sharma, A., Dorman, M., Finley, C. C., Panch, A. S., & Martin, K. (2006). Minimization of cochlear implant stimulus artifact in cortical auditory evoked potentials. *Clinical Neurophysiology, 117,* 1772–1782.

Gordon, K. A., Wong, D. D., Valero, J., Jewell, S. F., Yoo, P., & Papsin, B. C. (2011). Use it or lose it? Lessons learned from the developing brains of children who are deaf and use cochlear implants to hear. *Brain Topography, 24*(3–4), 204–219.

Gorga, M. P., Beauchaine, K. A., & Reiland, J. K. (1987). Comparison of onset and steady-state responses of hearing aids: Implications for use of the auditory brainstem response in the selection of hearing aids. *Journal of Speech and Hearing Research, 30,* 130–136.

Gravel, J., Kurtzberg, D., Stapells, D. R., Vaughan, H. G., & Wallace, I. F. (1989). Case studies. *Seminars in Hearing, 10,* 272–287.

Hall III, J. W. (1992). *Handbook of auditory evoked responses.* Needham Heights, MA. Allyn & Bacon.

Halliday, L. F., & Moore, D. R. (2010). Auditory basis of language and learning disorders. In C. J. Plack (Ed.), *Hearing. OUP handbook of auditory science* (pp. 349–374). Oxford, UK: Oxford University Press.

Harris, J. A., Iguchi, F., Seidl, A. H., Lurie, D. I., & Rubel, E. W (2008). Afferent deprivation elicits a transcriptional response associated with neuronal survival after a critical period in the mouse cochlear nucleus. *Journal of Neuroscience, 28,* 10990–11002.

Hecox, K. E. (1983). Role of the auditory brain stem response in the selection of hearing aids. *Ear and Hearing, 4,* 51–55.

Hogan, S. C. M., & Moore, D. R. (2003). Impaired binaural hearing in children produced by a threshold level of middle ear disease. *Journal of the Association for Research in Otolaryngology, 4,* 123–129.

Humes, L. E., Halling, D., & Coughlin, M. (1996). Reliability and stability of various hearing-aid outcome measures in a group of elderly hearing-aid wearers. *Journal of Speech, Language, and Hearing Research, 39,* 923–935.

Humes, L. E., & Wilson, D. L. (2003). An examination of the changes in hearing-aid performance and benefit in the elderly over a 3-year period of hearing-aid use. *Journal of Speech, Language, and Hearing Research, 46,* 137–145.

Humes, L. E., Wilson, D. L., Barlow, N. N., & Garner, C. B. (2002). Measures of hearing-aid benefit following 1 or 2 years of hearing-aid use by older adults. *Journal of Speech, Language, and Hearing Research, 45,* 772–782.

Hyde, M. (1997). The N1 response and its applications. *Audiology and Neurotology, 2,* 281–307.

Irvine, D. R. F., & Rajan, R. (1996). Injury- and use-related plasticity in the primary sensory cortex of adult mammals: Possible relationship to perceptual learning. *Clinical and Experimental Pharmacology and Physiology, 23,* 939–947.

Irving, S., & Moore, D. R. (2011). Training sound localisation in normal hearing listeners with and without a unilateral ear plug. *Hearing Research, 280,* 100–108.

Jakobson, L. S., Lewycky, S. T., Kilgour, A. R., & Stoesz, B. M. (2008). Memory for verbal and visual material in highly trained musicians. *Music Perception, 26,* 41–55.

Kaas, J. H., Krubitzer, L. A., Chino, Y. M., Langston, A. L., Polley, E. H., & Blair, N. (1990). Reorganization of retinotopic cortical maps in adult mammals after lesions of the retina. *Science, 248,* 229–23.

Kaas, J. H., Merzenich, M. M., & Killackey, H. P. (1983). The reorganization of somatosensory cortex following peripheral nerve damage in adult and developing mammals. *Annual Review of Neuroscience, 6,* 325–356.

Kacelnik, O., Nodal, F. R., Parsons, C. H., & King, A. J. (2006). Training-induced plasticity of auditory localization in adult mammals. *PLoS Biology, 4,* e71.

Kates, J. M. (2005). Principles of digital dynamic-range compression. *Trends in Amplifications, 9,* 45–76.

Kathmann, N., Soyka, M., Bickel, R., & Engel, R. R. (1996). ERP changes in alcoholics with and without alcohol psychosis. *Biological Psychiatry, 39,* 873–881.

Keidser, G., Convery, E., & Dillon, H. (2008). The effect of a self-adjustable and trainable hearing aid: A consumer survey. *Journal of the Acoustical Society of America, 124,* 1668–1681.

Kiessling, J. (1982). Hearing aid selection by brainstem audiometry. *Scandanavian Audiology, 11,* 269–275.

Kileny, P. (1982). Auditory brainstem responses as indicators of hearing aid performance. *Annals of Otology, 91,* 61–64.

Kim, J. R., Brown, C. J., Abbas, P. J., Etler, C. P., & O'Brien, S. (2009). The effect of changes in stimulus level on electrically evoked cortical auditory potentials. *Ear and Hearing, 30,* 320–329.

Kitzes, L. M. (1984). Some physiological consequences of cochlear destruction in the inferior colliculus of the gerbil. *Brain Research, 306,* 171–178.

Kochkin, S. (2002). MarkeTrak, V: "Why my hearing aids are in the drawer": The consumer perspective. *Hearing Journal, 53,* 34–42.

Kolb, B. (1995). *Brain plasticity and behaviour.* Mahwah, NJ: Erlbaum.

Korczak, P. A., Kurtzberg, D., & Stapells, D. R. (2005). Effects of sensorineural hearing loss and personal hearing aids on cortical event-related potential and behavioral measures of speech sound processing. *Ear and Hearing, 26,* 165–185.

Kral, A., & Eggermont, J. J. (2007). What's to lose and what's to learn: development under auditory deprivation, cochlear implants and limits of cortical plasticity. *Brain Research Reviews, 56,* 259–269.

Kraus, N., & Skoe, E. (2009). New directions: Cochlear implants. *Annals of the New York Academy of Sciences: The Neurosciences and Music III. Disorders and Plasticity, 1169,* 516–517.

Kraus, N., Skoe, E., Parbery-Clark, A., & Ashley, R. (2009). Experience-induced malleability in neural encoding of pitch, timbre, and timing implications for language and music. The neurosciences and music III—disorders and plasticity. *Annals of the New York Academy of Sciences, 1169,* 543–557.

Kricos, P. B., & McCarthy, P. (2007) From ear to there: A historical perspective on auditory training. *Seminars in Hearing, 28,* 89–98.

Kujawa, S. G., & Liberman, M. C. (2009). Adding insult to injury: Cochlear nerve degeneration after "temporary" noise-induced hearing loss. *Journal of Neuroscience., 29,* 14077–14085.

Kumpik, D. P., Kacelnik, O., & King, A. J. (2010). Adaptive reweighting of auditory localization cues in response to chronic unilateral earplugging in humans. *Journal of Neuroscience, 30,* 4883–4894.

Levi, D. M., & Li, R. W. (2009a). Improving the performance of the amblyopic visual system. *Philosophical Transactions of the Royal Society B: Biological Sciences, 364,* 399–407.

Levi, D. M., & Li, R. W. (2009b). Perceptual Learning as a potential treatment for amblyopia. *Vision Research, 21,* 2535–2549.

Levi-Montalcini, R. (1949). The development of the acoustico-vestibular centers in the chick embryo in the absence of afferent root fiber and of descending fiber tracts. *Journal of Comparative Neurology, 91,* 209–241.

Li, R. W., Levi, D. M., & Klein, S. A. (2004). Perceptual learning improves efficiency by re-tuning the "template" for position discrimination. *Nature Neuroscience, 7,* 178–183.

Liepert, J., Storch, P., Fritsch, A., & Weiller, C. (2000). Motor cortex disinhibition in acute stroke. *Advances in Clinical Neurophysiology, 111,* 671–676.

Lightfoot, G., & Kennedy, V. (2006). Cortical electric response audiometry hearing threshold estimation: Accuracy, speed, and the effects of stimulus presentation features. *Ear and Hearing, 27,* 443–456.

Mahoney, T. M. (1985). Auditory brainstem response hearing aid applications. In J. T. Jacobson (Ed.), *The auditory brainstem response.* Boston, MA: College-Hill.

Martin, B. A. (2007). Can the acoustic change complex be recorded in an individual with a cochlear implant? Separating neural responses from cochlear implant artifact. *Journal of the American Academy of Audiology, 18,* 126–140.

Martin, B. A., Korczak, P., & Tremblay, K. L. (2008). Speech-evoked potentials: From the laboratory to the clinic. *Ear and Hearing, 29,* 285–313.

Marynewich, S. L. (2010). *Slow cortical potential measures of amplification.* Master of Science thesis, University of British Columbia, Vancouver, Canada.

Maurage, P., Campanella, S., Philippot, P., Charest, I., Martin, S., & de Timary, P. (2009). Impaired emotional facial expression decoding in alcoholism is also present for emotional prosody and body postures. *Alcohol and Alcoholism, 44,* 476–485.

Maurage, P., Campanella, S., Philippot, P., Martin, S., & de Timary, P. (2008). Face processing in chronic alcoholism: A specific deficit for emotional features. *Alcoholism: Clinical and Experimental Research, 32,* 600–606.

McGraw, P. V., Webb, B. M., & Moore, D. R. (2009). Sensory learning: From neural mechanisms to rehabilitation. *Philosophical Transactions of the Royal Society B., 364,* 277–420.

Meredith, M. A., Kryklywy, J., McMillan, A. J., Malhotra, S., Lum-Tai, R., & Lomber, S. G. (2011). Crossmodal reorganization in the early deaf switches sensory, but not behavioral roles of auditory cortex. *Proceedings of the National Academy of Sciences of the United States of America, 108,* 8856–8861.

Merzenich, M. M., Jenkins, W. M., Johnson, P., Scheiner, C., Miller, S. L., & Tallal, P. (1996). Temporal processing deficits of language-learning impaired children ameliorated by training. *Science, 271,* 77–81.

Micheyl, C., McDermott, J. H., & Oxenham, A. J. (2009). Sensory noise explains auditory frequency discrimination learning induced by training with identical stimuli. *Perception and Psychophysics, 71,* 5–7.

Moncrieff, D. W., & Wertz, D. (2008). Auditory rehabilitation for interaural asymmetry: Preliminary evidence of improved dichotic listening performance following intensive training. *International Journal of Audiology, 47,* 84–97.

Moore, D. R. (1990). Auditory brainstem of the ferret: Bilateral cochlear lesions in infancy do not affect the number of neurons projecting from the cochlear nucleus to the inferior colliculus. *Developmental Brain Research, 54,* 125–130.

Moore, D. R. (1990). Effects of early binaural experience on development of binaural pathways in the brain. *Seminars in Perinatology, 14,* 294–298.

Moore, D. R., & Aitkin, L. M. (1975). Rearing in an acoustically unusual environment: Effects on neural auditory responses. *Neuroscience Letters, 1,* 29–34.

Moore, D. R., Ferguson, M. A., Edmondson-Jones, A. M., Ratib, S., & Riley, A. (2010). The nature of auditory processing disorder in children. *Pediatrics, 126,* e382–e390.

Moore, D. R., Halliday, L.F., & Amitay, S. (2009), Use of auditory learning to manage listening problems in children. *Philosophical Transactions of the Royal Society B., 364,* 409–420.

Moore, D. R., Hutchings, M. E., King, A. J., & Kowalchuk, N. E. (1989). Auditory brainstem of the ferret: Some effects of rearing with a unilateral ear plug on the cochlea, cochlear nucleus and projections to the inferior colliculus. *Journal of Neuroscience, 9,* 1213–1222.

Moore, D. R., & Irvine, D. R. F. (1981). Development of responses to acoustic interaural intensity differences in the cat inferior colliculus. *Experimental Brain Research, 41,* 301–309.

Moore, D. R., & Shannon, R. V. (2009). Beyond cochlear implants—awakening the deafened brain. *Nature Neuroscience, 12,* 686–691.

Munro, K. J., Pisareva, N., Parker, D., & Purdy, S. (2007a). Asymmetry in the auditory brainstem response following experience of monaural amplification. *NeuroReport, 18,* 1871–1874.

Munro, K. J., Purdy, S. C., Ahmed, S., Begum, R., & Dillon, H. (2011). Obligatory cortical auditory evoked-potential waveform detection and differentiation using a commercially available clinical system: HEARLab. *Ear and Hearing, 32*(6), 782–786.

Munro, K. J., Walker, A., & Purdy, S. (2007b). Evidence for adaptive plasticity in elderly monaural hearing aid users. *NeuroReport, 18,* 1237–1240.

Musacchia, G., Sams, M., Skoe, E., & Kraus, N. (2007). Musicians have enhanced subcortical auditory and audiovisual processing of speech and music. *Proceedings of the National Academy of Sciences of the United States of America, 104,* 15894–15898.

Näätänen, R., & Picton, T. (1987). The N1 wave of the human electric and magnetic response to sound: A review and an analysis of the component structure. *Psychophysiology, 24,* 375–425.

National Institute on Deafness and Other Communication Disorders. (2002). *Otitis media (ear infection)* (NIH Publication No. 974216). Bethesda, MD: Author.

Nordmann, A. S., Bohne, B. A., & Harding, G. W. (2000). Histopathological differences between temporary and permanent threshold shift. *Hearing Research, 139*, 13–30.

Palmer, C., Nelson, C., & Lindley, G. (1998). The functionally and physiologically plastic adult auditory system. *Journal of the Acoustical Society of America, 103*, 1705–1721.

Pantev, C., Lütkenhöner, B., Hoke, M., &. Lehnertz, K. (1986). Comparison between simultaneously recorded auditory-evoked magnetic fields and potentials elicited by ipsilateral, contralateral and binaural tone burst stimulation. *Audiology, 25*, 54–61.

Parbery-Clark, A., Skoe, E., Lam, C., & Kraus, N. (2009). Musician enhancement for speech-in-noise. *Ear and Hearing, 30*, 653–661.

Pascual-Leone, A., Amedi, A., Fregni, F., & Merabet, L. B. (2005). The plastic human brain cortex. *Annual Review of Neuroscience, 28*, 377–401.

Philibert, B., Collet, L., Vesson, J. F., & Veuillet, E. (2005). The auditory acclimatization effect in sensorineural hearing-impaired listeners: Evidence for functional plasticity. *Hearing Research, 205*, 131–142.

Phillips, D. P., & Kelly, J. B. (1992). Effects of continuous noise maskers on tone-evoked potentials in cat primary auditory cortex. *Cerebral Cortex, 2*, 134–140.

Pichora-Fuller, M. K. (2006). Perceptual effort and apparent cognitive decline: Implications for audiologic rehabilitation. *Seminars in Hearing, 27*, 284–293.

Picton, T. W., Durieux-Smith, A., Champagne, S. C., Whittingham, J., Moran, L. M., Giguere, C., & Beauregard, Y. (1998). Objective evaluation of aided thresholds using auditory steady-state responses. *Journal of the American Academy of Audiology, 9*, 315–331.

Ponton, C. W., Don, M, Eggermont, J. J., Waring, M. D., Kwong, B., & Masuda, A. (1996). Auditory system plasticity in children after long periods of complete deafness. *NeuroReport, 8*, 61–65.

Ponton, C. W., & Eggermont, J. J. (2001). Of kittens and kids: Altered cortical maturation following profound deafness and cochlear implant use. *Audiology and Neurotology, 6*, 1729–1733.

Ponton, C. W., Vasama, J. P., Tremblay, K. L., Khosla, D., Kwong, B., & Don, M. (2001). Plasticity in the adult human central auditory system: Evidence from late-onset profound unilateral deafness. *Hearing Research, 154*, 32–44.

Popelar, J., Eire, J. P., Aran, J. M., & Cazals, Y. (1994). Plastic changes in ipsi-contralateral differences of auditory cortex and inferior colliculus evoked potentials after injury to one ear in the adult guinea pig. *Hearing Research, 72*, 125–134.

Preminger, J. E., & Ziegler, C. H. (2008). Can auditory and visual speech perception be trained within a group setting? *American Journal of Audiology, 17*, 80–97.

Purdy, S. C., Kelly, A. S., & Thorne, P. R. (2001). Auditory evoked potentials as measures of plasticity in humans. *Audiology and Neurotology, 6*, 211–215.

Ramirez-Inscoe, J., & Moore, D. R. (2011). Evidence for inheritance of communicative impairments in deaf children using cochlear implants. *Ear and Hearing.* [Epub ahead of print] PMID: 21637101.

Rapin, I., & Graziani, L. J. (1967). Auditory-evoked responses in normal, brain-damaged, and deaf infants. *Neurology, 17*, 881–894.

Reale, R. A., Brugge, J. F., & Chan, J. C. (1987). Maps of auditory cortex in cats reared after unilateral cochlear ablation in the neonatal period. *Brain Research, 192*, 281–290.

Rebillard, G., & Rubel, E. W. (1981). Electrophysiological study of the maturation of auditory responses from the inner ear of the chick. *Brain Research, 229*, 15–23.

Roberts, J. E., Rosenfeld, R. M., & Zeisel, S. A. (2004). Otitis media and speech and language: A meta-analysis of prospective studies. *Pediatrics, 113*, 237–247.

Robertson, D., & Irvine, D. R. F. (1989). Plasticity of frequency organization in auditory cortex of guinea pigs. *Journal of Comparative Neurology, 282*, 456–471.

Robinson, K., & Summerfield, A. Q. (1996). Adult auditory learning and training. *Ear and Hearing, 17*, 51S–65S.

Ross, B., & Tremblay, K. L. (2009). Stimulus experience modifies auditory neuromagnetic responses in young and older listeners. *Hearing Research, 248*, 48–59.

Ruffin, C. V., Tyler, R. S., Witt, S. A., Dunn, C. C., Gantz, B. J., & Rubinstein, J. T. (2007). Long-term performance of Clarion 1.0 Cochlear Implant users. *Laryngoscope, 117*, 1183–1190.

Rye, M. S., Bhutta, M. F., Cheeseman, M. T., Burgner, D., Blackwell, J. M., Brown, S. D., & Jamieson, S. E. (2011). Unraveling the genetics of otitis media: From mouse to human and back again. *Mammalian Genome, 22*, 66–82.

Ryugo, D. K., Baker, C. A., Montey, K. L., Chang, L., Coco, A., Fallon, J. B., & Shepherd, R. K. (2010). Synaptic plasticity after chemical deafening and electrical stimulation of the auditory nerve in cats. *Journal of Comparative Neurology, 518*, 1046–1063.

Sanes, D. H., & Constantine-Paton, M. (1985a). The development of stimulus following in the cochlear nerve and inferior colliculus of the mouse. *Experimental Brain Research, 354*, 255–267.

Sanes, D. H., & Constantine-Paton, M. (1985b). The sharpening of frequency tuning curves requires patterned activity during development in the mouse, Mus musculus. *Journal of Neuroscience, 5*, 1152–1166.

Saunders, G. H., & Cienkowski, K. M. (1997). Acclimatization to hearing aids. *Ear and Hearing, 18*, 129–139.

Scheffler, K., Bilecen, D., Schmid, N., Tschopp, K., & Seelig, J., (1998). Auditory cortical responses in hearing subjects and unilateral deaf patients as detected by functional magnetic resonance imaging. *Cerebral Cortex, 8*, 156–163.

Scherer, S. S., Xu, Y. T., Nelles, E., Fischbeck, K., Willecke, K., & Bone, L. J. (1998). Connexin32-null mice develop a demyelinating peripheral neuropathy. *Glia, 24*, 8–20.

Schön, D., Magne, C., & Besson, M. (2004). The music of speech: Electrophysiological study of pitch perception in language and music. *Psychophysiology, 41*, 341–349.

Schow, R. L., Balsara, N., Smedley, T. C., & Whitcomb, C. (1993). Aural rehabilitation by ASHA audiologists. 1980–1990. *American Journal of Audiology, 2,* 28–37.

Shahin, A., Roberts, L. E., Pantev, C., Trainor, L. J., & Ross, B. (2005). Modulation of P2 auditory-evoked responses by the spectral complexity of musical sounds. *NeuroReport, 16,* 1781–1785.

Sharma, A., Dorman, M. F., & Spahr, A. J. (2002) A sensitive period for the development of the central auditory system in children with cochlear implants: Implications for age of implantation. *Ear and Hearing, 23,* 532–539.

Sharma, M., Purdy, S. C., & Kelly, A. S. (2009). Comorbidity of auditory processing, language, and reading disorders. *Journal of Speech, Language, and Hearing Research, 52,* 706–722.

Skoe, E., & Kraus, N. (2010). Auditory brainstem response to complex sounds: A tutorial. *Ear and Hearing, 31,* 302–324.

Souza, P. E., & Tremblay, K. L. (2006). New perspectives on assessing amplification effects. *Trends in Amplification, 10,* 119–143.

Stapells, D. R., & Kurtzberg, D. (1991). Evoked potential assessment of auditory system integrity in infants. *Clinics in Perinatology, 18,* 497–518.

Steinschneider, M., Schroeder, C. E., Arezzo, J. C., & Vaughan, Jr., H. G. (1994). Speech-evoked activity in primary auditory cortex: Effects of voice onset time. *Electroencephalography Clinical Neurophysiology, 92,* 30–43.

Stone, M. A., & Moore, B. C. J. (1999). Tolerable hearing aid delays. I. Estimation of limits imposed by the auditory path alone using simulated hearing losses. *Ear and Hearing, 20,* 182–192.

Strait, D., Kraus, N., Parbery-Clark, A., & Ashley, R. (2010). Musical experience shapes top-down auditory mechanisms: Evidence from masking and auditory attention performance. *Hearing Research, 261,* 22–29.

Surr, R. K., Cord, M. T., & Walden, B. E. (1998). Long-term versus short-term hearing aid benefit. *Journal of the American Academy of Audiology, 9,* 165–171.

Sweetow, R., & Palmer, C. V. (2005). Efficacy of individual auditory training in adults: A systematic review of the evidence. *Journal of the American Academy of Audiology, 16,* 494–504.

Sweetow, R. W., & Sabes, J. H. (2006). The need for and development of an adaptive Listening and Communication Enhancement (LACE) Program. *Journal of the American Academy of Audiology, 17,* 538–858.

Taylor, K. S. (1993). Self-perceived and audiometric evaluations of hearing aid benefit in the elderly. *Ear and Hearing, 14,* 390–394.

Tervaniemi, M., Kruck, S., Baene, W. D., Schröger, E., Alter, K., & Friederici, A. D. (2009). Top-down modulation of auditory processing: Effects of sound context, musical expertise and attentional focus. *European Journal of Neuroscience, 30,* 1636–1642.

Tremblay, K. L. (2006). Acoustic information and auditory learning in the adult auditory system: Implications for auditory rehabilitation. In C. Palmer & R. Seewald (Eds.), *Hearing care for adults 2006, Proceedings of the First International Adult Conference* (pp. 307–315). Switzerland: Phonak AG.

Tremblay, K. L., (2007). Training-related changes in the brain: Evidence from human auditory-evoked potentials. *Seminars in Hearing, 28,* 120–132.

Tremblay, K. L., Billings, C. J., Friesen, L. M., & Souza, P. E. (2006a). Neural representation of amplified speech sounds. *Ear and Hearing, 27,* 93–103.

Tremblay, K. L., Inoue, K., McClannahan, K., & Ross, B. (2010). Repeated stimulus exposure alters the way sound is encoded in the human brain. *Public Library of Science One, 5,* e10283.

Tremblay, K. L., Kalstein, L., Billings, C. J., & Souza, P. E. (2006b). The neural representation of consonant vowel transitions in adults who wear hearing aids. *Trends in Amplification, 10,* 155–162.

Tremblay, K. L., Kraus, N., & McGee, T. (1998). The time course of auditory perceptual learning: Neurophysiological changes during speech-sound training. *NeuroReport, 9,* 3557–3560.

Tremblay, K. L., McClannahan, K., Inoue, K., Ross, B., & Collet, G. (2011). *Auditory training: Stimulus exposure, task execution, and response feedback affect the neural detection of sound.* Acoustical Society of America, Abstract. Seattle. WA.

Tremblay, K. L., Piskosz, M., & Souza, P. (2002). Aging alters the neural representation of speech cues. *NeuroReport, 13,* 1865–1870.

Tremblay, K. L., Piskosz, M., & Souza, P. (2003). Effects of age and age-related hearing loss on the neural representation of speech cues. *Clinical Neurophysiology, 114,* 1332–1343.

Turner, C. W., & Bentler, R. A. (1998). Does hearing aid benefit increase over time? *Journal of the Acoustical Society of America, 104,* 3673–3674.

Turner, C., Humes, L., Bentler, R., & Cox, R. (1996). A review of past research on changes in hearing aid benefit over time. *Ear and Hearing, 17,* 14S–28S.

Tye-Murray, N., Purdy, S. C., & Woodworth, G. G. (1992). Reported use of communication strategies by SHHH members. Client, talker, and situational variables. *Journal of Speech and Hearing Research, 35,* 708–717.

Tyler, R. S., Fryauf-Bertschy, H., Kelsay, D. M., Gantz, B. J., Woodworth, G. P., & Parkinson, A. (1997). Speech perception by prelingually deaf children using cochlear implants. *Otolaryngology — Head and Neck Surgery, 117,* 180–187.

Vernon-Feagans, L., Hurley, M., & Yont, K. (2002). The effect of otitis media and daycare quality on mother/child bookreading and language use at 48 months of age. *Journal of Applied Developmental Psychology, 22,* 1–21.

Wall, P. D., & Egger, M. D. (1971). Formation of new connections in adult rat brains after partial deafferentation. *Nature, 232,* 542–545.

Ward, N. S., & Cohen, L. G. (2004). Mechanisms underlying recovery of motor function after stroke. *Archives of Neurology, 61,* 1844–1848.

Watson, C. S. (1991). Auditory perceptual learning and the cochlear implant. *American Journal of Otology, 12,* 73–79.

Wiesel, T. N. (1982). Postnatal development of the visual cortex and the influence of the environment. *Nature, 299,* 583–592.

Willott, J. F. (1996). Physiological plasticity in the auditory system and its possible relevance to hearing aid use, deprivation effects, and acclimatization. *Ear and Hearing, 17*(Suppl. 3), 66S–77S.

Wolpaw, R., & Penry, J. K. (1975). A temporal component of the auditory evoked response. *Electroencephalography and Clinical Neurophysiology, 39,* 609–620.

Wong, D. D., & Gordon, K. A. (2009). Beamformer Suppression of cochlear implant artifacts in an electroencephalography dataset. *IEEE Transactions on Bio-Medical Engineering, 56,* 2851–2857.

Wong, P. C. M., Skoe, E., Russo, N. M., Dees, T., & Kraus, N. (2007). Musical experience shapes human brainstem encoding of linguistic pitch patterns. *Nature Neuroscience, 10,* 420–422.

Xiaoxia, Li., Kaibao, Nie., Karp, F., Tremblay, K. L., & Rubinstein, J. T. (2010). Characteristics of stimulus artifacts in EEG recordings induced by electrical stimulation of cochlear implants. *Biomedical Engineering and Informatics, 2,* 799–803.

Index